HEALTH OF HIV INFECTED PEOPLE

HEALTH OF HIV INFECTED PEOPLE

FOOD, NUTRITION AND LIFESTYLE WITHOUT ANTIRETROVIRAL DRUGS

VOLUME II

Edited by

RONALD ROSS WATSON
University of Arizona, Tucson, AZ, USA

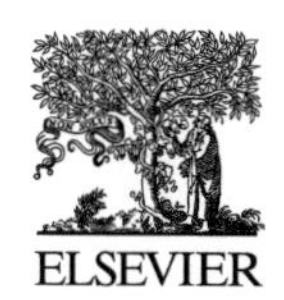

AMSTERDAM • BOSTON • HEIDELBERG • LONDON
NEW YORK • OXFORD • PARIS • SAN DIEGO
SAN FRANCISCO • SINGAPORE • SYDNEY • TOKYO
Academic Press is an imprint of Elsevier

Academic Press is an imprint of Elsevier
125, London Wall, EC2Y 5AS, UK
525 B Street, Suite 1800, San Diego, CA 92101-4495, USA
225 Wyman Street, Waltham, MA 02451, USA
The Boulevard, Langford Lane, Kidlington, Oxford OX5 1GB, UK

ISBN: 978-0-12-800767-9

British Library Cataloguing-in-Publication Data
A catalogue record for this book is available from the British Library

Library of Congress Cataloging-in-Publication Data
A catalog record for this book is available from the Library of Congress

For information on all Academic Press publications
visit our website at http://store.elsevier.com/

Typeset by MPS Limited, Chennai, India
www.adi-mps.com

Printed and bound in the United States of America

Contents

I

OVERVIEW AND FOOD

3. Infant Feeding Policies and HIV

LOUISE KUHN

4. Alcohol Use and Food Insecurity in HIV Disease Management

SETH C. KALICHMAN, JENNIFER A. PELLOWSKI AND DOMINICA HERNANDEZ

5. Carotid Intima–Media Thickness and Plaque in HIV-Infected Patients on the Mediterranean Diet

KLAUDIJA VIŠKOVIĆ AND JOSIP BEGOVAC

II

NUTRITION AND LIFESTYLE

6. Nutritional Treatment Approach for ART-Naïve HIV-Infected Children

MARIANNE DE OLIVEIRA FALCO AND ERIKA APARECIDA DA SILVEIRA

11. HIV AIDS in India: A Nutritional Panorama

DEEPIKA ANAND AND SEEMA PURI

12. Undernutrition, Food Insecurity, and Antiretroviral Outcomes: An Overview of Evidence from sub-Saharan Africa

PATOU MASIKA MUSUMARI, TEERANEE TECHASRIVICHIEN, S. PILAR SUGUIMOTO, ADOLPHE NDARABU, AIMÉ MBOYO, BARON NGASIA, CHRISTINA EL-SAAIDI, BHEKUMUSA WELLINGTON LUKHELE, MASAKO ONO-KIHARA AND MASAHIRO KIHARA

13. How the HIV Epidemic Carved an Indelible Imprint on Infant Feeding

HOOSEN COOVADIA AND HEENA BRAHMBHATT

14. Nutrition Care of the HIV-Exposed Child

ANJU SETH AND ROHINI GUPTA

18. Exercise Treadmill Test for the Assessment of Cardiac Risk Markers in HIV

ANDREA DE LORENZO AND FILIPE PENNA DE CARVALHO

19. Measures of Physical Function in the Management of Individuals Living with HIV/AIDS

VAGNER RASO AND ROY JESSE SHEPHARD

IV

MODELS OF HIV: LESSONS TO BE LEARNED FROM ANIMAL VIRUSES

20. Animal Lentiviruses: Models for Human Immunodeficiency Viruses and Nutrition

MITCHEL GRAHAM STOVER AND RONALD ROSS WATSON

Preface

When the HIV/AIDS epidemic began in the 1980s and 1990s outside of Africa, there was great concern because of the absence of a cure or effective therapy. People have historically used dietary plants, herbal extracts, and nutrients as potential therapies for incurable diseases. Thus, they were used in AIDS to compensate for physical changes such as wasting and nutritional deficiencies by the retroviral infection. Treatment of nutritional problems could compensate for some of the effects of the retroviral infection. Each plant has approximately 10,000 different chemical entities, and many have been used for therapy of different diseases and may reduce the HIV burden. Impoverished people as well as those who dislike pharmaceutical treatments and their side effects continue to search for methods within their control, such as dietary plants, herbal extracts, and nutrients as potential therapies, to compensate for and regulate adverse effects of retroviral therapy.

Section I: Overview and food. Pellowski and Kalichman review the role of dietary supplements used by AIDS patients and the Internet as a source of medical misinformation. Gibbs follows with specific examples of food and HIV risk via its use at funerals. Kuhn describes infant feeding policies for those with AIDS. Kalichman and Pellowski describe the role of significant alcohol use and abuse in food insecurity and, ultimately, health in AIDS patients. Višković and Begovac discuss carotid intima-media thickness and plaque in HIV-infected patients on the Mediterranean diet.

Section II: Nutrition and lifestyle. Falco and da Silveira describe an approach to treat HIV-infected children not using HAART. Thereafter, Falco and da Silveira describe an approach to treat HIV-infected adults not using HAART. Sunguya, Urassa, Yasuoka, and Jimba discuss poor feeding habits of AIDS patients in developing countries. They describe the nutrition training of health care workers who help patients without much knowledge of nutrition and their special needs as AIDS patients. Całyniuk, Kokot, Nowakowska-Zajdel, Grochowska-Niedworok, and Muc-Wierzgoń review nutrition and food in AIDS patients. Zhang, Zeng, Duan, and Gui review the role of zinc in health and nutritional requirements of HIV-infected people. Anand and Puri review the course of and nutrition for AIDS in India. Musumari and a large group of experienced researchers review undernutrition induced by food insecurity and HIV and its treatment with antiretroviral drugs based on their long clinical experiences in sub-Saharan Africa. Coovadia and Brahmbhatt describe the effects of AIDS on infant feeding practices in Southern Africa, thus changing the practices of other pediatricians around the world. Seth and Gupta review the role of nutrition on HIV-exposed but not necessarily HIV-infected infants. Burini, Moreto, and Yu review the effects of glutamine and cysteine for health promotion in HIV-infected individuals. Pinzone and Nunnari describe micronutrients for HIV-infected patients.

Section III: Exercise and behavioral lifestyle changes in the prevention and treatment of HIV/AIDS nutritional changes. Yahioui and Voss discuss changes due to aging. They discuss the role of exercise in the management of body weight. De Lorenzo reviews exercise using the treadmill test to assess cardiac risk markers in HIV patients who have special assessment needs. Raso and Shephard review the special measures of physical function in those with AIDS.

Section IV: Models of HIV: lessons to be learned from animal viruses. Stover and Watson discuss animal models of AIDS that allow many studies, including those involving dietary supplements that are not easily possible in humans. The authors discuss animal lentiviruses as models of immunodeficiency viruses. Guerra and Porbén review the Cuban experience regarding provision of food and nutrition care for people with AIDS, focusing on T-cell number, nutritional status, and HIV load.

List of Contributors

Deepika Anand Department of Food and Nutrition, Institute of Home Economics, University of Delhi, New Delhi, India

Josip Begovac University Hospital for Infectious Diseases, The University of Zagreb, School of Medicine, Šalata, Zagreb, Croatia

Heena Brahmbhatt Johns Hopkins Bloomberg School of Public Health, Department of Population, Family and Reproductive Health, Baltimore, MD, USA

Roberto Carlos Burini Centre for Nutritional and Physical Exercise Metabolism, Department of Public Health, Botucatu Medical School, Sao Paulo State University—UNESP, Botucatu, SP, Brazil

Bruno Cacopardo Department of Clinical and Molecular Biomedicine, Division of Infectious Diseases, University of Catania, Catania, Italy

Beata Całyniuk Department of Human Nutrition, Silesian Medical University, Zabrze, Poland

Hoosen Coovadia MatCH Health Systems a Division of the University of the Witwatersrand, Emeritus Professor of Paediatrics and Child Health, University of KwaZulu-Natal Commissioner, National Planning Commission at the Presidency, Republic of South Africa

Erika Aparecida da Silveira Researcher, teacher of Postgraduate Studies Program in Health Sciences, Department of Surgery, Medical School, Federal University of Goiás, GO, Brazil

Marianne de Oliveira Falco Department of Nutrition, Society Intensive Care, Goiás, Brazil, Postgraduate Studies Program Ph. D. in Health Sciences, Medical School, Federal University of Goiás, GO, Brazil

Andrea De Lorenzo Instituto Nacional de Cardiologia, Rio de Janeiro, RJ, Brazil; Universidade Federal do Rio de Janeiro, Rio de Janeiro, RJ, Brazil; Clinica de Diagnostico por Imagem, Rio de Janeiro, RJ, Brazil

Yanjun Duan College of Pharmacy, University of Nebraska Medical Centre; West China School of Pharmacy, Sichuan University, Chengdu, China

Christina El-Saaidi Department of Global Health and Socio-epidemiology, Kyoto University School of Public Health, Yoshida-Konoe-cho, Sakyo-ku, Kyoto, Japan

Philip Gibbs School of Culture, History and Language, Canberra, Australia

Elżbieta Grochowska-Niedworok Department of Human Nutrition, Silesian Medical University, Zabrze, Poland

Elisa Maritza Linares Guerra Universidad de Ciencias Médicas de Pinar del Río, Pinar del Río. Cuba

Ge Gui Evidence-Based Pharmacy Center, West China Second University Hospital, Sichuan University, Chengdu, China; West China School of Pharmacy, Sichuan University, Chengdu, China; Department of Pharmacy, West China Second University Hospital, Sichuan University, Chengdu, China

Rohini Gupta Pediatric Center of Excellence in HIV Care, Lady Hardinge Medical College, New Delhi, India

Dominica Hernandez Department of Psychology, University of Connecticut, Storrs, CT, USA

Zhiqiang Hu Department of Pharmacy, West China Second University Hospital, Sichuan University, Chengdu, China; West China School of Pharmacy, Sichuan University, Chengdu, China; Evidence-Based Pharmacy Center, West China Second University Hospital, Sichuan University, Chengdu, China

Masamine Jimba Department of Community and Global Health, Graduate School of Medicine, The University of Tokyo, Hongo, Bunkyo-ku, Tokyo, Japan

Seth C. Kalichman Department of Psychology, University of Connecticut, Storrs, CT, USA

Masahiro Kihara Department of Global Health and Socio-epidemiology, Kyoto University School of Public Health, Yoshida-Konoe-cho, Sakyo-ku, Kyoto, Japan

Teresa Kokot Department of Internal Diseases, Silesian Medical University, Bytom, Poland

Louise Kuhn Gertrude H. Sergievsky Center, College of Physicians and Surgeons, New York, NY, USA

Bhekumusa Wellington Lukhele Department of Global Health and Socio-epidemiology, Kyoto University School of Public Health, Yoshida-Konoe-cho, Sakyo-ku, Kyoto, Japan

Aimé Mboyo Multisectoral program of the fight against HIV/AIDS (PNMLS), Ex-Fonames bld, Kasa-Vubu, Kinshasa, Democratic Republic of Congo

Fernando Moreto Centre for Nutritional and Physical Exercise Metabolism, Department of Public Health, Botucatu Medical School, Sao Paulo State University—UNESP, Botucatu, SP, Brazil

Małgorzata Muc-Wierzgoń Department of Internal Diseases, Silesian Medical University, Bytom, Poland

Patou Masika Musumari Department of Global Health and Socio-epidemiology, Kyoto University School of Public Health, Yoshida-Konoe-cho, Sakyo-ku, Kyoto, Japan

Adolphe Ndarabu Centre Hospitalier Monkole, Masangambila, Mont-Ngafula, Kinshasa 817 Kinshasa XI, Democratic Republic of Congo

Baron Ngasia Centre Hospitalier Lumbulumbu-Clinique MAPON, Kindu, Maniema, Democratic Republic of Congo

Ewa Nowakowska-Zajdel Department of Internal Diseases, Silesian Medical University, Bytom, Poland

Giuseppe Nunnari Department of Clinical and Molecular Biomedicine, Division of Infectious Diseases, University of Catania, Catania, Italy

Masako Ono-Kihara Department of Global Health and Socio-epidemiology, Kyoto University School of Public Health, Yoshida-Konoe-cho, Sakyo-ku, Kyoto, Japan

Jennifer A. Pellowski Department of Psychology, University of Connecticut, Storrs, CT, USA

Filipe Penna de Carvalho Clinica de Diagnostico por Imagem, Rio de Janeiro, RJ, Brazil

Marilia Rita Pinzone Department of Clinical and Molecular Biomedicine, Division of Infectious Diseases, University of Catania, Catania, Italy

Sergio Santana Porbén Hermanos Ameijeiras Hospital, Havana, Cuba

Seema Puri Department of Food and Nutrition, Institute of Home Economics, University of Delhi, New Delhi, India

Vagner Raso School of Medicine of the University of Western Sao Paulo, UNOESTE, Brazil Masters Program on Body Balance Rehabilitation of the Anhanguera University, UNIAN, Brazil

Anju Seth Pediatric Center of Excellence in HIV Care, Lady Hardinge Medical College, New Delhi, India

Roy Jesse Shephard Faculty of Kinesiology and Physical Education of the University of Toronto, Toronto, ON, Canada

S. Pilar Suguimoto Department of Global Health and Socio-epidemiology, Kyoto University School of Public Health, Yoshida-Konoe-cho, Sakyo-ku, Kyoto, Japan

Mitchel Graham Stover Department of Veterinary Science and Microbiology, University of Arizona, Tucson, AZ, USA

Bruno F. Sunguya Department of Community and Global Health, Graduate School of Medicine, The University of Tokyo, Hongo, Bunkyo-ku, Tokyo, Japan

Teeranee Techasrivichien Department of Global Health and Socio-epidemiology, Kyoto University School of Public Health, Yoshida-Konoe-cho, Sakyo-ku, Kyoto, Japan

David P. Urassa School of Public Health and Social Sciences, Muhimbili University of Health and Allied Sciences, Dar es Salaam, Tanzania

Klaudija Višković Head of Department of Radiology and Ultrasound, University Hospital for Infectious Diseases, Zagreb, Croatia

Joachim G. Voss University of Washington, School of Nursing, Biobehavioral Nursing and Health Systems, Seattle, WA, USA

Ronald Ross Watson Mel and Enid Zuckerman College of Public Health, School of Medicine, University of Arizona, Tucson, AZ, USA

Heather Worth School of Public Health and Community Medicine, University of New South Wales, Sydney, NSW, Australia

Anella Yahiaoui University of Washington, School of Nursing, Biobehavioral Nursing and Health Systems, Seattle, WA, USA

Junko Yasuoka Department of Community and Global Health, Graduate School of Medicine, The University of Tokyo, Hongo, Bunkyo-ku, Tokyo, Japan

Yong-Ming Yu Massachusetts General Hospital, Department of Surgery, Shriners Burns Hospital, Harvard Medical School, Boston, MA, USA

Linan Zeng Evidence-Based Pharmacy Center, West China Second University Hospital, Sichuan University, Chengdu, China; Key Laboratory of Birth Defects and Related Diseases of Women and Children (Sichuan University), Ministry of Education, Chengdu, China; Department of Pharmacy, West China Second University Hospital, Sichuan University, Chengdu, China

Lingli Zhang Evidence-Based Pharmacy Center, West China Second University Hospital, Sichuan University, Chengdu, China; Key Laboratory of Birth Defects and Related Diseases of Women and Children (Sichuan University), Ministry of Education, Chengdu, China; Department of Pharmacy, West China Second University Hospital, Sichuan University, Chengdu, China

Acknowledgement

The work of Dr. Watson's editorial assistant, Bethany L. Stevens, in communicating and working with authors on the manuscripts was critical to the successful completion of these two books. It is very much appreciated. The encouragement, advice and support of Jill Leonard and Elizabeth Gibson at Elsevier was very helpful. Support for Ms. Stevens's and Dr. Watson's work was graciously provided by the Natural Health Research Institute (www.naturalhealthresearch.org) and Southwest Scientific Editing & Consulting, LLC. Finally the work of the librarian at the Arizona Health Sciences Library, Mari Stoddard, was vital and very helpful in identifying key researchers who participated in the book.

SECTION I

OVERVIEW AND FOOD

CHAPTER

1

Dietary Supplements Among People Living with HIV and Vulnerability to Medical Internet Misinformation

Jennifer A. Pellowski and Seth C. Kalichman

Department of Psychology, University of Connecticut, Storrs, CT, USA

1.1 SECTION 1: COMPLEMENTARY AND ALTERNATIVE MEDICINE USE AMONG PEOPLE LIVING WITH HIV

According to the National Center for Complementary and Alternative Medicine [1], complementary and alternative medicine (CAM) includes a number of things that are not considered part of "conventional" or Western medicine. CAM includes natural products, dietary supplements, mind–body medicine, and traditional healing practices [1,2]. Complementary medicine describes patient use of "nonconventional" approaches to healing in conjunction with Western medical treatments. For example, a person living with HIV may take high-dose vitamins along with antiretroviral therapy (ART), both with the end goal of protecting and boosting the immune functioning. Alternative medicine describes patient use of nonconventional approaches in place of Western medical treatments. For example, a person living with HIV may take a combination of antioxidants,

Health of HIV Infected People, Volume 2.
DOI: http://dx.doi.org/10.1016/B978-0-12-800767-9.00001-7

multivitamins, and probiotics to manage the HIV infection without using any antiretrovirals.

In general, CAM use among people living with HIV is quite common. In a review of recent international research, Littlewood and Vanable [3] found that in resource-poor areas, people living with HIV have a higher rate of CAM use. In their review they found that all studies conducted in resource-poor settings (i.e., Africa, China, and India) reported rates of 50% or higher. The authors argue that these individuals take a more pluralistic approach because of the limited access to ART in these areas. In the absence of ART, individuals naturally turn to their traditional methods for treating and managing the symptoms of HIV infection. When ART becomes available, patients continue to use their traditional medicines as a complement to biomedical treatment.

Other studies have also found similarly high levels of CAM use among people living with HIV. Among a sample of people living with HIV in Malaysia, 78.2% of the sample indicated that they used some form of CAM [4]. In this sample, the most frequently used CAM were vitamins, supplements, and herbal products. Among men living with HIV in California, Florida, and Georgia, 69% reported CAM use, most frequently supplements and spiritual therapies [5]. In a sample of 293 patients at HIV outpatient clinics in London, 61% of patients were using supplements or herbal remedies [6]. Overall, Lorenc and Robinson [7] estimate averages of CAM use among people living with HIV in Western countries to be approximately 55% based on their systematic review of the literature.

These rates are similar to those found in the general population [2]. Two National Health Information Survey (NHIS) studies found rates of CAM use in the average adult population to vary between 38.3% and 62%, depending on the definition of CAM used [2,8]. These prevalence rates among people living with HIV, however, do not follow the general trend between socioeconomic status (SES) and CAM use. In the general population literature, a positive relationship exists such that CAM use increases as SES increases, particularly when considering education level [9]. Given this, we might expect people living with HIV to have lower than average rates of CAM use because many people living with HIV have low income levels and often below average education levels [1,10]. However, chronic illness status may moderate the relationship between SES and CAM use. In general, previous literature has found that individuals living with chronic illnesses are two- to five-times more likely to report using CAM than nonchronically ill individuals [11]. Although the moderation of the SES and CAM use relationship by chronic illness status has not been statistically tested (to our knowledge), it seems to be one of the more plausible explanations for the increased CAM use among people living with HIV.

1.2 SECTION 2: CORRELATES OF CAM USE AMONG PEOPLE LIVING WITH HIV

Given the high levels of CAM use among people living with HIV, it becomes imperative to study why, and under what circumstances, an individual may be more likely to use them. Individuals who use dietary supplements or other types of herbal treatments as an alternative to biomedicine do so for vastly different reasons than do individuals who use them in conjunction with or as a complement to biomedicine.

As discussed, Littlewood and Vanable [3] found that when access to ART was limited, particularly in resource-poor settings, patients turn to traditional medicine in the interim. These patients use traditional forms of medicine to manage HIV-related symptoms and to boost their immune systems; however, as Littlewood and Vanable [3] found, this type of use does not lead to this individuals rejecting ART when it does become available. Instead, they tend to use both forms of medicine in a complementary fashion.

Quite different are individuals who have access to ART but choose not to use it. Choosing not to use ART when it is available can stem from a number of reasons, including not feeling ready to start what can be a burdensome regimen, the patient feeling good so he/she makes the conclusion that medications are unnecessary, and, most troubling, skepticism about the safety of biomedicine, in general, and HIV medications, specifically.

Medical mistrust is not uncommon, especially among racial minorities with histories of maltreatment, particularly African-Americans. Often this mistrust is attributed to historical instances of maltreatment by medical and research institutions. The Tuskegee Syphilis Study is often pointed to as just one example of mistreatment [12]. In addition to historical instances of mistreatment by medical institutions, individual experiences of perceived racism and discrimination of minority patients within patient–provider interactions also impact an individual's mistrust of their provider as well as the institution in general [13,14].

AIDS denialism is a specific form of medical mistrust. AIDS denialists believe that HIV does not cause AIDS; rather, AIDS is caused by any number of environmental factors such as poverty, malnutrition, contaminated drinking water, poor sanitation, illicit drug abuse, and even antiretroviral medications [15]. Mistrust and denialism are rooted in conspiracy theories. These beliefs are not that uncommon among people living with HIV; Bogart and Thorburn [16] found that 53.4% of their sample agreed with the statement "there is a cure for AIDS, but it is being withheld from the poor" and 6% agreed with the statement "the medicine used to treat HIV causes people to get AIDS." Kalichman et al. [17] found that one in five of their participants endorsed statements such as "there is no proof that HIV causes AIDS" and "HIV treatments do more harm than good." Kalichman et al. [17] also found that those who endorsed these beliefs were significantly less likely to be using ART. Although that specific data analysis did not incorporate CAM use, from the wider literature we can assume that they are also the ones who are more likely to use dietary supplements in place of ART [18].

In addition to using CAM as an alternative to biomedical treatment, there are also several reasons for using CAM as an adjunct to biomedical treatment. For example, ART can have side effects that may cause discomfort to the patient such as nausea, diarrhea, headache, trouble sleeping, and lipodystrophy [19]. Some people living with HIV use CAM to treat the side effects that they experience from using ART and other HIV-related disease symptoms [20,21]. One multisite study found that CAM use rates during the current era of highly active antiretroviral therapy (HAART) were similar to usage rates pre-HAART [22]. This indicates that although people living with HIV use CAM to help treat side effects associated with antiretroviral medications, this usage has not increased over time due to changes in the types of medications available.

In addition to using CAM to help treat medication side effects, some people living with HIV believe that the use of CAM is important for the maintenance of their health [23]. The authors explained that in this Canadian sample, CAM use gave participants a very important sense of empowerment in their own health care. Another study conducted in the United States also found that CAM usage helped participants feel more in control of their illness [24]. This is particularly important for people living with HIV who often feel helpless, depressed, and stigmatized due to the disease [25,26]. Furthermore, others simply believe that their health is improved due to the use of CAM [4,27]. Sparber et al. [24] found that 61% of their sample believed that CAM was as effective as or more effective than biomedical treatments. Additionally, Sparber et al. [24], found that nearly all participants (94.2%) felt that using CAM enhanced their treatment outcomes.

It is clear that individuals use CAM for a multitude of reasons, both in conjunction with biomedical treatments and instead of them. Using CAM can provide patients with a wide variety of positive psychosocial benefits, including a sense of control and empowerment, and helps them become an active participant in their own health. In light of these clear psychosocial benefits, an important question that is often asked is how safe and effective these treatments are and, when used in conjunction with biomedical treatments such as ART, are there harmful interactions? This is particularly important in light of the common usage of ART among people living with HIV.

1.3 SECTION 3: EFFICACY AND UTILITY OF CAM FOR PEOPLE LIVING WITH HIV

The beginning of this chapter stated that far more research has been performed regarding biomedical treatments compared with CAM. With that in mind, we must consider the following findings with a grain of salt. There is more that we do not know about the efficacy and utility of CAM than we know.

In Lorenc and Robinson's [7] systematic review, they found nine empirical reviews that provided information about the efficacy of various treatments. In general, the reviews were positive toward the efficacy and potential use of CAM among people living with HIV. However, many of these reviews were conducted in the late 1990s or early 2000s. More current studies are also fairly positive. Olsen et al. [28] conducted a randomized controlled trial to test the impact of lipid-based nutritional supplements (whey or soy protein) on lean mass weight gain and grip strength in Ethiopia. They found that both types of nutritional supplements increased lean mass weight and grip strength over the 3-month period and were also associated with improved immune functioning. Among HIV-positive children in Agra, India, Gautam et al. [29] found that children who received probiotic supplements had higher CD4 cell counts at follow-up. Additionally, children who received micronutrient supplements showed a significant delay in the progression through WHO clinical stages.

In addition to efficacy of CAM treatments, there has been continued concern about interactions between herbal CAM and ART. Specifically, ART often uses a combination of a nucleoside reverse-transcriptase inhibitor (NRTI) and either a non-nucleoside reverse-transcriptase inhibitor (NNRTI) or a protease inhibitor (PI) [30]. PI and NNRTI classes of ART medications are metabolized through the cytochrome P450 pathway [6]. Thus, herbal CAM can interact with ART medications through the inhibition of the CYP3A4 enzyme [31]. Examples of herbal CAM that can cause a risk of this CYP3A4 enzyme inhibition include garlic, Kava, St. John's Wort, Ginko biloba, Ginseng, and milk thistle [6].

There are also several other herbal CAM known to have potential drug interactions with ART. Echinacea can be problematic for any HIV-positive individual because of the risk of stimulating the immune system that can result in an increase in HIV viral load [32]. Additionally, aloe vera can cause increased gastrointestinal transit that overmetabolizes every class of ART medications, leading to suboptimal absorption and subsequent failure of ART [33]. Overall, the herbal CAM interaction research literature is dense and not easily comprehended, particularly for those without backgrounds in nutrition.

In addition to harmful drug interactions, there is also evidence that CAM usage can negatively impact adherence to biomedical treatments. Among a cohort of HIV-positive women, Owen-Smith et al. [34] found that women who were using CAM, specifically immunity boosters and vitamins, were more likely to report missing one or more doses of ART medication in the past month. Jernewall et al. [35] also found a similar pattern among HIV-positive Latino gay and bisexual men. Eighty percent of their study population reported using CAM, and those who were Latino and used CAM were less likely to adhere to regular medical appointments and were less likely to adhere to their ART medication in the past 3 days. The inconsistencies in medication adherence that appear to be linked to CAM usage is problematic because of drug resistance. Parienti et al. [36] found that gaps in adherence as short at 2 days can cause loss of viral suppression. In this type of situation, the individual not only becomes more infectious but also there is the possibility that the individual can become resistant to that medication, rendering it useless for the medical management of HIV.

Although there is mounting evidence for the efficacy of some types of CAM, there are still issues that emerge when using CAM as a complement to biomedicine, including drug interactions and nonadherence. Previous research has suggested that it is a provider's obligation to encourage disclosure of CAM use by being nonjudgmental and to determine whether the CAM that the patient is using is harmful [37,38]. Patients often do not have the ability to read and fully comprehend research articles, limiting the full understanding of what they are using on their own.

1.4 SECTION 4: DISCLOSURE OF CAM USE TO STANDARD HIV CARE PROVIDERS

Given the high prevalence rates of CAM use and the possibility of drug interactions, disclosure of CAM use to providers is vitally important for people living with HIV. Unfortunately, the literature examining disclosure and patient–provider communication is somewhat limited. However, there is a trend in the literature that indicates that CAM use disclosure is suboptimal. One study found that although 79.7% of their sample reported using CAM, only half of these individuals had discussed their usage with their HIV care provider [39]. Among a sample of women, only 36% of participants had disclosed CAM use to their health care provider [40]. Given the possibility of drug interactions that could seriously undermine the standard HIV care for the patient, this lack of disclosure is alarming.

However, patients often have their own reasons for not disclosing their CAM use to their standard HIV care provider. A serious example appears among a sample of immigrants from Mexico. Shedlin et al. [21] found that people living with HIV who were of Mexican origin seeking care in the United States were afraid to disclose their CAM use for fear that their provider would stop treating them. Under these circumstances, patients felt that it was more important to continue with the standard HIV care they were getting and keep their CAM use a secret than to lose access to standard care completely. More generally, many people living with HIV are concerned that their provider will disapprove of their CAM use and/or make them stop [21]. Thus, they come to the conclusion that it is better to not disclose their CAM use than it would be to discuss it with their provider. Similarly, another reason that individuals may not disclose is if they strongly feel as though it is their body and their health, so they have the ultimate say in what happens regardless of their providers' suggestions and therefore there is no need to disclose use [41].

Providers can play a large role in the disclosure of CAM use among people living with HIV. Unfortunately, researchers have found that health care providers often feel uncomfortable discussing CAM use with their patients because they feel uncomfortable condoning its use [42]. In a sample of Mexico border US-based clinicians, almost half of the providers sampled disclosed that they did not routinely inquire about CAM usage among their patients with HIV infection [42]. Similarly, Sparber et al. [24] found that only 53% of their sample were explicitly asked by their providers about their CAM use. These examples perfectly mirror the fears that people who use CAM have in the possibility of disclosing; they correctly guess that their providers are uncomfortable condoning its use. As a result, providers fall short in delivering on Irish's [37] and Palmer's [38] suggestions of nonjudgmental approaches and, thus, do not inquire about it.

Much of providers' decisions not to inquire about an individual's use of CAM may be from their own lack of information. Muñoz et al. [42] also asked HIV care providers how knowledgeable they were about CAM for people living with HIV. Most of the HIV care providers sampled admitted to lacking adequate information about CAM use. Still, these providers were concerned about CAM–drug interactions and the relationship between CAM use and nonadherence. In general, providers were wary about CAM use among their patients [42]. Conversely, Wynia et al. [43] found that the majority (63%) of providers sampled felt that CAM therapies may be helpful for people living with HIV. Wynia et al. [43] also found that those who felt that CAM was helpful were also more likely to discuss CAM use with their patients. However, even in this sample, only approximately one-quarter of physicians actually discussed CAM therapies with their patients.

It is clear that, for people living with HIV, getting information about CAM use from their provider is not an efficient method, either because the patients do not want to disclose their use or because their provider feels uncomfortable discussing it, or both. Thus, people living with HIV must turn to other, possibly less credible sources in their quest to find information about different types of CAM.

1.5 SECTION 5: SEEKING INFORMATION ABOUT HERBAL SUPPLEMENTS AND OTHER CAM

Original sources of research often end up behind a pay wall and, even when accessible, the typical consumer cannot extract the meaning of complex scientific writing. When submitting a manuscript for publication, researchers are writing for fellow researchers who speak the same scientific language with little regard for the people who the article is actually written about. Additionally, although there is some research on the efficacy of some dietary supplements and other herbal types of CAM, there are far more products with health claims that have not been studied within a stringent scientific research framework.

Leonard et al. [23] found that the sources that participants used to seek information about CAM varied widely. Common sources of information were "their CAM providers, their physicians, books, resources from AIDS Service Organizations, the Internet, and health food stores" [23]. However, these sources of information vary in their accuracy and quality, and it can be difficult to decipher which information is correct. This study also found that although participants rated the safety of CAM as one of the most important issues, their actual knowledge of these safety issues was limited [23].

One place that a person living with HIV may go to learn about different types of CAM is a local health food store. However, health food stores may also be a particularly problematic place to seek information for people living with HIV. Mills et al. [44] conducted a study in which four male confederates posed as people living with HIV and sought information from 32 Canadian health food stores. The authors found that, in general, employees at these health food stores had limited training in CAM, particularly regarding CAM for people living with HIV. Disconcertingly, several employees recommended natural products that could be potentially harmful for people living with HIV. Although this is just one study, people living with HIV should be wary of the information provided about supplements and CAM at health food stores.

The other common place that a person may turn to is the Internet. Kalichman et al. [45] found that people living with HIV use the Internet for a broad range of health-related activities, such as searching for health information, searching for AIDS-specific information, and using the Internet to communicate with providers. Research also suggests that individuals who use the Internet, particularly to search for health information, are healthier in general. Kalichman et al. [46] found that individuals who used the Internet were more likely to have an undetectable HIV RNA viral load than those who did not use the Internet. Additionally, those who used the Internet for health-related purposes also had higher medication adherence [47]. Although these trends are promising, there are some caveats.

Incomplete and inaccurate health information is common on the Internet, and for some individuals it is indistinguishable from credible ones [48]. In a survey of 324 adults living with HIV, Benotsch et al. [49] found that participants rated a sample of online health information less critically than medical professionals did. Additionally, participants were less able to discriminate between high-quality and low-quality online information than medical professionals. This was particularly true for participants who had low health literacy, low income, lower educational attainment, and those who held irrational health beliefs. It appears that some subpopulations of people living with HIV are at increased vulnerability to medical misinformation on the Internet.

This is where problems with dietary supplements and other types of CAM may come into play. As stated, there is much more information about types of CAM that is not scientifically supported than there is for CAM that is scientifically supported; many claims about specific dietary supplements are not supported by scientific research. Thus, information available on the Internet can often be misleading or downright false. Kalichman et al. [18] conducted a study that controlled the credibility of health information presented to participants. Using example web sites that were either supported by scientific evidence or not supported by credible sources, the researchers tested how believable and interesting this information was for people living with HIV. They found that having greater interest in and believing in Internet medical misinformation predicted higher rates of dietary supplement use [18]. Individuals who used supplements were also more likely to endorse erroneous statements such as "vitamins and health foods can cure AIDS," "Traditional medicines can cure AIDS," and "Herbal and national remedies can cure AIDS in some people" [18]. Although several types of CAM have been shown to be beneficial to people living with HIV, none has been shown to cure AIDS.

The Internet can provide a wealth of information that can be essential for being an informed decision-maker and having a sense of control over one's own health. This is particularly true given the trend of providers not being comfortable or having enough information about CAM to discuss these issues with their HIV-positive patients. That being said, people living with HIV should think critically about all information related to their health, particularly when looking for information on the Internet.

1.6 SECTION 6: RECOMMENDATIONS FOR PATIENTS

Gaining appropriate and accurate information about CAM is essential to becoming an informed participant in one's own health. Information can empower a sense of control over one's health, which is an important psychological factor that predicts positive health outcomes. The Internet is a good source of information if one knows where to look. Web sites that contain .edu or .gov can often be the most reputable sources. These types of sites contain information that is supported by scientific evidence but may be easier to read and comprehend than primary journal sources. Additionally, these types of sites often incorporate information from multiple primary sources, making the information more comprehensive. The National Center for Complementary and Alternative Medicine web site is a good place to start (available at http://nccam.nih.gov). This site provides detailed information about a large variety of CAM and also provides information specific to individual diseases. Although fairly limited currently, the National Center for Complementary and Alternative Medicine site contains information specific to people living with HIV (available at http://nccam.nih.gov/health/hiv). There are also several nonacademic, nongovernmental web sites that also provide good, scientifically based information such as The Body (www.thebody.com), amfAR: The Foundation for AIDS Research (www.amfar.org), and POZ magazine (www.poz.com).

In addition to looking up reputable information on the Internet, another step is to disclose CAM use to their HIV care provider. This may be difficult given the literature on providers' knowledge and comfort level; however, starting the conversation is the key to safe and effective usage of CAM. The goal in this is for the patient to be an active participant in his/her own health care. By entering into the patient–provider relationship with a sense of self-advocacy, patients can begin to work with their health care provider in a collaborative way. A patient asking about these issues may cause the provider to read more of the literature, benefitting not only the initial patient but also subsequent patients as well. Although providers are often seen as being more powerful within patient–provider relationships, this does not have to be the case, and it starts with an informed patient that advocates for his/her own health.

1.7 SECTION 7: RECOMMENDATIONS FOR PROVIDERS

On the flip side of that relationship, there is also the obligation of the provider to offer patients the best, most accurate care possible. Based on the literature, it seems that some providers lack some of the necessary knowledge about the efficacy and utility of CAM to properly advise their patients on its use. It appears that providers who know a little bit about the research on drug interactions may generalize this knowledge to all herbal CAM or all CAM in general and may take the stance the CAM is always problematic and should not be used. Conversely, providers who believe that CAM may be of benefit to their patients are more open to discussing CAM use. In general, the problem of disclosure seems to stem from both sides of the patient–provider relationship.

Given the prevalence rates and potential for drug interactions, the trend in the literature that suggests CAM use is not discussed often with patients' providers is disconcerting. This may also speak to some more general problems with patient–provider relationships and communication for people living with HIV and their providers, in general. In accordance with the model of health care empowerment (HCE), patients' perceptions of their participation in health care is based on the dynamic interplay between contextual/environmental factors, personal resources, and intrapersonal processes and states [50]. Feeling more empowered has been associated with greater positive provider relationships and higher beliefs in biomedical treatments for people living with HIV [51]. Currently, there is work being done using this model to increase positive provider relationships, which may lead to increases in communication [51,52]. This would be particularly useful within the realm of CAM disclosure and discussion.

Another suggestion for assisting with the patient–provider relationship is Freeman and MacIntyre's [53] suggestion that the role of nurses may be a helpful point of discussion. Freeman and MacIntyre [53] suggest that nurses have a unique role in the treatment of people living with HIV. Nurses have expert medical knowledge in addition to interpersonal skills and a nurturing mindset. In combination, these could be useful in a patient feeling that the environment is nonjudgmental, a key component in the decision to disclose CAM use. Freeman and MacIntyre [53] also point out that more CAM knowledge on the part of nurses would be necessary for interventions in the management of HIV-related symptoms to be possible.

In addition to the possibility of nursing interventions, there still needs to be more research in the area of patient–provider relationships with regard to CAM use among people living with HIV. There are several other barriers that impede the disclosure of CAM use in addition to the patients' attitudes toward their provider, including the patients' attitudes about CAM, and the provider's attitudes about CAM. Pinpointing interventions for these issues is key. Research should explore whether CAM disclosure interventions are best at the provider level, the patient level, or both.

Additionally, it appears that providers lack sufficient knowledge about the safety and efficacy of individual CAM [42,53]. Providers need more knowledge about the specific types of CAM so that they can better assess a patient's safe usage. Part of this problem is the lack of rigorous trials examining the efficacy and safety of CAM for people living with HIV [2,54], which falls on the shoulders of researchers.

1.8 SECTION 8: RECOMMENDATIONS FOR RESEARCHERS

The lack of rigorous trials in the literature needs to be addressed to ascertain the safety and efficacy of individual CAM for people living with HIV. Although it is true that funding is limited for research focused on these issues, this does not have to be the case. Greater efforts can be made to show just how important studying CAM is to garner more financial support for research on this topic. CAM use among people living with HIV, in particular, is very high. This fact in and of itself necessities more research to be performed to determine the safety of these products, particularly in combination with antiretroviral therapies for people living with HIV.

Additionally, research on CAM has also been limited by methodology and changing definitions of CAM to draw clear conclusions about the efficacy and utility of these areas [2]. Specifically, the assessment of CAM use among people living with HIV has lacked instrument reliability and validity [54]. In a systematic review, Owen-Smith et al. [54] found that only six articles out of 32 reported reliability data of CAM measures for people living with HIV. This is an obvious hole in the research. Without reliable measures, it is impossible to know if the relationships being studied are truly there or just a statistical anomaly. Researchers must be more deliberate in testing the reliability and validity of these measures prior to their use in scientific work. Another hole identified in this systematic review was the lack of assessment regarding frequency, dose, and/or duration of CAM use [54]. As the authors point out, this information could be very important in the clinical implications that it has for patients. Obviously, more frequent use of herbal CAM known to interact with antiretrovirals would be more concerning than infrequent use of it.

Finally, testing interventions to increase CAM use disclosure among people living with HIV is necessary. As mentioned, one key factor to target is increasing the patient–provider relationship. There is a wide range of literature looking at this; however, nothing, to our knowledge, looks specifically at this relationship with the end outcome being disclosure of CAM use to HIV care providers. Although there are some effective interventions that already exist to increase the positive nature of the patient–provider relationship, we do not actually know if this will also increase CAM use disclosure. To test this, stringent research methodology, such as randomized controlled trials, must be used. It becomes the job of the researcher to weed out the interventions that are truly effective within and across different populations from interventions that are subpar.

1.9 SECTION 9: SUMMARY

In sum, prevalence rates of CAM are particularly high among people living with HIV and use is often not disclosed to HIV health care providers.

When seeking information among CAM from sources other than HIV care providers, patients may turn to health food stores and the Internet, which may provide inaccurate information. Some subpopulations may be particularly vulnerable to believing medical misinformation presented on the Internet as fact.

CAM use among people living with HIV is an issue that requires involvement from patients, providers, and researchers alike. The acquisition and dissemination of accurate knowledge are the keys across all of these roles. More methodologically sound research must be conducted to gain accurate information about the safety and efficacy of various types of CAM. This information must then be disseminated to both providers and patients through published scientific articles and then distilled down in more readable formats such as through .gov and .edu web sites. Providers can seek this information from the primary journal articles as well as from .gov and .edu web sites. Patients can also visit these web sites, but they can also discuss these issues with their providers. Figure 1.1 shows

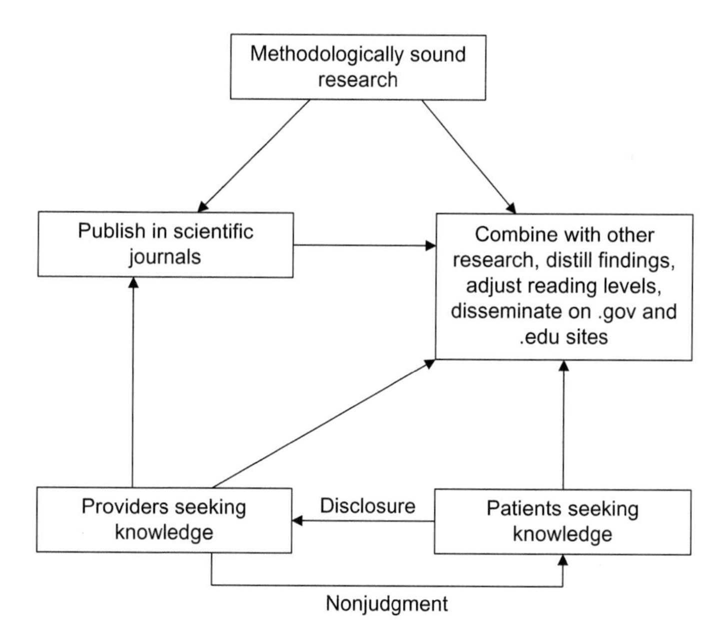

FIGURE 1.1 The acquisition and dissemination of knowledge regarding CAM.

an infographic of these paths of knowledge. The key point of this model, however, is the importance of the spread of knowledge through these different points and people. If specific pathways become weak, then the spread of knowledge also suffers. All of the paths are essential to solve issues presented in this chapter.

Acknowledgment

This research was supported by the National Institute of Mental Health Grant T32MH07487.

References

[1] National Center for Complementary and Alternative Medicine. CAM basics: what is complementary and alternative medicine? Retrieved from: <http://nccam.nih.gov/health/whatiscam>; 2001.

[2] Park C, Mind-body CAM. Interventions: current status and considerations for integration into clinical health psychology. J Clin Psychol 2013;69:45–63.

[3] Littlewood RA, Vanable PA. A global perspective on complementary and alternative medicine use among people living with HIV/AIDS in the era of antiretroviral treatment. Curr HIV/AIDS Rep 2011;8(4):257–68.

[4] Hasan SS, See CK, Choong CL, et al. Reasons, perceived efficacy, and factors associated with complementary and alternative medicine use among Malaysian patients with HIV/AIDS. J Altern Complement Med 2010;16(11):1171–6.

[5] Bormann JE, Uphold CR, Maynard C. Predictors of complementary/alternative medicine use and intensity of use among men with HIV infection from two geographic areas in the United States. J Assoc Nurses AIDS Care 2009;20(6):468–80.

[6] Ladenheim D, Horn O, Werneke U, et al. Potential health risks of complementary alternative medicines in HIV patients. HIV Med 2008;9(8):653–9.

[7] Lorenc A, Robinson N. A review of the use of complementary and alternative medicine and HIV: issues for patient care. AIDS Patient Care STDS 2013;27(9):503–10.

[8] Barnes PM, Powell-Griner E, McFann K, et al. Complementary and alternative medicine use among adults: United States, 2002. Adv Data 2004;27:1–19.

[9] Bishop FL, Lewith GT. Who uses CAM? A narrative review of demographic characteristics and health factors associated with CAM use. Evid Based Complement Alternat Med 2010;7(1):11–28.

[10] Song R, Hall HA, Harrison KM, et al. Identifying the impact of social determinants of health on disease rates using correlation analysis of area-based summary information. Public Health Rep 2011;126(Suppl. 3):70–80.

[11] Willison KD, Williams P, Andrews GJ. Enhancing chronic disease management: a review of key issues and strategies. Complement Ther Clin Pract 2007;13:232–9.

[12] Ball K, Lawson W, Alim T. Medical mistrust, conspiracy beliefs & HIV-related behavior among African Americans. J Psychol Behav Sci 2013;1:1–7.

[13] LaVeist TA, Nickerson KJ, Bowie JV. Attitudes about racism, medical mistrust, and satisfaction with care among African American and white cardiac patients. Med Care Res Rev 2000;57:146–61.

[14] López-Cevallos DF, Harvey SM, Warren JT. Medical mistrust, perceived discrimination, and satisfaction with health care among young-adult rural Latinos. J Rural Health 2014;30:344–51.

[15] Kalichman SC. Denying AIDS: conspiracy theories, pseudoscience, and human tragedy. copernicus. New York, NY: Springer; 2009.

[16] Bogart LM, Thorburn S. Are HIV/AIDS conspiracy beliefs a barrier to HIV prevention among African Americans? J Acquir Immune Defic Syndr 2005;38(2):213–8.
[17] Kalichman SC, Eaton L, Cherry C. There is no proof that HIV causes AIDS: AIDS denialism beliefs among people living with HIV/AIDS. J Behav Med 2010;33(6):432–40.
[18] Kalichman SC, Cherry C, White D, et al. Use of dietary supplements among people living with HIV/AIDS is associated with vulnerability to medical misinformation on the Internet. AIDS Res Ther 2012;9(1):1.
[19] Catz SL, Kelly JA, Bogart LM, et al. Correlates, and barriers to medication adherence among persons prescribed new treatments for HIV disease. Health Psychol 2000;19(2):124–33.
[20] Foot-Ardah CE. The meaning of complementary and alternative medicine practices among people living with HIV in the United States: strategies for managing everyday life. Sociol Health Illn 2003;25(5):481–500.
[21] Shedlin MG, Asnastai JK, Decena CU, et al. Use of complementary and alternative medicines and supplements by Mexican-origin patients in a U.S.–Mexico border HIV clinic. J Assoc Nurses AIDS Care 2013;24(5):396–410.
[22] Josephs JS, Fleishman JA, Gaist P, et al. Use of complementary and alternative medicines among a multistate, multisite cohort of people living with HIV/AIDS. HIV Med 2007;8(5):300–5.
[23] Leonard B, Huff H, Merryweather B, et al. Knowledge of safety and herb–drug interactions amongst HIV+ individuals: a focus group study. Can J Clin Pharmacol 2004;11(2):e227–31.
[24] Sparber A, Wootton JC, Baurer L, et al. Use of complementary medicine by adult patients participating in HIV/AIDS clinical trials. J Altern Complement Med 2000;6(5):415–22.
[25] Ciesla JA, Roberts JE. Meta-analysis of the relationship between HIV infection and risk for depressive disorders. Am J Psychiatry 2001;158:725–30.
[26] Herek GM. AIDS and stigma. Am Behav Sci 1999;42:1106–16.
[27] Furler MD, Einarson TR, Walmsley S, et al. Use of complementary and alternative medicine by HIV-infected outpatients in Ontario, Canada. AIDS Patient Care STDS 2003;17(4):155–68.
[28] Olsen MF, Abdissa A, Kæstel P, et al. Effects of nutritional supplementation for HIV patients starting antiretroviral treatment: randomized controlled trial in Ethiopia. BMJ 2014;348:g3187.
[29] Gautam N, Dayal R, Agarwal D, et al. Role of multivitamins, micronutrients and probiotics supplementation in management of HIV infected children. Indian J Pediatr 2014;81:1315–20.
[30] Wood R. Antiretroviral therapy. In: Abdool Karim SS, Abdool Karim Q, editors. HIV/AIDS in South Africa. South Africa: Cambridge University Press; 2010. pp. 529–50.
[31] Budzinski JW, Foster BC, Vandenhoek S, et al. An *in vitro* evaluation of human cytochrome P450 3A4 inhibition by selected commercial herbal extracts and tinctures. Phytomedicine 2000;7:273–82.
[32] Block KI, Mead MN. Immune system effects of echinacea, ginseng, and astragalus: a review. Integr Cancer Ther 2003;2:247–67.
[33] Fugh-Berman H. Herb–drug interaction. Lancet 2000;355:134–8.
[34] Owen-Smith A, Diclemente R, Wingood G. Complementary and alternative medicine use decreases adherence to HAART in HIV-positive women. AIDS Care 2007;19(5):589–93.
[35] Jernewall N, Zea MC, Reisen CA, et al. Complementary and alternative medicine and adherence to care among HIV-positive Latino gay and bisexual men. AIDS Care 2005;17(5):601–9.
[36] Parienti JJ, Das-Douglas M, Massari V, et al. Not all missed doses are the same: sustained NNRTI treatment interruptions predict HIV rebound at low-to-moderate adherence levels. PLoS One 2008;3(7):e2783.

[37] Irish AC. Maintaining health in persons with HIV infection. Semin Oncol Nurs 1989;5:302–7.
[38] Palmer R. Use of complementary therapies to treat patients with HIV/AIDS. Nurs Stand 2008;22:35–41.
[39] Owen-Smith A, McCarty F, Hankerson-Dyson D, et al. Prevalence and predictors of complementary and alternative medicine use in African-Americans with acquired immune deficiency syndrome. Focus Altern Complement Ther 2012;17(1):33–42.
[40] Liu C, Yang Y, Gange SJ, et al. Disclosure of complementary and alternative medicine use to health care providers among HIV-infected women. AIDS Patient Care STDS 2009;23(11):965–71.
[41] McDonald K, Slavin S. My body, my life, my choice: practices and meanings of complementary and alternative medicine among a sample of Australian people living with HIV/AIDS and their practitioners. AIDS Care 2010;22(10):1229–35.
[42] Muñoz FA, Servin AE, Kozo J, et al. A binational comparison of HIV provider attitudes towards the use of complementary and alternative medicine among HIV-positive Latino patients receiving care in the US–Mexico border region. AIDS Care 2013;25(8):990–7.
[43] Wynia MK, Eisenberg DM, Wilson IB. Physician–patient communication about complementary and alternative medical therapies: a survey of physicians caring for patients with human immunodeficiency virus infection. J Altern Complement Med 1999;5(5):447–56.
[44] Mills E, Singh R, Kawasaki M, et al. Emerging issues associated with HIV patients seeking advice from health food stores. Can J Public Health 2003;94:363–6.
[45] Kalichman SC, Weinhardt L, Benotsch E, et al. Internet access and Internet use for health information among people living with HIV–AIDS. Patient Educ Couns 2002;46(2):109–16.
[46] Kalichman SC, Benotsch EG, Weinhardt LS, et al. Internet use among people living with HIV/AIDS: association of health information, health behaviors, and status. AIDS Educ Prev 2002;14(1):51–61.
[47] Kalichman SC, Cain D, Cherry C, et al. Internet use among people living with HIV/AIDS: coping and health-related correlates. AIDS Patient Care STDS 2005;19(7):439–48.
[48] Berland GK, Elliott MN, Morales LS, et al. Health information on the Internet: accessibility, quality, and readability in English and Spanish. JAMA 2001;285(20):2612–21.
[49] Benotsch EG, Kalichman SC, Weinhardt LS. HIV–AIDS patients' evaluation of health information on the Internet: the digital divide and vulnerability to fraudulent claims. J Consult Clin Psychol 2004;72(6):1004–11.
[50] Johnson MO. The shifting landscape of health care: toward a model of health care empowerment. Am J Public Health 2011;101:264–70.
[51] Johnson MO, Sevelius JM, Dilworth SE, et al. Preliminary support for the construct of health care empowerment in the context of treatment for human immunodeficiency virus. Patient Prefer Adherence 2012;6:395–404.
[52] Sarafino EP, Smith TW. Health psychology: biopsychosocial interactions, 7th ed. Hoboken, NJ: Wiley; 2010.
[53] Freeman EM, MacIntyre RC. Evaluating alternative treatments for HIV infection. Nurs Clin North Am 1999;34(1):147–62.
[54] Owen-Smith A, DePadilla L, DiClemente R. The assessment of complementary and alternative medicine use among individuals with HIV: a systematic review and recommendations for future research. J Altern Complement Med 2011;1:789–96.

CHAPTER

2

Eating Coffee Candy: HIV Risk at Huli Funerals

Philip Gibbs[1] and Heather Worth[2]

[1]School of Culture, History and Language, Canberra, Australia,
[2]School of Public Health and Community Medicine, University of New South Wales, Sydney, NSW, Australia

Traditionally, sex and death have a symbiotic relationship in many cultures in Papua New Guinea (PNG). In a strange turn of fate, this relationship has been reinstated in PNG through human immunodeficiency virus (HIV) and AIDS. PNG is the epicenter of the HIV epidemic in the Pacific, with an estimated HIV prevalence among adults of approximately 1% [1] and double that in the Southern Highlands and Hela Provinces, where the data for this chapter were collected. The main route of HIV transmission in PNG is sex between men and women.

The Huli are a large cultural group of 140,000 people [2] occupying approximately 5,000 km^2 in the Southern Highlands of PNG.[1] Traditionally, Huli lived by hunting, gathering plants, and growing crops because they are exceptional farmers and much of the land is fertile. The Huli's first encounter with Westerners occurred in 1934–1935 [3,4], and continued with Government and Christian mission presence from the 1950s [5]. Many Huli men migrated out as indentured laborers on plantations in other parts of the country; opportunities opened up in and around Huli territory in the 1980s and 1990s with the Mt. Kare gold rush [6–8], and the establishment of resource development projects such as the Hides Garfield, Kutubu Petroleum, and the Porgera Gold Mine [4,9]. These developments

[1] We recognize that the Huli are not a totally homogenous group and that there are minor local, cultural, and social differences among the Huli-speaking people.

Health of HIV Infected People, Volume 2.
DOI: http://dx.doi.org/10.1016/B978-0-12-800767-9.00002-9

have brought opportunities for employment and access to money and other material items, but they have also been instrumental in facilitating rapid cultural and social change. Although there was an almost complete breakdown of law and order around the time of the failed 2002 national elections in the Southern Highlands Province (SHP), there has been a semblance of progress in recent years with the beginning of a multibillion dollar liquefied natural gas (LNG) project [10].

The Huli are known for their traditional cultural beliefs and practices that discouraged contact between men and women [11–15]. In what is now the generation of grandfathers, boys from the age of approximately 13 years and older were told not to eat food cooked or handled by women. Young men were secluded in the *haroli* initiation rites lasting over several years, where they lived separately and grew and cooked their own food. They were taught that any sort of contact with women, including their mothers and sisters, would impair their growth. In some places there were separate walking paths for men and women [16]. Married men used spells for protection during sex. To not do so would risk impairing their health, premature aging, or even death. Traditionally, sexual intercourse was considered highly dangerous to the man under three circumstances: during menstruation, after a woman had given birth, and with a woman approaching or beyond menopause [13]. Frankel describes at length men's illnesses deemed to be caused by contact with women.

Since the 1960s, exposure to social and cultural beliefs and practices from other parts of PNG and global processes has contributed to changing the Huli lifestyle. Initiation rites have long been abandoned and modern education has produced young men and women who have largely forgone the training that would equip them for life in the traditional society of their parents and grandparents [17]. Although "men's" houses still exist in many places, they are the place of primary residence only for some older men and unmarried male youth. Now, married men generally reside in family houses along with their wives, children, and perhaps other relatives.

HIV has hit people hard in the Highlands region, generally. In the SHP until the end of 2008, 738 people had been diagnosed with HIV, with more women than men testing HIV-positive (mostly due to antenatal surveillance) [18]. In 2008, a total of 11,139 people had been tested for HIV in SHP, with an HIV incidence of 1.7% [18]. There are a number of social and economic reasons why Huli are at risk for HIV. First, large-scale resource extraction has meant that many men have migrated for work at enclave sites. Wardlow [19] found that many villages in Tari had nearly half of all the adult men missing. Second, royalty payments for land use have put large amounts of cash in the hands of a few (male) landowners. Recent evidence has indicated that many of these landowners visit Port Moresby to pick up royalty payments and pay for sex while they are away from home [20].[2] Third, women, often alone and without money for periods of time, turn to transactional or paid sex [19,21].

Huli society is polygynist; men may take multiple wives but women may only have one husband at a time. However, extramarital liaisons are also common. Wardlow [22], referring to the "social construction of infidelity," argues that there are more socioeconomic structures that promote, enable, and normalize Huli men's extramarital sexuality—and thus increase women's HIV risk—than constrain or discourage it [22]. Social risks of extramarital sex are constructed so that husbands face few penalties as long as their liaisons are with women who are perceived as "not belonging," such as widows, divorcees, and women who engage in transactional sexual relations [22].

In this chapter, we examine the Huli funeral as an occasion of HIV risk. Using interview data collected in the Southern Highlands from Huli, we examine the ways in which traditional modes of thinking and behaving at funerals are being overturned and, in the process, sexual risk is heightened.

2.1 METHOD

The initial insight for this chapter came from research for the Sexually Transmitted Infections Management Program (STIMP)—part of the PNG Sexual Health Improvement Program (PASHIP).[3] The STIMP study involved focus group discussions and semi-structured in-depth interviews with key informants and others during 2008–2009 in Simbu and the SHPs. Interviews were conducted mostly in Tok Pisin,[4] but also in English, and in Huli with the assistance of a translator. Focus groups were desegregated by sex and age. Candidates for in-depth interviews were chosen either because of the quality of their contribution to the focus group discussions or because of their social position in the community. The interviews were transcribed and entered into NVivo 8 qualitative data

[2] The recent study by Kelly et al. [20] has found that "traditional landowners" are the most common clients of those who sell and/or exchange sex in the capital city, Port Moresby. It is common knowledge that with payments for the LNG project being negotiated and distributed in Port Moresby at the time of the study, the Huli are well-represented in that group of traditional landowners. Every likelihood indicates that these traditional landowners will return home, some unknowingly bringing sexually transmitted infections (STIs) with them. This will add to the source of infection already in circulation.

[3] The results of the STIMP research are published in the report *Sik Nogut o Nomol Sik* [23].

[4] Although PNG has more than 800 local languages, *Tok Pisin* is PNG's lingua franca.

management software.[5] Analysis of the data involved standard thematic coding and thoughtful interrogation of these. Approximately one-quarter of the STIMP research was in the Tari (Huli) District. During the 21 focus group discussions and 25 personal interviews conducted in the Huli-speaking regions (including 79 men and 90 women), there was frequent reference to funerals being the principal risk occasions for contracting HIV in the Tari area. This chapter takes some representative quotes from the STIMP interviews and pursues these with further literature research, updated data on HIV, follow-up interviews, and on-site observation to achieve an in-depth understanding of the topic.

Ethical approval for the STIMP research was gained from the Research Advisory Council (RAC) of the National AIDS Council (NAC) of PNG. Informed verbal consent was obtained before interviews and pseudonyms had been substituted for the actual names of those quoted in this chapter.

2.2 RESULTS: EATING COFFEE AND CANDY AT HULI FUNERALS

According to traditional custom, funerals were women's space. Men would take no part in the mourning. Their only formal tasks were the provision of firewood and preparing a platform on which the body was placed. In recent decades, it would involve the construction of a coffin and digging of the grave. Then, the men would retire and return for the actual burial and filling of the grave. Frankel and Smith describe a traditional Huli funeral in the 1970s. "When someone dies the women who have been in attendance begin to keen. In this area of scattered settlements the news is thus carried to the whole neighborhood, and so scores of women, or even hundreds if the deceased was a prominent person, gather at the *duguanda* (literally 'crying house') where the body is laid out on a platform. The women crush around the platform. They weep freely, rock from leg to leg, clutch at the body, embrace it, caress the feet, and bewail their loss" [14]. One or two women lead in singing a lament for the dead (*kiabudugu*), with the other women joining in the death wail [24,25]. The women continue to mourn with the body through the night until interment, usually the next day.

Today, women still lead the mourning at funerals; however, modern-day funerals are very different from before. The following from Mbira, a senior man in the focus group, is typical of what older people are saying about funerals around Tari today.

[5] One male interviewer coded the interviews with men and one woman interviewer coded the interviews with women. The data for this article come principally from the material coded under the node "funerals."

> Funerals are different now. Before the women would stay in the funeral house during the night and the men would go and sleep elsewhere. Now at funerals the men and women stay together until dawn. That is why there is so much sex at funerals. It seems that the funeral house has taken the place of the *daweanda*. We have abandoned the *daweanda* and the duguanda has taken its place.

Mbira makes two important points here. First, the expression "stay together" calls for clarification. Traditionally, women occupied different spaces at funerals than did men. Mbira's concern is that now these spaces are no longer separate, and to stay together involves sex. Second, he is arguing that the funeral house (the duguanda) has morphed into another Huli institution (the *daweanda*). The *daweanda* traditionally was an occasion for a feast to honor the dead, or a memorial for the dead if there were no recent deaths. But the daweanda was also reputed to be an occasion of sexual excess because young or unattached women were permitted to mingle with the older men. The sexual connotation of the daweanda is apparent in a play on words in which it was covertly called a *tauanda*. *Tau* refers to sexual organs and *anda* refers to a house; young men were forbidden to participate in events at the daweanda for fear that they would participate in a "feast of the genitals," which according to social norms would endanger their health and growth.

By the 1990s when Wardlow, an ethnographer who has written extensively on Huli and sexual practices, was in Tari, the aspect of a feast for the dead had diminished as men paid an entrance fee and competed by singing courtship songs. She notes that the daweanda "are also somewhat like brothels" [19]. Some men were content with the sexual joking and the camaraderie of the event, but many others were chosen by women present to have sex at the end of the night. Wardlow notes how daweanda were said to be "*gonolia pulap*" (full of sexually transmitted infections [STIs]) and that the Tari hospital was paying the police to burn them down [19]. Recently, the daweanda has, for the most part, been discontinued due to pressure from churches and the local leaders who considered it a health hazard, although there are currently moves to revive them again.

In contrast to the daweanda, which was held occasionally, the duguanda mourning house is mandatory as soon as a person dies. Mbira says that practices from funerals are now taking the place of the daweanda because funerals now include activities that formerly were part of the feasting, courting, and sexual activity associated with the daweanda. The logic expressed is that funerals have replaced the daweanda, when in fact the contrary appears to be the case.

Mende, during a focus group for middle-aged men, clarifies as follows:

> Many go there and they say, "We are going to eat coffee candy." One time I went and witnessed at the funeral house for an old woman who had died, how all of Tari came, and I saw how they were paired off, and one man said, "Not three or four together, it must be two-two." They had a Coleman lamp and then they turned off

the lamp. I asked, "What sort of behavior is this?" And they said, "Now it is the way we do things." I went there and saw it.

The expression "eat coffee candy" literally refers to a type of candy flavored with coffee syrup in the middle and sold in PNG under the brand name Jack 'n Jill XO Coffee and Butter Caramel Candy. At one time people would provide cups of coffee to help those staying overnight at a funeral to stay awake. Now the coffee candy is replacing the cup of coffee. Young people started using the Tok Pisin expression "*kaikai kofi kendi*" (eat coffee candy) in approximately 2006 [26]. However, there is more to coffee candy than staying awake—the expression "eat coffee candy" is a metaphor for sexual intimacy at Huli funerals. The way he questioned the events he witnessed at the funeral for an old woman, Mende appears to have found it a shocking novelty when a man was telling people to pair off before the lamp was extinguished. Moreover, Mende notes how "all of Tari was there" to emphasize the size of the crowd gathering during the night at the funeral. Formerly, depending on the status of the person who had died, funerals might not gather large crowds. Now, the crowd is expanded through ties associated with the Huli cognatic kinship system, and those looking for sex take advantage of the occasion. Tebone, during a focus group for young men, explained, "When a girl gives me that look and I make a sign with my eyes, then we agree. When we hear of a funeral we will attend, and the girl will be there and we will have sex during the night."

Market places are an alternative venue for people to meet; however, most markets are held during daylight hours, which limits the possibilities for intimacy. Night markets, movie nights, and "discos" usually finish well before midnight. However, funerals offer the chance for people to be together "*six tu six*" (Tok Pisin: literally "from 6 p.m. to 6 a.m."), and some funerals extend over 2 or even 3 nights. During the day a small group of women will remain mourning with the body, but at night large crowds assemble.

Some informants said that a couple would consent to meet at the mourning house, but then go outside in the bushes or long grass for sex. However, Mende insinuates that in some places sexual activity occurs at the funeral site itself after people have paired off and under the cover of darkness once the lamp has been extinguished. Those most upset by the changing customary meaning of the mourning house are older people who consider it offensive both morally (people having sex "*nating nating*" [Tok Pisin: literally "nothing nothing"—promiscuously]) and practically (it spreads diseases such as HIV).

2.3 DISCUSSION: "EAT AND DIE"

How could sex on such a public occasion enter into a society that appears to expend much time and energy keeping men and women apart?

In his article on Mortuary Rites on Tanga Island, Foster [27] points out the cultural logic wrapping death, sex, and food.[6] Mortuary symbolism converts death into life by reconstituting social relations through eating in opposition to commonly held beliefs about female sexuality and death. Also, there is a common expression in Huli, *nalu homabe* (literally: "eat [and] die"), that has both traditional and modern meanings. According to tradition, women bring forth new life and are also responsible for bringing death to humankind. Goldman [28] relates the Huli myth of the woman who gave birth to the first child and who did not respond when a man carrying the water of life addressed her as "Mother of life." Through her silence she became "Mother of death." As a result, as noted earlier in this chapter, Huli believed that contact with women could cause a man to become ill and/or die. This idea was and is used to warn boys and young men about the dangers of eating food contaminated by menstrual blood. For a young man to have sex without knowing and practicing the protective rituals used by married men would be to risk illness and even death. Today, with the presence of HIV, the expression has taken on new meaning. Young men apply the expression to the risk in having sex when there is the chance of being infected by the HIV virus, which, prior to the availability of antiretroviral therapy, was thought to mean a sure death.[7]

The sentiment is expressed by Mane, a middle-aged male respondent during an in-depth interview, saying, "I heard the young people say 'Eat and die, eat and die.' They want to eat coffee candy and die." Here "eating" is not just consuming a small piece of candy, it is a metaphor for consuming in a wider sense. Coffee candy with its sweet, sugary taste that makes the mouth water for a short time is a euphemism for sex. It is about the sweetness and pleasure of sexual excitement.[8]

Wardlow says that the daweanda "is a site of contradiction" because women there are potential wives, but also "free food" [19]. Now, the duguanda also exhibits signs of contradiction with mourning in one part and sex in another. Eating coffee candy has more to do with sex than

[6] "Death and sex comprise two forms of a generalized process of consumption, the archetype of which is eating…" [27].

[7] Antiretroviral therapy (ART) in Tari is available principally through St. Joseph's VCT Centre run by Catholic Health Services. As of July 2011, the Centre provides ART for 290 people.

[8] The image of "eating" does not necessarily imply oral sex. The verb "eat" in Huli (verb stem: *ne*, purposive form—in order to eat: *nole*) is a "proverb" that Lomas glosses as "to ingest." One hears *tomo naju* (he/she ate food), *mundu naja* (he/she ate tobacco [smoked]), *taga naja* (he/she ate [was consumed by] shame), or *ita naja* (fire ate [burned] him/her). The verb "to eat" takes particular social significance when, as Wardlow notes, accepting money for sex, and the women are sometimes said to "eat their own bridewealth" or even to "eat their own vaginas" [29].

mourning. Older people find this appalling: "They don't go to mourn, they go to have sex!" (Nogowali, in a focus group for married women). For the younger people and the unattached, "eating coffee candy" is appealing as a modern transgressive event. Such occasions are not without their consequences. If a young woman becomes pregnant after such an event, then people might say, *kendi najagome ge nde lajada* (by eating candy her leg was twisted/betrayed). They use a euphemism, but the meaning is clear to the listeners.

One might ask why pregnancies happen and why STIs are spread. Typical of PNG Highlands behavior, many people engage "skin to skin" (unprotected sex), with the attendant risks, including that of being infected with HIV.[9] A health worker in the Tari district told of the following case.

> A married man came for testing the other day. He appeared quite worried and said before the test, "Sister, you have to help me. Please give me some drugs to limit my chances of getting infected. I'm quite worried. I attended this funeral last week and had sex with three women. My wife is at home and I haven't slept with her yet." I told him that it is too late to do anything now but I could help him after he tested. I counseled him and ran an HIV test. His test came out reactive. He was very regretful but I told him to come back for confirmatory tests and provided post-test counseling.

No doubt the man was infected previously, but his behavior at this particular event illustrates how funerals are a space in which there is HIV risk. This is not an isolated case. One health worker in Tari tells how young people use mobile phones to facilitate their encounter.

> In Tari customary law proscribes young men and women going around together in public. But there is no law to prohibit them going to a funeral. A boy and girl will decide to go to a funeral and they have their mobile phones with them. When she decides to leave and go home the girl will send a text to her boyfriend to let him know. When she leaves, he will follow. This is how girls get pregnant or how young people get infected. I know of some who are HIV-positive and that is how they got infected.

The Huli world is changing rapidly. This is particularly the case for young people, especially those who have been to school and who are dissatisfied with a subsistence agriculture-based lifestyle. Even in the mid-1990s among the Kewa—Highland neighbors of the Huli—Lisette Josephides (1999) [30] noticed significant changes in the lives and attitudes of young women who were seeking new forms of personal space, lifestyles, and aesthetic expression. Clark and Hughes note how in the early 1990s there were radical changes in gender relations among the

[9] Condoms are available in Tari through health centers or are sold in some stores. However, some find it embarrassing to request them and not all people choose to use them [22]. Use by some at funerals is obvious from the empty wrappers seen in the vicinity after the event.

Huli [31]. They note how Huli beliefs about female contamination are "dynamic and flexible" [31]. Rather than being the source of pollution, women started to accuse men of acting like "pigs" and "dogs," and of being responsible for the spread of STIs. In the decade and a half since those studies, the changes have continued and even accelerated. Mobile phones and movies/DVDs are two of many globalizing influences.

Huli are also experiencing changing power relations. Previously, older men controlled young men through initiation rites and the culture of fear associated with women and sexuality [13]. Young men were forbidden to attend the daweanda. However, that control could not be sustained when young men no longer participated in traditional initiation rites when they went to work on coastal plantations or went to school or just did not want to participate any more. The churches also encouraged nuclear family living arrangements and opposed beliefs that appeared to lower the status of women.[10] These and other factors contributed to lessening of fears about pollution, disempowering the older men, and providing new avenues for the young.

Huli funerals today are part of the changing social behavior in present day Huli life. "Feasting for the dead"—the daweanda—which has been discontinued, has been inculcated into the duguanda—the "crying house." However, these transformations also date back to traditional beliefs in the interstices of sexuality, pollution, sickness, and death. The daweanda and duguanda appear to have morphed to form a hybrid characterized by the ambiguity of modernity and freedom from tradition, new meanings for funerals, and the dangers and responsibilities of remaining healthy in the midst of an HIV epidemic.

The Huli funeral is part of a globalized world led by young people who have had to reinvent themselves in the shifting environment. There are new meanings for funerals, having less to do with mortality and the end of everything and having more to do with social life and sexual life. HIV presents very real challenges for health and well-being. Anxieties about the connection between illness and sexuality in traditional society, with little empirical basis in fact, now have some substance [31]. All of these are symbolized in sharing, unwrapping, and savoring the imported sticky sweetness of "coffee candy."

2.4 RESPONSES

Community and church leaders and health workers are attempting to deal with the situation. Mogome, a community leader, told how at the

[10] Wardlow notes how, ironically, some men say that the church made the daweanda more necessary, because many men no longer had their men's houses to escape to [19].

time of her mother's funeral she and her family simply assumed control and told the men and other visitors to go home at night and come back the next day for the burial: "No one can come eat coffee candy or whatever here—most certainly not (Tok Pisin: '*nogat na nogat olgeta*'). We were tough about it and no one came for that." Others have suggested that funerals be curtailed. Dauni, a young married church worker, during a focus group discussion suggested, "if someone dies in the morning we could bury them in the afternoon of the same day, then they would not need to stay overnight." A listener added, "What is the use of keeping a dead body, it is of no use, so bury it quickly." During a meeting of church leaders at one Catholic Church, there was discussion regarding whether the body could be moved from the duguanda to the church building overnight. We were told that village court magistrates have threatened to charge men and women four or five pigs for having sex at a funeral—if they are caught.

However, attempts focusing on funerals miss the point, unless they take into account the deeper issues identified in this chapter, such as Huli gender ideology, the changing meaning of social structures, and healthy sexual intimacy in the context of an HIV epidemic.

References

[1] National Department of Health PNG Papua New Guinea HIV prevalence: 2009 estimates. Waigani, Papua New Guinea: NDOH and PNGNACS; 2010.
[2] Haley N, May RJ, editors. Conflict and resource development in the Southern Highlands of Papua New Guinea. Canberra, Australia: ANU Epress; 2007.
[3] Hides J. Papuan wonderland. London: Blackie and Son; 1936.
[4] Ballard C. A history of Huli society and settlement in the Tari region. PNG Med J 2002;45:8–14.
[5] Meshanko R. The gospel amongst the Huli. MA Thesis. Washington Theological Union: Washington, DC; 1985.
[6] Biersack A. The Mount Kare python and his gold: totemism and ecology in the Papua New Guinea highlands. Am Anthropol 1999;101:68–87.
[7] Clark J. Gold, sex, and pollution: male illness and myth at Mt Kare, Papua New Guinea. Am Ethnol 1993;20:742–57.
[8] Vail J. All that glitters: the Mt Kare gold rush and its aftermath. In: Biersack A, editor. Papuan borderlands. Huli, Duna, and Ipili perspectives on the Papua New Guinea Highlands. Ann Arbor, MI: University of Michigan Press; 1995. pp. 343–74.
[9] Biersack A, editor. Papuan borderlands: Huli, Duna, and Ipili perspectives on the Papua New Guinea Highlands. Ann Arbor, MI: University of Michigan Press; 1995.
[10] PNG LNG Project overview. <http://www.pnglng.com/media/pdfs/publications/137425_Mar2010_PNG_Fact_Sheets_V3_FS1.pdf>; 2010 [accessed 03.04.11].
[11] Glasse R. The Huli of the Southern Highlands. In: Lawrence P, Meggitt M, editors. Gods, ghosts and men in Melanesia: some religions of Australian New Guinea and the New Hebrides. Melbourne, Australia: Oxford University Press; 1965. pp. 27–49.
[12] Glasse R. Huli of Papua: a cognatic descent system. The Hague, the Netherlands: Mouton; 1968.
[13] Frankel S. The Huli response to illness. Cambridge: Cambridge University Press; 1986.
[14] Frankel S, Smith D. Conjugal bereavement amongst the Huli people of Papua New Guinea. Br J Psychiatry 1982;141:302–5.

[15] Hughes J. Impurity and danger: the need for new barriers and bridges in the prevention of sexually-transmitted disease in the Tari Basin, Papua New Guinea. Health Transit Rev 1991;1:131–40.
[16] Wardlow H. Economy, and female agency: problematizing "prostitution" and "sex work" among the Huli of Papua New Guinea. Signs 2004;29:1017–40.
[17] Lomas G. The Huli language of Papua New Guinea. PhD dissertation. School of English and Linguistics, Macquarie University; 1988; Retrieved 2 April 2011 from <http://hdl.handle.net/1959.14/22313>.
[18] National Department of Health STI, HIV and AIDS Surveillance Unit The 2008 STI, HIV and AIDS annual surveillance report. Waigani, Papua New Guinea: NDOH; 2009.
[19] Wardlow H. Wayward women: sexuality and agency in a New Guinea Society. Berkeley and Los Angeles, CA: University of California Press; 2006.
[20] Kelly A, Kapul M, Man WYN, Nosi S, Lote N, Rawstorne P, et al. Askim na save (ask and understand): people who sell and/or exchange sex in Port Moresby. Key quantitative findings. Sydney, Australia: Papua New Guinea Institute of Medical Research and the University of New South Wales; 2011.
[21] Lepani K. Mobility, violence, and the gendering of HIV in Papua New Guinea. Special issue on modern men: continuities and ruptures in Australia and the Pacific. J.P. Taylor (Ed.). Austr J Anthropol, 2008;19:150–64.
[22] Wardlow H. Men's extramarital sexuality in rural Papua New Guinea. Am J Public Health 2007;97:1006–14.
[23] Gibbs P., Mondu M. Sik Nomol o Nogut Sik: a study into the socio-cultural factors contributing to sexual health in the Southern Highlands and Simbu Provinces, Papua New Guinea. Caritas Australia, 2010.
[24] Pugh J. Communication, language and Huli music. BA (Hons) thesis. Department of Music, Monash University, Australia. 1975.
[25] Peters B. Huli music: its cultural context, musical instruments and *gulupobe* music. BA (Hons) thesis. Department of Music, Monash University, Australia. 1975.
[26] Personal communication Matthew Timbalu, Tari, 27 March, 2011.
[27] Foster R. Nurture and force-feeding: mortuary feasting and the construction of collective individuals in New Ireland society. Am Ethnol 1990;17:431–48.
[28] Goldman L. Talk never dies: the language of Huli disputes. London: Tavistock Publications; 1983.
[29] Wardlow H. Giving birth to *gonolia*: "culture" and sexually transmitted disease among the Huli of Papua New Guinea. Med Anthropol Q 2002;16:151–75.
[30] Josephides L. Disengagement and desire: the tactics of everyday life. Am Ethnol 1999;26:139–59.
[31] Clark J, Hughes J. A history of sexuality and gender in Tari. In: Biersack A, editor. Papuan borderlands. Huli, Duna, and Ipili perspectives on the Papua New Guinea Highlands. Ann Arbor, MI: University of Michigan Press; 1995. pp. 315–40.

CHAPTER

3

Infant Feeding Policies and HIV

Louise Kuhn

Gertrude H. Sergievsky Center, College of Physicians and Surgeons, New York, NY, USA

3.1 INTRODUCTION

The observation that human immunodeficiency virus (HIV) infection can be transmitted via breastfeeding was made soon after the first cases of the unusual and fatal disease that would later become known as HIV were first identified in New York City and San Francisco [1]. Before the likelihood of transmission of HIV via breastfeeding was known, the Centers for Disease Control had already issued recommendations prohibiting breastfeeding for any HIV-infected woman [1]. In the ensuing almost three decades, infant feeding policy for HIV-infected women in sub-Saharan Africa would become one of the most contentious issues on the global health agenda.

In this chapter, the key dimensions of the policy debates around breastfeeding and HIV are described. The focus of the chapter is on sub-Saharan Africa because this is the region most severely affected by the HIV epidemic, with massive epidemics in countries in the southern region of the continent. For example, in South Africa, HIV prevalence rates among women presenting at antenatal care clinics have stabilized at approximately 30% [2]. Thus, the burden of HIV and the influence of the infant feeding policies are most acutely felt by the women and children in sub-Saharan Africa, particularly in the southern sections.

The chapter first introduces the concept of competing risks that underlies the polarized debate around whether HIV-infected women should breastfeed at all. Next, the chapter outlines three "middle-ground concepts" that attempt to steer policies away from simple "all-or-nothing" thinking. These are (i) exclusive breastfeeding; (ii) early weaning; and

Health of HIV Infected People, Volume 2.
DOI: http://dx.doi.org/10.1016/B978-0-12-800767-9.00003-0

(iii) informed choice. The chapter then reviews the game-changing scientific breakthroughs in how antiretroviral drugs can be used to prevent breastfeeding-associated HIV transmission and how these have become integrated into policies. Finally, the chapter considers some key gaps that have not yet been addressed by infant feeding policies in the context of HIV.

3.2 TO BREASTFEED OR NOT TO BREASTFEED? IS THAT THE RIGHT QUESTION?

The Centers for Disease Control in the United States was quick to advise against breastfeeding for HIV-infected women [1]. The World Health Organization was slow to even acknowledge that HIV was an issue that needed to be taken into account for its infant feeding policies, particularly in sub-Saharan Africa. This led to a disturbing situation early in the epidemic of an apparent "double-standard" with breastfeeding recommended for HIV-infected women in Africa and avoidance of all breastfeeding recommended for HIV-infected women in the United States and Europe [3]. To understand the basis for this disparity, it is necessary to appreciate the competing risks that need to be taken into account.

The dilemma that lies at the heart of the policy debate is that HIV infection can be transmitted via breastfeeding and, at the same time, avoidance of all breastfeeding is associated with increased risk of morbidity and mortality. In other words, there is no good alternative. The only rational approach is to estimate the magnitude of the risk with each alternative to compare these estimates and to recommend the alternative with the least amount of harm.

3.2.1 Quantifying the Magnitude of Breastfeeding-Associated HIV Infection

Current estimates of the magnitude of breastfeeding-associated HIV infection indicate that, in the absence of any antiretroviral drug interventions, there is an approximately 1% additional risk of HIV infection with each month of breastfeeding when an HIV-infected woman breastfeeds her child [4]. This risk is in addition to the risk of an HIV-infected woman transmitting to the unborn infant during pregnancy (intrauterine-acquired infection) and transmitting to the infant during delivery (intrapartum-acquired infection) [4]. In the absence of any antiretroviral drug interventions, there is an approximately 20% risk of an infant acquiring HIV intrauterine or intrapartum. If an HIV-infected woman breastfeeds her infant for 10 months, then the cumulative risk of HIV infection acquired through all vertical or mother-to-child routes is approximately 30%. If she breastfeeds until 15 months, then the total vertical transmission rate is 35%, and so on [4].

It took some time to establish reasonably robust estimates of the magnitude of breastfeeding-associated transmission. Initial approaches simply compared the total amount of mother-to-child HIV transmission observed in populations where breastfeeding was the norm (sub-Saharan African populations) with that observed in populations where breastfeeding was rare (US and European populations). A meta-analysis taking this approach reported a risk of acquiring HIV via breastfeeding of 14% (95% confidence interval, 7–21%) as early as 1992 [5]. Despite the methodological limitations of this approach, a randomized trial in Nairobi confirmed this rate of transmission [6].

With the development of polymerase chain reaction (PCR) technology which is able to detect HIV DNA, it was possible to quantify the magnitude of breastfeeding-associated HIV transmission more directly. Sequential blood tests could be conducted in breastfed infants and the steady accumulation of HIV infections described. It was through these methods that our current estimates of breastfeeding-associated transmission risks are derived [7]. PCR technology also allowed for appreciation that the duration of breastfeeding needs to be taken into account in describing risks of transmission. Given the inefficiency of HIV transmission and the large sample sizes required for precise quantification, even with PCR technology it has proven difficult to determine whether the risk of postnatal transmission is constant over the full duration of breastfeeding or whether the risk declines as the child ages [4,8].

3.2.2 Quantifying the Magnitude of Risks Associated with Not Breastfeeding

In the nutrition and child health literature, there are many risks associated with avoidance of breastfeeding. These include, from the child's point of view, increased risk of infectious disease including pneumonia and diarrhea, increased risk of poor growth, long-term risks of obesity and metabolic disorders, and worse cognitive outcomes [9]. From the mother's point of view, these include worse recovery from pregnancy and delivery, sooner risk of a subsequent pregnancy, and long-term risks of certain diseases including breast cancer [9]. For the purposes of considering competing risks in the context of HIV, only one outcome has ever been considered sufficiently severe to weigh against the risk of HIV transmission. This is all-cause mortality in infants (younger than 12 months) or children (2 to 5 years).

Quantifying risks of infant or child all-cause mortality associated with avoidance of breastfeeding requires knowledge of two additional parameters: (i) the absolute magnitude of the mortality risk among *breastfed* children in the population of interest and (ii) the *relative* increase in this mortality likely to occur if there is a shift away from breastfeeding. Both of these parameters are heavily influenced by context.

Routine statistics are maintained regarding infant and child mortality rates for all countries as a fundamental part of vital statistics and global health indicator data. For countries where breastfeeding is the norm, these statistics essentially provide an estimate of background rates of mortality among breastfed infants (parameter 1). There are glaring disparities in infant and child mortality rates between richer and poorer countries, with sub-Saharan African countries having considerably higher rates than that observed in the United States and Europe [10]. For example, in 2010, less than 5-year mortality was estimated to be 5/1,000 live births in the United Kingdom, 7/1,000 in the United States, 51/1,000 in South Africa, and 119/1,000 in Zambia [10]. Thus, a critical dimension to weighing the competing risks requires taking background mortality into account.

The relative risk of mortality if breastfeeding is avoided (parameter 2) has to be estimated from observational epidemiological studies. Although there is overwhelming consistency across studies demonstrating at least some increased risk associated with shifts away from breastfeeding, there is a great deal of variability across studies on the actual size of this risk. These studies differ in their rigor and the extent to which they adequately deal with the methodological challenges inherent in observational epidemiology such as confounding, measurement error, and reverse causality [11]. Few studies have focused on all-cause mortality specifically, and most focus on specific causes of death such as diarrhea and pneumonia or examine morbidity only [12]. These studies have also been conducted in a range of different settings. Higher relative risks (3- to 5-fold increases) are generally observed in studies conducted in more impoverished settings where infectious diseases make a bigger contribution to child mortality, with more modest relative risks (1.5- to 2-fold increases) observed in high-resource settings in the United States and Europe [12]. Thus, poverty exacerbates risks associates with avoidance of breastfeeding.

3.2.3 How Do the Numbers Stack Up?

There are several published competing risks models quantifying risks of breastfeeding-associated HIV transmission and weighing these risks against child mortality due to avoidance of breastfeeding by HIV-infected women [13–15]. All of these models reach the same conclusion: it depends! These models reach the conclusion that the choice between breastfeeding and not breastfeeding for HIV-infected women depends on the background infant or child mortality rates for the setting of interest. Generally, when infant mortality exceeds approximately 25/1,000, breastfeeding is a better option to maximize outcomes even in the absence of antiretroviral drugs [13–15]. All settings with mortality rates below this cutoff (i.e., all of North America and Europe) would have better outcomes if HIV-infected women avoided all breastfeeding. All settings with mortality rates above this cutoff (i.e., all of sub-Saharan Africa) would have better outcomes if all HIV-infected women breastfed.

In sum, the competing risks model provides a rational (in terms of least amount of harm) justification for the "double-standard" policy. But it is a bitter pill to swallow for most advocates, scientists, and clinicians concerned with maternal and child health in sub-Saharan Africa.

3.3 HARM REDUCTION APPROACHES

Given this unsatisfactory state of affairs, attention turned to potential harm reduction strategies focusing on reducing risks of HIV transmission via breastfeeding and/or reducing risks of mortality associated with avoiding breastfeeding. Harm reduction possible with the use of antiretroviral drugs during lactation was able to finally provide a path out of this dilemma (discussed in the final section of the chapter). At this point, two nonpharmaceutical options for reduction of postnatal transmission are discussed, exclusive breastfeeding and early weaning. Harm reduction on the other side of the scale (to reduce mortality) took a complex form that argued that women should make informed choices to avoid breastfeeding if an alternative to breastfeeding was affordable, feasible, acceptable, stainable, and safe (AFASS).

3.3.1 Exclusive Breastfeeding

The first almost 15 years of debate around infant feeding policies for HIV-infected women in sub-Saharan Africa largely considered breastfeeding as a simple dichotomy: some breastfeeding versus no breastfeeding. Breastfeeding practices were not differentiated in terms of either duration or quality. Widely accepted characteristics of healthy lactation in the first few months of life, such as *exclusive* breastfeeding, or hotly debated topics in the nutrition field, such as the optimal *duration* of exclusive breastfeeding, were unfamiliar to most HIV-focused practitioners providing services for HIV-infected women in sub-Saharan Africa [16]. This was to change with the report from Durban, South Africa, suggesting that exclusive breastfeeding conveyed a lower risk of HIV transmission than nonexclusive breastfeeding [17].

In the Durban study, HIV-infected women were recruited during pregnancy and counseled about their infant feeding options. Those women who chose to initiate some breastfeeding were counseled to exclusively breastfeed until at least 4 months. Detailed information was collected over time regarding women's actual feeding practices and infants were tested at regular intervals for HIV using PCR tests. In the analysis, rates of mother-to-child HIV transmission were compared across three groups: (i) those who never breastfed; (ii) those who breastfed exclusively until at least 3 months; and (iii) those who breastfed but the period of exclusive breastfeeding, if any, was less than 3 months. Rates of infection detectable by 6 weeks were the same across the three groups. This is to be expected because this describes intrauterine or intrapartum infection and would not be expected to differ by postnatal feeding practices. After 6 weeks, there were essentially no new infections through 3 months in those who were not breastfeeding or among those who were exclusively breastfeeding through this time [17]. This study prompted a series of further studies and analyses that also reported that risks of postnatal transmission of HIV were lower if breastfeeding was exclusive compared with nonexclusive breastfeeding in the first few months of life [18–20].

It was a straightforward policy decision to recommend exclusive breastfeeding for 6 months for HIV-infected women. This simply made breastfeeding recommendations for HIV-infected women consistent with standard recommendations for general population women who intended to breastfeed. However, motivation for exclusive breastfeeding emphasized its benefits for HIV transmission rather than clearly contextualizing the policy in the context of lactation advice designed to optimize non-HIV-related health benefits for mother and child. The latter is a more standard reason for recommending exclusive breastfeeding in the absence of HIV.

The HIV risk associated with breastfeeding continued to dominate thinking. Because exclusive breastfeeding did not entirely stop all breastfeeding-associated HIV transmission, exclusive breastfeeding was pitted against avoidance of all breastfeeding. By definition, avoidance of all breastfeeding avoids all breastfeeding-associated transmission. In this comparison, exclusive breastfeeding is an inferior option. Taken outside of the competing risks framework, the mortality and other downsides of avoidance of all breastfeeding become invisible.

Strangely, policy in support of *exclusive* breastfeeding also began to be used as an argument against breastfeeding itself. Two polarized options were promoted: exclusive breastfeeding or exclusive formula feeding. If women did not adhere to exclusive breastfeeding, then they were encouraged to switch to exclusive formula feeding. How the "logic" of this was reached is unclear but appears to be driven by HIV transmission concerns. In presenting these two "all-or-nothing" choices, non-HIV implications of shifts away from breastfeeding were ignored. Nowhere within HIV programs was there a clear recommendation that some breastfeeding was better than no breastfeeding with regard to non-HIV-related outcomes such as infant mortality.

3.3.2 Early Weaning

During the same time that associations between exclusive breastfeeding and lower rates of postnatal HIV transmission relative to nonexclusive breastfeeding were being described, nutrition policy around the optimal duration of exclusive breastfeeding for the general population was being debated [16]. This debate finally settled on recommending 6 months as the optimal duration of exclusive breastfeeding in contrast to the "4–6 months" advised in prior iterations of policy. Given the strong messaging around the importance of avoiding any nonexclusive breastfeeding from an HIV transmission point of view, the transition to complementary feeding after 6 months posed a challenge for policies for HIV-infected women. It was taken as inconsistent to be recommending exclusive breastfeeding until 6 months and nonexclusive breastfeeding thereafter. Thus, the only apparent internally consistent option was to recommend stopping all breastfeeding as soon as breastfeeding could no longer be exclusive (i.e., early weaning).

It is unfortunate that the observations that risks of postnatal HIV transmission were lower among exclusive than among nonexclusive breastfeeders during the first 4 months of life and were extrapolated to argue for early weaning, because this extrapolation manifests flawed reasoning. The first flaw pertains to the lack of biological plausibility of generalizing the HIV-related benefits of exclusive breastfeeding during the period when this practice is developmentally appropriate, that is, before 6 months to the period after 6 months when this practice is no longer developmentally appropriate. In addition to lack of biological plausibility, there are no studies reporting that risks of postnatal transmission *increase* in the period of complementary feeding after 6 months. Studies that have reported changes in the rates of breastfeeding-associated transmission rates over time have observed static or declining rates of HIV transmission as the child ages [8].

Utilization of data demonstrating benefits of exclusive breastfeeding for HIV transmission as an argument to support early weaning is also flawed because it ignores the competing risks of non-HIV adverse outcomes. An argument in support of early weaning needs to weigh the magnitude of postnatal HIV transmission that can be avoided with early weaning against the magnitude of non-HIV-related adverse outcomes that will result when breastfeeding is truncated before its usual duration. Early models predicted that early weaning may be beneficial [13,21]. Like the simpler scenario of some versus no breastfeeding described at the beginning of the chapter, the competing risks of stopping breastfeeding earlier than usual compared with breastfeeding for a usual duration need to be quantified.

The magnitude of postnatal HIV transmission that can be avoided with early weaning is less than with no breastfeeding because some period of breastfeeding is already tolerated. In other words, for example, if we expected to avoid transmission in 15% of infants who would have been breastfed for 15 months but who now receive no breastfeeding at all, then we advise early weaning at 6 months, and we can now expect to avoid infection in only 9% of infants. From a competing risks point of view, to justify this smaller amount of benefit, only smaller risks of non-HIV adverse outcomes can be tolerated.

Like in the original competing risks model using some versus no breastfeeding, only HIV-exposed uninfected infant or child mortality has been considered to be of sufficient severity to be weighed against risks of HIV transmission. In terms of child mortality, the strongest argument in support of early weaning comes from data suggesting that benefits of breastfeeding are greatest for younger infants [22]. Both absolute risks of mortality and relative benefits of breastfeeding have been shown to be greater for the younger the child [22]. Based on these assumptions, competing risks models predicted that early weaning (at approximately 4–6 months of age) would optimally balance risks of HIV transmission and uninfected child mortality [13,21].

One randomized clinical trial was set up to directly test this model prediction—the Zambian Exclusive Breastfeeding Study (ZEBS) [23]. In ZEBS, HIV-infected women were randomized either to early weaning at 4 months or to continued breastfeeding for a duration of their own choice. Women in the continuing breastfeeding arm of this study breastfed for a median of 16 months. Postnatal HIV transmission was quantified using repeat testing of children for HIV DNA by PCR through 24 months. Mortality among HIV-exposed children with no positive PCR results was described through 24 months. These two adverse outcomes were counted as equivalent to yield an estimate of HIV-free survival. This primary endpoint describes the probability of surviving free of HIV infection from 4 to 24 months.

In contrast to model predictions, ZEBS reported no difference in HIV-free survival between the two randomized arms [23]. The lack of benefit of early weaning was not explained by poor adherence to the intervention. ZEBS also reported that early weaning was not enthusiastically embraced in this population. Further analyses of the data from this trial revealed that the lack of net benefit of early weaning was explained by increases in uninfected child mortality associated with early weaning that cancelled out the small benefits in terms of postnatal HIV infections averted [24,25]. Further, in contrast to what had been expected in terms of declining risks of mortality as the child aged, ZEBS observed persisting high relative risks of mortality when breastfeeding was withdrawn that persisted until the child was approximately 15 months of age [25].

At the same time that this trial was being undertaken, most programs shifted to recommending early weaning for HIV-infected women. Studies published after this unfortunate natural experiment demonstrated that mortality in these populations increased [26,27].

3.3.3 When Is Avoidance of Breastfeeding AFASS?

It is challenging to support an infant feeding policy purely on the basis of the rational least amount of harm point of view when the amount of harm remains considerable. As a result of this uncomfortable policy position, one solution is to enter into denial about the accuracy of the information. It proved impossible to deny the reality of HIV transmission via breastfeeding, which left the question of whether avoidance of breastfeeding is actually dangerous. It may seem surprising that the benefits of breastfeeding would be called into question. Yet such is the power of concerns about HIV transmission. At the extreme end of the continuum were those who felt that there were no risks associated with avoidance of breastfeeding and that the only policy issue at stake was cost. Access to infant formula was argued to be a "human right" and passionate advocacy for the provision of formula was undertaken. Many programs started offering free infant formula for HIV-infected women despite criticism of the safety of this approach [28].

In this fractious climate, the World Health Organization attempted a compromise position that would support avoidance of all breastfeeding for HIV-infected women if they chose this option after counseling that allowed them to make an informed choice. The basis of their informed choice was to hinge on what became known as the AFASS criteria. AFASS stands for "affordable, feasible, acceptable, sustainable, and safe." If an HIV-infected woman was of the opinion that avoidance of all breastfeeding was AFASS for herself, then she was to be supported in her choice not to breastfeed. If a woman did not feel that she met the AFASS criteria, then she was to be encouraged to breastfeed.

The intention of this policy was to contextualize risks associated with avoidance of breastfeeding and to make palatable the reality that, in sub-Saharan African countries, mortality associated with avoidance of breastfeeding is larger than that associated with postnatal HIV transmission. In practice, it led to a great deal of confusion and concern within programs [29].

The flaw in this approach is that the only solution it offers to reduce risks associated with avoidance of breastfeeding is to confine formula use to populations where the absolute risk of mortality is low. Implied in the approach is the assumption that if AFASS criteria are met, then formula feeding is safe. Although it is true that socioeconomic characteristics exacerbate adverse consequences of shifts away from optimal breastfeeding [30], it is an incorrect assumption that avoidance of breastfeeding is equivalently healthy in wealthier populations. The health benefits of breastfeeding have been consistently demonstrated in both low and high socioeconomic circumstances [31].

3.4 ANTIRETROVIRAL INTERVENTIONS TRANSFORM THE POLICY ARENA

It was established in 1994 that antiretroviral drugs can be used to prevent mother-to-child HIV transmission [32]. Steadily over time, antiretroviral drug regimens were refined and modified to make them more applicable to low-resource settings. However, despite being used in populations where breastfeeding was the norm, the design of these interventions continued to focus only on the intrauterine and intrapartum period. Antiretroviral drugs were given to the mother from variable amount of times during pregnancy and then for relatively short periods to mothers and infants during the postpartum period [33]. As a result, it became quite concerning that these interventions reduced the risks of prenatal and perinatal infection but that breastfeeding added new infections during the postnatal period [34].

There are two ways in which antiretroviral drugs can be used during the postnatal period to prevent breastfeeding-associated HIV transmission: (i) antiretroviral drugs can be given to the mother and (ii) antiretroviral drugs can be given to the infant. Currently, strategies to reduce risks of transmission combine maternal and infant components.

The antiretroviral drugs that are used for prevention of vertical transmission are the same drugs that are used for treatment of HIV disease. In the case of treatment, these drugs are almost always used in triple drug combinations and, once started, are required indefinitely. In the case of prevention, these drugs initially were used in short courses of generally only one drug. However, this began to change to the point that the drug regimens used for treatment and those used for prevention are essentially indistinguishable. A complication in the simple conclusion that access to *treatment* for women will provide *prevention* for infants is that not all HIV-infected adults necessarily *need* treatment for their own health. Which HIV-infected adults need treatment has been a matter for debate and study. Generally, CD4 counts, as a marker of immunosuppression caused by HIV, have been used to set the dividing line between those HIV-infected adults considered to need treatment and those considered suitable to defer treatment until later. Clinical trials have indicated clearly that those HIV-infected adults with CD4 counts less than 350 require antiretroviral treatment for their own health [35].

From the infant point of view, if the mother needs and receives treatment, then this will also act as prevention. Because this treatment will need to continue indefinitely, the full duration of breastfeeding is covered. But for those infants whose mothers do not require treatment, these same drugs need to be given for the purpose of prevention. However, in this case, the duration of the regimen needs some consideration. Finally, clinical trials focusing on this latter group of women demonstrated that continuing antiretroviral drugs through 6 months reduced breastfeeding-associated transmission occurring through 6 months [36].

The choice of 6 months was based on the recommendations in place at the time the studies were performed that encouraged early weaning. Hence, the debates about whether to stop breastfeeding just shifted to the 6-month time point. In 2010 guidelines, the World Health Organization offered a compromise of 12 months of breastfeeding, recommending that maternal triple drug antiretroviral prophylaxis could continue for as long 12 months. This was based on logistical considerations about provision of drugs.

It also became increasingly clear that having to provide CD4 tests to determine which HIV-infected pregnant women needed antiretroviral therapy and which needed antiretroviral prophylaxis was a barrier in some settings to getting the women most in need (those with low CD4 counts) the antiretroviral treatment that they needed for their own health [37]. The national program in Malawi opted for what, at the time, was considered a rather radical approach that was to simply initiate lifelong antiretroviral treatment in all HIV-infected pregnant women [37]. This approach of universal antiretroviral therapy for pregnant women began to be called B+. This was a riff on the previously named Option B, which referred to providing the same drugs for a shorter period of time and then stopping when breastfeeding was to end. In 2013, the World Health Organization endorsed the B+ strategy as one of the preferred options for low-resource settings. At the same time, they expanded criteria for initiating antiretroviral therapy in adults to all those with CD4 counts less than 500 [38].

Infant antiretroviral prophylaxis was administered as part of regimens to prevent HIV transmission and was modeled from the first regimens that were studied. A type of "postexposure prophylaxis" was added to minimize the risks associated with intrapartum HIV exposure. Eventually, however, studies were performed extending the antiretroviral drugs administered to the infant during the breastfeeding period, providing a type of periexposure prophylaxis (pre-exposure and postexposure prophylaxis). This also proved to be highly effective in preventing postnatal transmission through breastfeeding [39,40]. Again, because of accidents of history (or coincidence), these studies were also planned and undertaken at the same time as early weaning was recommended, and thus evaluated only a maximum of 6 months of infant prophylaxis. Nevertheless, it appeared as if either maternal or infant antiretroviral drug interventions were used during the breastfeeding period, and the World Health Organization supported either one of these two approaches for preventing infections in infants of women who did not yet meet criteria for treatment. Infant prophylaxis was named Option A and maternal treatment was named Option B.

With the necessity for programs to provide antiretroviral therapy, Option B+ has come to dominate thinking about how to prevent infection in infants, but the role of infant prophylaxis is less clear [38]. Nevertheless, infant prophylaxis continues to be administered for at least some period of time in most settings, even when antiretroviral treatment is advised for women. Infant prophylaxis may play an important role when maternal antiretroviral therapy is started too late [40].

3.5 KEY GAPS IN INFANT FEEDING POLICIES AND HIV

Universal antiretroviral treatment for HIV-infected women reduces risks of postnatal HIV transmission through breastfeeding to very low levels. This renders moot the continued debated about whether to avoid breastfeeding, because even slight increases in mortality associated with reduced breastfeeding are larger than the small risks of transmission. Unfortunately, several gaps in policy remain, with a crucial one being implementation.

There has been marked neglect of the topic of how to support breastfeeding for HIV-infected women. A review of the literature could locate only one study that specifically considered the question of how to improve breastfeeding practices among HIV-infected women. This study evaluated a community-based intervention to support exclusive breastfeeding in four African countries. The intervention was successful in increasing the uptake of exclusive breastfeeding across all settings but revealed how far short of optimal breastfeeding practices were among many HIV-infected women [41]. There is an urgent need for more intervention-oriented research to help improve lactation practices among HIV-infected women.

References

[1] Centers for Disease Control Recommendations for assisting in the prevention of perinatal transmission of human T-lymphotropic virus type III/lymphadenopathy-associated virus and acquired immunodeficiency syndrome. MMWR Morb Mortal Wkly Rep 1985;34:721–6. 31–2.

[2] United Nations Children's Fund (UNICEF) Sixth Stocktaking Report ed. Towards an AIDS-free generation—children and AIDS. New York, NY: UNICEF; 2013.

[3] Kuhn L, Aldrovandi G. Pendulum swings in HIV-1 and infant feeding policies: now halfway back. Adv Exp Med Biol 2012;743:273–87.

[4] Rollins N, Mahy M, Becquet R, Kuhn L, Creek T, Mofenson L. Estimates of peripartum and postnatal mother-to-child transmission probabilities of HIV for use in spectrum and other population-based models. Sex Transm Infect 2012;88(Suppl. 2):i44–51.
[5] Dunn DT, Newell ML, Ades AE, Peckham CS. Risk of human immunodeficiency virus type 1 transmission through breastfeeding. Lancet 1992;340:585–8.
[6] Nduati R, John G, Mbori-Ngacha D, Richardson B, Overbaugh J, Mwatha A, et al. Effect of breastfeeding and formula feeding on transmission of HIV-1: a randomized clinical trial. JAMA 2000;283:1167–74.
[7] Coutsoudis A, Dabis F, Fawzi W, Gaillard P, Haverkamp G, Harris DR, et al. Late postnatal transmission of HIV-1 in breast-fed children: an individual patient data meta-analysis. J Infect Dis 2004;189:2154–66.
[8] Miotti PG, Taha TE, Kumwenda NI, Broadhead R, Mtimavalye LA, Van der Hoeven L, et al. HIV transmission through breastfeeding: a study in Malawi. JAMA 1999;282:744–9.
[9] Labbok MH, Clark D, Goldman AS. Breastfeeding: maintaining an irreplaceable immunological resource. Nat Rev Immunol 2004;4:565–72.
[10] Rajaratnam JK, Marcus JR, Flaxman AD, Wang H, Levin-Rector A, Dwyer L, et al. Neonatal, postneonatal, childhood, and under-5 mortality for 187 countries, 1970–2010: a systematic analysis of progress towards millennium development goal 4. Lancet 2010;375:1988–2008.
[11] Golding J, Emmett PM, Rogers IS. Breast feeding and infant mortality. Early Hum Dev 1997;49(Suppl.):S143–55.
[12] Bhutta ZA, Ahmed T, Black RE, Cousens S, Dewey K, Giugliani E, et al. What works? Interventions for maternal and child undernutrition and survival. Lancet 2008;371:417–40.
[13] Kuhn L, Stein Z. Infant survival, HIV infection and feeding alternatives in less developed countries. Am J Public Health 1997;87:926–31.
[14] Ross JS, Labbok MH. Modeling the effects of different infant feeding strategies on infant survival and mother-to-child transmission of HIV. Am J Public Health 2004;94:1174–80.
[15] Hu DJ, Heyward WL, Byers Jr. RH, Nkowane BM, Oxtoby MJ, Holck SE, et al. HIV infection and breast-feeding: policy implications through a decision analysis model. AIDS 1992;6:1505–13.
[16] Kramer MS, Kakuma R. The optimal duration of exclusive breastfeeding: a systematic review. Adv Exp Med Biol 2004;554:63–77.
[17] Coutsoudis A, Pillay K, Kuhn L, Spooner E, Tsai WY, Coovadia HM. Method of feeding and transmission of HIV-1 from mothers to children by 15 months of age: prospective cohort study from Durban, South Africa. AIDS 2001;15:379–87.
[18] Kuhn L, Sinkala M, Kankasa C, Semrau K, Kasonde P, Scott N, et al. High uptake of exclusive breastfeeding and reduced early post-natal HIV transmission. PLOS ONE 2007;2:e1363.
[19] Iliff PJ, Piwoz EG, Tavengwa NV, Zunguza CD, Marinda ET, Nathoo KJ, et al. Early exclusive breastfeeding reduces the risk of postnatal HIV-1 transmission and increases HIV-free survival. AIDS 2005;19:699–708.
[20] Coovadia HM, Rollins NC, Bland RM, Little K, Coutsoudis A, Bennish ML, et al. Mother-to-child transmission of HIV-1 infection during exclusive breastfeeding in the first 6 months of life: an intervention cohort study. Lancet 2007;369:1107–16.
[21] Nagelkerke NJ, Moses S, Embree JE, Jenniskens F, Plummer FA. The duration of breastfeeding by HIV-1-infected mothers in developing countries: balancing benefits and risks. J Acquir Immune Defic Syndr Hum Retrovirol 1995;8:176–81.
[22] Effect of breastfeeding on infant and child mortality due to infectious diseases in less developed countries: a pooled analysis. Who Collaborative Study Team on the Role of Breastfeeding on the Prevention of Infant Mortality. Lancet 2000;355:451–5.
[23] Kuhn L, Aldrovandi GM, Sinkala M, Kankasa C, Semrau K, Mwiya M, et al. Effects of early, abrupt weaning on HIV-free survival of children in Zambia. N Engl J Med 2008;359:130–41.

[24] Kuhn L, Aldrovandi GM, Sinkala M, Kankasa C, Semrau K, Kasonde P, et al. Differential effects of early weaning for HIV-free survival of children born to HIV-infected mothers by severity of maternal disease. PLOS ONE 2009;4:e6059.

[25] Kuhn L, Sinkala M, Semrau K, Kankasa C, Kasonde P, Mwiya M, et al. Elevations in mortality associated with weaning persist into the second year of life among uninfected children born to HIV-infected mothers. Clin Infect Dis 2010;50:437–44.

[26] Taha TE, Hoover DR, Chen S, Kumwenda NI, Mipando L, Nkanaunena K, et al. Effects of cessation of breastfeeding in HIV-1-exposed, uninfected children in Malawi. Clin Infect Dis 2011;53:388–95.

[27] Jamieson DJ, Chasela CS, Hudgens MG, King CC, Kourtis AP, Kayira D, et al. Maternal and infant antiretroviral regimens to prevent postnatal HIV-1 transmission: 48-week follow-up of the BAN randomised controlled trial. Lancet 2012;379:2449–58.

[28] Coutsoudis A, Goga AE, Rollins N, Coovadia HM. Free formula milk for infants of HIV-infected women: blessing or curse? Health Policy Plan 2002;17:154–60.

[29] Chopra M, Rollins N. Infant feeding in the time of HIV: rapid assessment of infant feeding policy and programmes in four African countries scaling up prevention of mother to child transmission programmes. Arch Dis Child 2008;93:288–91.

[30] Habicht JP, DaVanzo J, Butz WP. Mother's milk and sewage: their interactive effects on infant mortality. Pediatrics 1988;81:456–61.

[31] Section on Breastfeeding Breastfeeding and the use of human milk. Pediatrics 2012;129:e827–41.

[32] Connor EM, Sperling RS, Gelber R, Kiselev P, Scott G, O'Sullivan MJ, et al. Reduction of maternal–infant transmission of human immunodeficiency virus type 1 with zidovudine treatment. Pediatric AIDS clinical trials group protocol 076 study group. N Engl J Med 1994;331:1173–80.

[33] Mofenson LM. Advances in the prevention of vertical transmission of human immunodeficiency virus. Semin Pediatr Infect Dis 2003;14:295–308.

[34] Mofenson LM. Antiretroviral drugs to prevent breastfeeding HIV transmission. Antivir Ther 2010;15:537–53.

[35] Severe P, Juste MA, Ambroise A, Eliacin L, Marchand C, Apollon S, et al. Early versus standard antiretroviral therapy for HIV-infected adults in Haiti. N Engl J Med 2010;363:257–65.

[36] Shapiro RL, Hughes MD, Ogwu A, Kitch D, Lockman S, Moffat C, et al. Antiretroviral regimens in pregnancy and breast-feeding in Botswana. N Engl J Med 2010;362:2282–94.

[37] Schouten EJ, Jahn A, Midiani D, Makombe SD, Mnthambala A, Chirwa Z, et al. Prevention of mother-to-child transmission of HIV and the health-related millennium development goals: time for a public health approach. Lancet 2011;378:282–4.

[38] Ahmed S, Kim MH, Abrams EJ. Risks and benefits of lifelong antiretroviral treatment for pregnant and breastfeeding women: a review of the evidence for the option B+ approach. Curr Opin HIV AIDS 2013;8:474–89.

[39] Coovadia HM, Brown ER, Fowler MG, Chipato T, Moodley D, Manji K, et al. Efficacy and safety of an extended nevirapine regimen in infant children of breastfeeding mothers with HIV-1 infection for prevention of postnatal HIV-1 transmission (HPTN 046): a randomised, double-blind, placebo-controlled trial. Lancet 2012;379:221–8.

[40] Chasela CS, Hudgens MG, Jamieson DJ, Kayira D, Hosseinipour MC, Kourtis AP, et al. Maternal or infant antiretroviral drugs to reduce HIV-1 transmission. N Engl J Med 2010;362:2271–81.

[41] Tylleskar T, Jackson D, Meda N, Engebretsen IM, Chopra M, Diallo AH, et al. Exclusive breastfeeding promotion by peer counsellors in sub-Saharan Africa (PROMISE-EBF): a cluster-randomised trial. Lancet 2011;378:420–7.

CHAPTER

4

Alcohol Use and Food Insecurity in HIV Disease Management

Seth C. Kalichman, Jennifer A. Pellowski and Dominica Hernandez

Department of Psychology, University of Connecticut, Storrs, CT, USA

The global human immunodeficiency virus (HIV) pandemic is characterized by multiple layers of diversity, from the populations most afflicted, to the behaviors that confer transmission of the virus, to the genetic variations of the virus itself. For all of their variation, HIV subepidemics share a common underlying thread of impoverishment and social disadvantage. The ills of HIV subepidemics represent one of many interconnected facets of poverty. HIV is just one of multiple co-occurring epidemics, or syndemics, in which HIV infection is associated with economic disadvantage, unstable housing, lack of transportation, food insecurity, traumatic experiences, social distress, mental illness, and substance abuse [1]. Poverty serves to isolate individuals within communities and to distance communities from a broad array of resources. Fueled by substance abuse and gender inequality, HIV spreads within closed social and sexual networks. Studies show that symptoms of depression are associated with food insecurity and that one in five people with HIV who are food insecure are also active drug users [2,3]. Thus, in even the most resource-rich countries of the world, including the United States, Canada, and Western Europe, HIV infections are most prevalent in the places of greatest poverty.

Health inequalities that characterize HIV epidemics emerge in the context of social discrimination and disadvantaged economic opportunity.

Health of HIV Infected People, Volume 2.
DOI: http://dx.doi.org/10.1016/B978-0-12-800767-9.00004-2

These disparities occur at the individual and social–structural levels [4]. At the individual level, factors such as affective regulation, decision-making skills, and behaviors have direct effects on health, whereas characteristics such as gender, sexual orientation, race, and education have indirect effects through socioeconomic opportunity and access to supportive resources. In addition, multiple personal characteristics moderate the influence of psychological factors such as negative effect, trauma, social support, and resilience. These individual-level psychological factors, in turn, influence decision processes, health behaviors, and physical states that directly impact HIV disease trajectories and health outcomes. At the social–structural level, economic conditions and distribution of resources affect adjustment, behaviors, immune functioning, and other dimensions of health.

In this chapter, we examine food insecurity and alcohol misuse as two common features of poverty that are known to complicate the course of HIV disease. Food insecurity, defined as limited access to nutritious food to meet dietary needs for an active and healthy life, diminishes the health of anyone, but the adverse effects of food insecurity are pronounced in people living with HIV infection. Similarly, the health consequences of alcohol misuse are also amplified in people living with HIV. In addition to their direct health effects, both food insecurity and alcohol use have indirect behavioral consequences, particularly on the management of HIV infection. Although considered distinct challenges, food insecurity and alcohol misuse may synergize to impede the health of people living with HIV. We therefore discuss food insecurity and alcohol use in relation to HIV disease management as well as the inter-relationships of food insecurity and alcohol misuse. We also consider the implications of the co-occurrence of food insecurity and alcohol misuse for interventions aimed at improving the health and treatment of people living with HIV infection.

4.1 FOOD INSECURITY AND HIV DISEASE

Hunger and lacking reliable access to nutritious food, or food insecurity, are reliable markers of poverty. And yet food insecurity is unique among the many facets of poverty in its direct effects on health and its association with medication nonadherence. Food insecurity in resource-rich countries is every bit as impactful as that seen in resource-poor countries. For example, in a study of homeless and marginally housed people living with HIV in San Francisco, Weiser et al. [5] found that more than half of the study participants were food-insecure, with one in three being defined as severely food-insecure. Among those persons receiving antiretroviral therapy, more than half were food-insecure, and food insecurity was associated with poorer health, particularly incomplete medication adherence and unsuppressed HIV replication [6]. Not having sufficient food was also related to poor adherence and was independently associated with poor treatment outcomes. Food insecurity itself appears to complicate HIV infection beyond its role in medication nonadherence. Food insecurity independently predicts emergency department visits, hospitalizations, and acute care outpatient visits [7]. Ultimately, food insecurity in combination with being underweight can contribute to the mortality of people living with HIV. In a study of HIV-infected individuals in Vancouver, 48% were experiencing food insecurity and 14% were underweight—defined as having a body mass index less than 18.5. In prospective analyses, with a median of 8.2 years of follow-up, the researchers found that 14% of their cohort had died from nonaccidental causes. In analyses that controlled for multiple confounding factors, the combination of being food insecure and underweight predicted mortality; individuals who were both food-insecure and underweight were nearly twice as likely to die in comparison with their food-secure or nonunderweight counterparts [8]. There was also a trend toward individuals who were food-insecure and not underweight having greater mortality, whereas those who were underweight but not food-insecure were not at greater risk for death. What was not considered in this study was the possibility that alcohol use may contribute to lower body mass index. Research from the Women's Interagency HIV Study found that alcohol use as well as tobacco use were independently associated with low body mass index in women living with HIV [9].

Although low body mass, or wasting, is most commonly considered a manifestation of food insecurity, malnutrition can also lead to high body mass and obesity when foods that are accessed have excessive low-nutrient energy. The increased prevalence of overweight and obesity in persons living with HIV runs in parallel to the general population, albeit with more dire health consequences [9,10]. Some studies have identified the prevalence of obesity within their sample to be as high as 29% in women and 13% in men [11], with the prevalence of overweight reaching 40% in both men and women. One study found that over the course of the participant's HIV infection (11 years), 72% gained weight, and 80% gained even greater amounts of weight if the participant was found to be overweight at the previous visit [12].

In a recent study of individuals living with HIV in Atlanta, Georgia, body composition and body weight were collected from a sample of men and women residing in impoverished neighborhoods [13]. In this sample, 27% of the participants were overweight (BMI $\geq 25\,kg/m^2$) and 29.1% were obese (BMI $\geq 30\,kg/m^2$). In addition, more females were overweight and obese than males, and the percentage of body fat was comparable for both men and women. However, men had a higher intake of fiber and servings of fruits and vegetables than women. Overall, all of the participants had daily fat intake percentages that were above the recommended daily allowances, with particularly low fiber and insufficient servings of fruits and vegetables. These results suggest that overweight and obesity are significantly impacting people living with HIV in impoverished settings. The study's nutritional analysis suggests people living with HIV may not be meeting minimal recommended nutritional standards, a situation that may be particularly detrimental to the care of these individuals.

Persons living with HIV are also burdened by life-threatening health conditions precipitated by reduction in critical immune functions, placing these individuals in vulnerable health circumstances. With overweight and obesity come multiple life-threatening health risks, such as type II diabetes, hypertension, coronary heart disease, and some cancers [14]. A person living with any one of these chronic health conditions faces numerous health risks, and the presence of dangerous comorbidities, such as obesity and HIV infection, may be even more life-threatening to this population because of their impaired immune function. The intersection of overweight/obesity and HIV likely compounds the severity of health risks to a greater extent than either HIV infection or any of the other chronic conditions alone.

4.2 ALCOHOL MISUSE AND HIV DISEASE

Alcohol misuse includes the broad spectrum of drinking patterns that increase risks for adverse outcomes from moderate drinking all the way to alcohol dependence. Within this spectrum, alcohol abuse is defined by the consequences that can incur from drinking, including disruptions in work, school, social obligations, interpersonal relationships, legal problem, and physical hazards of drinking. Alcohol dependence is the most severe gradation of alcohol abuse, the hallmark of which is physiological need for alcohol that, when unmet, results in withdrawal symptoms. However, even drinking in limited quantities and frequencies can impede HIV treatment and complicate HIV disease processes. The adverse effects of drinking on people living with HIV are known to span the entire range of alcohol consumption. In a carefully conducted study, Braithwaite et al. [15] found that even nonhazardous alcohol use of once per week or more can reduce survival of HIV-infected persons. The effects of alcohol on morbidity are even more pronounced in patients who are co-infected with HIV and hepatitis C virus. Alcohol use is a significant predictor of HIV transmission risks and, as such, most people infected with HIV have a history of alcohol misuse. Although many people stop drinking in an effort to remain healthy after they are diagnosed with HIV infection, alcohol use and misuse remain prevalent in people living with HIV. Data from the US Department of Veterans Affairs show that between 35% and 40% of patients receiving HIV clinical care have an alcohol use disorder.

Alcohol use has been discussed as a contributing factor in HIV disease progression since the early years of the epidemic. Alcohol has toxic effects at the cellular as well as organ and systemic levels [16]. Multiple components of the immune system are adversely impacted by alcohol misuse, including release of cytokines, host defenses, nutritional status, and oxidative stress, and these effects may be amplified in people who are immune-compromised from HIV infection [17]. Thus, the immunosuppressive effects of alcohol use have long been thought to be a contributing factor to developing AIDS. More recently, there is mounting evidence that alcohol accelerates HIV disease progression by directly affecting CD4 cells, the very immune cells that are targeted by HIV. Baum et al. [18] conducted a 30-month prospective study of alcohol use among people living with HIV who were receiving antiretroviral therapy and in comparison with individuals not receiving treatment. Results showed that individuals who drank two or more drinks daily were nearly three-times more likely to experience a clinically significant decline in CD4 cells independent of baseline health, treatment, and other relevant factors. Furthermore, Wu et al. [19] similarly reported that daily alcohol drinkers showed greater declines in CD4 cells and that they had nearly a four-fold increase in the likelihood of unsuppressed HIV replication. Importantly, the association between alcohol use and HIV suppression was not accounted for by medication adherence. There are several possible explanations for these findings, including the potential for alcohol and medications to interact in the liver and disrupt the metabolism and, therefore, clinical efficacy of antiretrovirals. It should also be noted that most of these studies have relied on self-reported adherence. In the absence of a more reliable and objective measures of adherence, it is possible that some of the well-established influences of alcohol use on medication adherence account for the failure to suppress HIV replication in drinkers.

As already noted, alcohol use has emerged as a significant complicating factor in people who are co-infected with HIV and hepatitis C virus. Liver disease is a common cause of death in HIV-infected persons, with liver-related mortality closely associated with hepatitis C virus co-infection. An estimated four to five million people in the world are living with HIV–hepatitis C virus co-infection [20]. Furthermore, antiretroviral therapy and substance use are both toxic to the liver, placing added strain on the liver with the potential to exacerbate liver damage. For example, alcohol use can amplify the hepatotoxicity of antiretroviral therapy and can accelerate the hepatitis disease trajectory [15]. Thus, combining antiretroviral medications and substance use will contribute to liver disease in people living with HIV, making antiretroviral medications, substance use, and hepatitis C virus co-infection a particularly lethal combination. Of those with low levels of alcohol use and HIV infection, 8% have developed advanced liver fibrosis and cirrhosis, and such is the case for 13% of people with hepatitis C virus infection only, compared with 31% among people living with HIV–hepatitis C virus co-infection [21]. The impact of alcohol use on antiretroviral therapy therefore extends beyond its contributions to treatment nonadherence, with hepatotoxicity interfering with the metabolism of antiretrovirals and, therefore, viral suppression. HIV–hepatitis C virus co-infected patients frequently report substance use, with nearly 1 in 10 abusing alcohol [22]. Studies suggest that frequency and quantity of alcohol consumption in co-infected patients may not differ in HIV mono-infected patients. In addition, co-occurring use of other drugs predicts greater alcohol consumption in HIV–hepatitis C virus co-infected patients, suggesting that multiple substances may be abused in people with co-infection.

Alcohol consumption is also related to multiple nutritional deficiencies that can contribute to impaired immune functioning. In part, alcohol itself has high-caloric intake value while offering no nutritional benefits. In addition, alcohol decreases the absorption of nutrients and interferes with nutrient metabolism [16]. Alcohol use further complicates health by impeding linkage and retention to care, undermining provider relationships and potentially creating pharmacological interactions with multiple treatments. In the context of limited personal resources, the cost of accessing alcohol further impacts health by diverting money and other limited resources toward obtaining and consuming alcohol and away from accessing food. For individuals who are alcohol-dependent, drinking is experienced as a biologically based survival need that can ultimately compete with the need for food and compromise health. Thus, a possible explanation for the linkage between alcohol misuse and food insecurity among the poor is the diversion of limited resources away from accessing food toward obtaining alcohol and other substances.

4.3 FOOD AND ALCOHOL AS COMPETING NEEDS

Under conditions of limited resources, alcohol use can have added adverse impacts by diverting resources away from accessing food. In a study of women in Rwanda, for example, alcohol use was strongly associated with food insecurity, such that women who used alcohol were three-times more likely to be food-insecure relative to women who did not drink alcohol [23]. The authors concluded that by controlling for income in their model, their results suggest that disposable income among women in their study was used to obtain alcohol rather than to obtain food; this was not a reflection of having more money available to purchase alcohol. In this sense, alcohol use can be considered a contributing factor to food insecurity. These results mirror research in resource-rich countries. A study in Vancouver, Canada, found that 63% of HIV-positive drug users reported experiencing recent hunger, 24% of those who were hungry consumed more than three alcoholic drinks daily, and more than half of individuals spent as much as $60 per day on drugs [24].

Further evidence that alcohol may divert limited resources away from accessing food comes from research involving men and women living with HIV infection in Atlanta, Georgia. Participants in one study were provided with a $30 grocery gift card for completing a survey, and the grocery receipts were returned and coded for how participants spent the funds. The study found that nearly one in four participants who returned receipts had purchased alcohol or tobacco products with their grocery gift cards. Among individuals who did purchase alcohol or tobacco, these participants spent more than 25% of their grocery gift card on alcohol or tobacco products. Overall, a greater proportion of gift card expenditures went toward tobacco than toward alcohol products. A multivariable logistic model showed that food insecurity was independently associated with unsuppressed HIV, and purchasing alcohol or tobacco products did not moderate this association. Results suggest a primary role of food insecurity in relation to HIV-related health outcomes that may be exacerbated by alcohol and tobacco use.

4.4 FOOD INSECURITY, ALCOHOL MISUSE, AND HIV DISEASE

Food insecurity is detrimental to the health of individuals at every point along the HIV continuum of care. In one study of adults in southern Africa, where one in three women did not have enough food to eat over a 12-month period, food insecurity was related to inconsistent condom use, sexual exchange, and other factors that confer sexual risks for HIV infection [25]. The relationship between food insecurity and sexual risks observed in women were attenuated in men, indicating the role of gender inequality, including in the link between food insecurity and sexual risks. This pattern of association is also observed in resource-rich countries. For example, in a study of homeless and marginally housed people living with HIV in San Francisco, both food insecurity and alcohol use were closely associated with engaging in unprotected sex, and food insecurity and drug use were related to having multiple sexual partners [3]. Food insecurity is also a barrier to HIV testing. For example, in a study in Uganda, where 36% of people living with HIV were defined as severely food-insecure and 31% were currently drinking alcohol, both food insecurity and alcohol use in women predicted never having been tested for HIV [26]. These associations were not observed in men, again indicating gender disparities in how food insecurity impacts HIV risk, transmission, diagnosis, and disease.

People living with HIV who are food-insecure and drink alcohol have more medical complications that result in greater medical service utilization. In a study of homeless and marginally housed people living with HIV, Weiser et al. [7] found that 24% experienced mild to moderate food insecurity and 31% were severely food-insecure. Only 5% were heavy drinkers, and yet both severity of food insecurity and heavy drinking predicted emergency department visits and hospitalizations for acute medical conditions. The HIV-related and co-occurring health problems in patients who drink are even further exacerbated by the central role that alcohol misuse plays in promoting medication and treatment nonadherence.

4.5 HIV TREATMENT ADHERENCE

As discussed, alcohol use and poor nutrition appear independently and interactively associated with HIV disease progression. These processes are also complicated by the significant influences of both drinking alcohol and food insecurity on medication adherence.

There is general agreement that patients should be told to take every dose of their medications and that those with adherence less than 85% can risk development of HIV viral resistance [27]. Prolonged treatment interruptions are more concerning than sporadic missed doses [28]. Parienti et al. showed that the predicted and observed HIV control, or viral suppression, is directly influenced by the duration of intervals of treatment discontinuation. This landmark study showed that medication interruptions of 10 days were associated with a 20% probability of antiretroviral therapy failure and interruptions of 15 days were associated with a 50% probability of failure. Periodic disruptions in meeting basic survival needs, such as access to food or extended periods of alcohol use and its aftereffects, may therefore be more detrimental to treatment than forgetting to take a dose of medication.

Alcohol use is among the most reliable predictors of medication nonadherence. Alcohol use can impair memory, disrupt organizational skills, disturb sleep patterns, and interfere with managing medications [29]. Alcohol consumption also has its own adverse health effects and is associated with malnutrition in its own right. Alcohol use and food insecurity therefore pose significant threats to the health of people living with HIV, including impacts on medication adherence. In what has become a classic meta-analysis in HIV treatment research, Hendershot et al. [29] examined 40 studies of antiretroviral therapy adherence, representing more than 25,000 research participants, and found that alcohol drinkers were more than half as likely to be medication-adherent than their nondrinking counterparts. Analyses further showed that formally defined problem drinkers were less adherent than persons who drank occasionally, who were less adherent than abstainers, suggesting a dose–response relationship between quantities of alcohol consumed and nonadherence to HIV medications, a pattern that is now well-established [30].

Food insecurity is also known to correlate with HIV treatment nonadherence [2]. Nearly half of HIV-positive individuals receiving drug treatment in British Columbia are food-insecure, a rate that is five-times greater than that of the general Canadian population [31]. As noted, food scarcity and malnutrition can contribute to HIV disease progression by compromising health in general and complicating HIV wasting in particular [32]. And, like alcohol, a lack of adequate food can interfere with the absorption of medications and pharmacokinetics of antiretroviral therapies [33]. There is also a close association between food insecurity and HIV medication adherence. In a study of homeless and marginally housed people living with HIV/AIDS in San Francisco, Weiser et al. [5] found that one in three people were severely food-insecure. Among those persons receiving antiretrovirals, more than half were food-insecure and food insecurity was associated with incomplete medication adherence and unsuppressed HIV [6]. Thus, not having sufficient food was related to poor adherence and was independently associated with poor treatment outcomes. Studies consistently show that food insecurity is a substantial barrier to medication adherence, and there is evidence that providing people with access to food improves adherence [34].

Food insecurity interferes with medication adherence by disrupting daily routines, impeding adherence strategies, and reducing motivation. In essence, the immediacy of accessing food to meet survival needs can understandably take priority over adhering to medication schedules. In addition to the direct effects of food insecurity on antiretroviral adherence, lacking food will further challenge the efficacy of antiretroviral therapy when medications are required to be taken with food for maximum absorption and clinical benefit [35]. Some patients may forego taking their medications when they are without food if they have been instructed that their medications should always be taken with food to work or to avoid side effects.

Food is required for processing, absorption, and optimal clinical benefits for certain antiretroviral regimens [36], with pharmacokinetic studies showing as much as a 38% increase in the availability of some antiretrovirals when taken with food [37]. The protease inhibitor darunavir (Prezista), for example, is rapidly absorbed and systemic exposure is increased by 30% when this medication is taken with a meal [38]. Similarly, administration of atazanavir (Reyataz) with a light meal results in a 70% increase in the drug's plasma concentration [39]. The bioavailability of ritonavir (Norvir), which itself is used to boost the bioavailability of other critical protease inhibitors, is also reduced when the medication is taken without food. People who are food-insecure must therefore periodically choose to either take their medications knowing they are not following directed use or skip their medications altogether when food is unavailable. People living with HIV who experience food insecurity may have poorer clinical outcomes as a result of both nonadherence and insufficient drug absorption. One study found that a significant number of people living with HIV who are food-insecure are prescribed HIV medications that should be taken with food, and these individuals had more HIV symptoms, lower CD4 cell counts, and poorer HIV suppression than their counterparts who were not prescribed medications that require food [40]. These results show a complex interplay between food and medication adherence that cuts across multiple levels, including daily habits and routines, competing priorities, and patient beliefs about the proper use of medications.

Individuals who drink alcohol and lack access to food are confronted by two of the most robust barriers to medication adherence, suggesting a confluence of challenges to maintaining the viral-suppressive effects of antiretroviral therapy. Because alcohol abuse and food insecurity co-occur in relation to poverty, they may not be independently associated with nonadherence. Researchers have therefore aimed to determine the primacy of alcohol use relative to food insecurity in determining medication nonadherence. Studies that have examined both alcohol use and food insecurity as predictors of medication adherence generally show that both factors are associated with nonadherence even when confounding influences are taken into account. For example, a study of men and women living with HIV in Atlanta found that food insecurity and alcohol use were both significantly associated with medication nonadherence after controlling for multiple facets of poverty, including education, employment status, income, housing stability, depression symptoms, social support, and nonalcohol drug use [41]. These cross-sectional analyses were replicated in a prospective study that also controlled for many of the same poverty markers [42]. In another prospective study, Franke et al. [43] examined the relationship between alcohol use, food insecurity, and medication adherence in a prospective cohort study of people living with HIV in Peru. Results showed that one in four participants was diagnosed with alcohol abuse or dependence, and this diagnosis was not associated with medication adherence. In contrast to alcohol use, food insecurity did predict medication nonadherence over the prospective study period.

Another prospective study of people living with HIV in a major US city examined monthly assessments of food insecurity and medication adherence [44]. The study observed that in any given month, one in three HIV-positive alcohol drinkers achieved less than 85% antiretroviral adherence. During every month of observation, individuals who had experienced food insecurity were less likely to achieve clinically optimal adherence. The rates of poor adherence were also reflected in the health status observed among those who were food-insecure in that food insecurity was associated with poorer HIV viral suppression, a greater likelihood of clinically significant low CD4 cell counts, and more HIV-related symptoms. Importantly, multivariate models were conducted to examine the primacy of factors associated with adherence and found that food insecurity predicted medication nonadherence and HIV viral nonsuppression over and above demographic characteristics and indicators of mental health problems as well as alcohol misuse and other drug use. Thus, food insecurity represents a marker for severe risk of medication nonadherence and poor viral suppression in people living with HIV, even to a greater extent than alcohol use.

4.6 IMPLICATIONS FOR INTERVENTIONS

Competing survival needs, including addictive substances such as alcohol use, should be addressed in programs that aim to alleviate poverty to enhance the health and well-being of people with HIV infection. One theoretical perspective that may help explain the underlying mechanisms of food insecurity, alcohol use, and adherence is the Conservation of Resources Theory of Stress and Coping [45,46]. This conceptual model states that health behaviors and health status are undermined in resource-constrained settings. Figure 4.1 shows an adaptation of the Conservation of Resources theoretical framework, which posits that gains in resources, including basic survival resources, protect individuals from stress and free internal resources for effective coping with everyday challenges. In contrast, loss of resources strain internal coping systems and disrupt what would normally be adaptive coping behaviors. Gained and lost resources, including threatened resources, therefore serve causal roles in coping and stress management, which in turn relate directly to adaptive health behaviors (e.g., medication adherence). Resources are broadly conceptualized in the model and extend beyond monetary resources and food to include factors such as housing, services, and support [47].

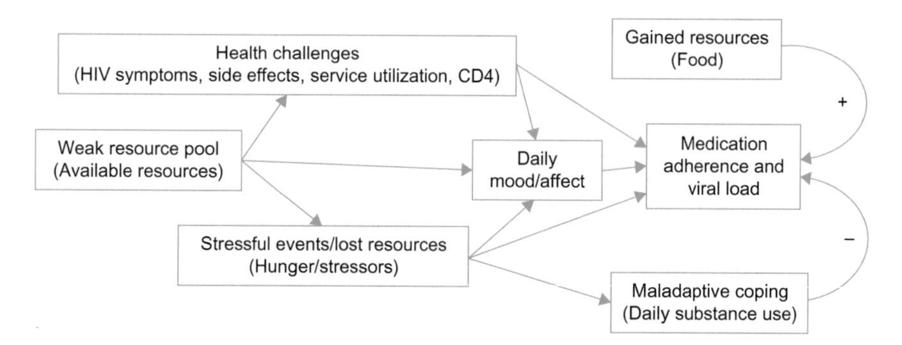

FIGURE 4.1 Conservation of resources theory of stress and coping [46] adapted to highlight the roles of food insecurity and substance use in medication adherence.

Consistent with Conservation of Resources Theory, there is evidence that increasing access to food improves treatment adherence among people living with HIV in resource-impoverished places [48]. A study conducted in Honduras found that providing monthly food baskets to people living with HIV who were experiencing food insecurity improved their adherence by 20% compared with patients who received nutrition education without food assistance [49]. In Haiti, Ivers et al. [50] showed marked improvements in body mass index and medication adherence when food was provided. Similarly, a small-scale randomized trial conducted with women living with HIV in India tested the effects of protein-supplemented diets and nutrition education about body composition and health [51]. Results showed that women who received protein supplements embedded within a nutrition education program significantly gained muscle mass, increased their body mass, and improved other health indicators, including increased CD4 cell counts compared with a control condition that received standard care. Importantly, women who received the protein supplement intervention also improved their medication adherence relative to women who received standard care. These findings mirror those of other research demonstrating an enabling effect of providing food assistance and increased treatment adherence for antiretroviral therapy [52].

The linkage between basic needs and health behaviors therefore may be explained by access to sustainable resources. However, access to resources can inadvertently increase access to alcohol and drugs and therefore undermine adherence [53]. The complex matrix of resources that can enhance as well as impede adherence remains virtually unknown and may be particularly important in understanding the impact of food insecurity in populations where alcohol and other drug use is prevalent. Few studies have examined interventions aimed to address the intersection of food insecurity and alcohol use in HIV-affected populations. In an effort to bridge this gap, Rotheram-Borus et al. [54] tested the effects of a visiting community health worker intervention on maternal and infant health outcomes. The intervention targeted pregnant women at risk for HIV infection with specific components of the intervention directed toward health factors, including nutritional support, alcohol use, and mental health. The study was conducted at the neighborhood level in impoverished South African townships. HIV-positive women were recruited from the communities and trained to serve as community peer interventionists, or mentors, and performed four prenatal and four postnatal home intervention visits. In their sample of 1,200 HIV-positive pregnant women, 17% drank alcohol prior to realizing they were pregnant and 5% continued drinking after recognizing their pregnancy. Results showed that 87% of women in the experimental condition received at least one intervention visit from a peer mentor, and that there were significant overall benefits in the mentor intervention condition compared with the standard care control group. In addition, compared with women who received standard care, those who were mentored were more likely to ask their sex partners to get tested for HIV, better protected their infants from HIV transmission, and had healthier infants. Although postnatal adherence to clinic groups was low, benefits for maternal and infant health persisted for more than 1 month after birth. Results also showed a marked difference in depression symptoms, with women who received mentoring significantly reducing their rates of depression compared with women who received standard care. Unfortunately, women who received the mentoring were significantly less likely to adhere to their antiretroviral therapy during pregnancy compared with women who received standard care [55,56].

4.7 CONCLUSIONS

HIV epidemics are concentrated in places of poverty and therefore intersect with multiple co-occurring health problems. Although antiretroviral therapy has changed the course of HIV infection, thereby transforming the disease from a virtual death sentence to a chronic manageable condition, a majority of people infected with HIV are at risk for not reaping the benefits of antiretrovirals. Food insecurity and alcohol misuse pose significant challenges to HIV treatment, including diverting resources away from accessing medications, impacts on medication adherence, impairing drug absorption, and compromising health. The relationship between food insecurity and alcohol use in people with HIV is now well-established. Although the need for interventions to improve treatment, adherence, and health by addressing food insecurity and alcohol misuse is compelling, few interventions have been developed and tested for this population. Because the effects of food insecurity and alcohol misuse on HIV treatment and health are quite robust, interventions aimed at these factors and their interaction will need to be intense and sustained. Priority should be placed on establishing interventions to address the direct and indirect effects of food insecurity and alcohol misuse in people living with HIV.

Acknowledgment

Preparation of this chapter was supported by National Institute of Alcohol Abuse and Alcoholism Grant R01-AA021471 and National Institute of Drug Abuse Grant R01-DA017399.

References

[1] Singer M. Pathogen–pathogen interaction: a syndemic model of complex biosocial processes in disease. Virulence 2010;1(1):10–18. [Epub 2010/12/24].
[2] Ivers LC, Cullen KA, Freedberg KA, Block S, Coates J, Webb P. HIV/AIDS, undernutrition, and food insecurity. Clin Infect Dis 2009;49(7):1096–102. [Epub 2009/09/04].

[3] Vogenthaler NS, Kushel MB, Hadley C, Frongillo Jr. EA, Riley ED, Bangsberg DR, et al. Food insecurity and risky sexual behaviors among homeless and marginally housed HIV-infected individuals in San Francisco. AIDS Behav 2013;17(5):1688–93. [Epub 2012/10/23].
[4] D'Amico R. How HIV does its dirty work. Posit Aware 1996;7(6):29. [Epub 1996/11/01].
[5] Weiser SD, Bangsberg DR, Kegeles S, Ragland K, Kushel MB, Frongillo EA. Food insecurity among homeless and marginally housed individuals living with HIV/AIDS in San Francisco. AIDS Behav 2009. [Epub 2009/08/01].
[6] Weiser SD, Frongillo EA, Ragland K, Hogg RS, Riley ED, Bangsberg DR. Food insecurity is associated with incomplete HIV RNA suppression among homeless and marginally housed HIV-infected individuals in San Francisco. J Gen Intern Med 2009;24(1):14–20. [Epub 2008/10/28].
[7] Weiser SD, Hatcher A, Frongillo EA, Guzman D, Riley ED, Bangsberg DR, et al. Food insecurity is associated with greater acute care utilization among HIV-infected homeless and marginally housed individuals in San Francisco. J Gen Intern Med 2012. [Epub 2012/08/21].
[8] Weiser SD, Fernandes KA, Brandson EK, Lima VD, Anema A, Bangsberg DR, et al. The association between food insecurity and mortality among HIV-infected individuals on HAART. J Acquir Immune Defic Syndr 2009;52(3):342–9. [Epub 2009/08/14].
[9] Boodram B, Plankey MW, Cox C, Tien PC, Cohen MH, Anastos K, et al. Prevalence and correlates of elevated body mass index among HIV-positive and HIV-negative women in the women's interagency HIV study. AIDS Patient Care STDs 2009;23(12):1009–16. [Epub 2009/11/17].
[10] Crum-Cianflone NF, Roediger M, Eberly LE, Vyas K, Landrum ML, Ganesan A, et al. Obesity among HIV-infected persons: impact of weight on CD4 cell count. AIDS 2010;24(7):1069–72. [Epub 2010/03/11].
[11] Hendricks KM, Willis K, Houser R, Jones CY. Obesity in HIV-infection: dietary correlates. J Am Coll Nutr 2006;25(4):321–31. [Epub 2006/09/01].
[12] Crum-Cianflone N, Tejidor R, Medina S, Barahona I, Ganesan A. Obesity among patients with HIV: the latest epidemic. AIDS Patient Care STDs 2008;22(12):925–30. [Epub 2008/12/17].
[13] Hernandez D. Nutritional intake, overweight and obesity among persons living with HIV in Atlanta Georgia. Under Rev 2014.
[14] Kopelman P. Health risks associated with overweight and obesity. Obes Rev 2007;8(Suppl. 1):13–17. [Epub 2007/02/24].
[15] Braithwaite RS, Conigliaro J, Roberts MS, Shechter S, Schaefer A, McGinnis K, et al. Estimating the impact of alcohol consumption on survival for HIV+ individuals. AIDS Care 2007;19(4):459–66. [Epub 2007/04/25].
[16] Watzl B, Watson RR. Role of alcohol abuse in nutritional immunosuppression. J Nutr 1992;122(Suppl. 3):733–7. [Epub 1992/03/01].
[17] Wang GT, Li S, Wideburg N, Krafft GA, Kempf DJ. Synthetic chemical diversity: solid phase synthesis of libraries of C2 symmetric inhibitors of HIV protease containing diamino diol and diamino alcohol cores. J Med Chem 1995;38(16):2995–3002. [Epub 1995/08/04].
[18] Baum MK, Rafie C, Lai S, Sales S, Page JB, Campa A. Alcohol use accelerates HIV disease progression. AIDS Res Hum Retroviruses 2010;26(5):511–8. [Epub 2010/05/12].
[19] Wu ES, Metzger DS, Lynch KG, Douglas SD. Association between alcohol use and HIV viral load. J Acquir Immune Defic Syndr 2011;56(5):e129–30. [Epub 2011/05/03].
[20] Schoonen WG, Lambert JG. Steroid metabolism in the seminal vesicles of the African catfish, clarias gariepinus (Burchell), during the spawning season, under natural conditions, and kept in ponds. Gen Comp Endocrinol 1986;61(3):355–67. [Epub 1986/03/01].
[21] Justice A, Sullivan L, Fiellin D. HIV/AIDS, comorbidity, and alcohol: Can we make a difference? Alcohol Res Health 2010;33(3):258–66. [Epub 2010/01/01].
[22] Constantinides A, Kappelle PJ, Lambert G, Dullaart RP. Plasma lipoprotein-associated phospholipase A2 is inversely correlated with proprotein convertase subtilisin–kexin type 9. Arch Med Res 2012;43(1):11–14. [Epub 2012/02/04].

[23] Sirotin N, Hoover D, Segal-Isaacson CJ, Shi Q, Adedimeji A, Mutimura E, et al. Structural determinants of food insufficiency, low dietary diversity and BMI: a cross-sectional study of HIV-infected and HIV-negative Rwandan women. BMJ open 2012;2(2):e000714. [Epub 2012/04/17].

[24] Anema A, Kerr T, Milloy MJ, Feng C, Montaner JS, Wood E. Relationship between hunger, adherence to antiretroviral therapy and plasma HIV RNA suppression among HIV-positive illicit drug users in a Canadian setting. AIDS Care 2014;26(4):459–65. [Epub 2013/09/11].

[25] Weiser SD, Leiter K, Bangsberg DR, Butler LM, Percy-de Korte F, Hlanze Z, et al. Food insufficiency is associated with high-risk sexual behavior among women in Botswana and Swaziland. PLoS Med 2007;4(10):1589–97. [discussion 98, Epub 2007/10/26].

[26] Fatch R, Bellows B, Bagenda F, Mulogo E, Weiser S, Hahn JA. Alcohol consumption as a barrier to prior HIV testing in a population-based study in rural Uganda. AIDS Behav 2013;17(5):1713–23. [Epub 2012/08/11].

[27] Bangsberg D, Kroetz DL, Deeks S. Adherence–resistance relationships to combination HIV antiretroviral therapy. Curr HIV/AIDS Rep 2007;4:65–72.

[28] Parienti JJ, Das-Douglas M, Massari V, Guzman D, Deeks SG, Verdon R, et al. Not all missed doses are the same: sustained NNRTI treatment interruptions predict HIV rebound at low-to-moderate adherence levels. PLoS One 2008;3(7):e2783. [Epub 2008/07/31].

[29] Hendershot CS, Stoner SA, Pantalone DW, Simoni JM. Alcohol use and antiretroviral adherence: review and meta-analysis. J Acquir Immune Defic Syndr 2009;52(2):180–202. [Epub 2009/08/12].

[30] Braithwaite RS, McGinnis KA, Conigliaro J, Maisto SA, Crystal S, Day N, et al. A temporal and dose–response association between alcohol consumption and medication adherence among veterans in care. Alcohol Clin Exp Res 2005;29(7):1190–7. [Epub 2005/07/28].

[31] Normen L, Chan ES, Braitstein P, Annema A, Bondy G, Montaner J. Food insecurity and hunger are prevalent among HIV-positive individuals in British Columbia, Canada. J Nutr 2005;135:820–5.

[32] van der Sande MA, Schim van der Loeff MF, Aveika AA, Sabally S, Togun T, Sarge-Njie R, et al. Body mass index at time of HIV diagnosis: a strong and independent predictor of survival. J Acquir Immune Defic Syndr 2004;37(2):1288–94. [Epub 2004/09/24].

[33] Alghamdi AA, Sheth T, Manowski Z, Djoleto OF, Bhatnagar G. Utility of cardiac CT and MRI for the diagnosis and preoperative assessment of cardiac paraganglioma. J Card Surg 2009. [Epub 2009/08/18].

[34] Singer AW, Weiser SD, McCoy SI. Does food insecurity undermine adherence to antiretroviral therapy? A systematic review. AIDS Behav 2014. [Epub 2014/08/07].

[35] Zhu W, Chong Y, Choo H, Mathews J, Schinazi RF, Chu CK. Synthesis, structure–activity relationships, and mechanism of drug resistance of D- and L-beta-3′-fluoro-2′,3′-unsaturated-4′-thionucleosides as anti-HIV agents. J Med Chem 2004;47(7):1631–40. [Epub 2004/03/19].

[36] Klarmann GJ, Smith RA, Schinazi RF, North TW, Preston BD. Site-specific incorporation of nucleoside analogs by HIV-1 reverse transcriptase and the template grip mutant P157S. Template interactions influence substrate recognition at the polymerase active site. J Biol Chem 2000;275(1):359–66. [Epub 2000/01/05].

[37] Manouilov KK, Xu ZS, Boudinot FD, Schinazi RF, Chu CK. Lymphatic targeting of anti-HIV nucleosides: distribution of 2′,3′-dideoxyinosine after intravenous and oral administration of dipalmitoylphosphatidyl prodrug in mice. Antiviral Res 1997;34(3):91–9. [Epub 1997/05/01].

[38] Wang P, Schinazi RF, Chu CK. Asymmetric synthesis and anti-HIV activity of L-carbocyclic 2′,3′-didehydro-2′,3′-dideoxyadenosine. Bioorg Med Chem Lett 1998;8(13): 1585–8. [Epub 1999/01/05].

[39] Lin YM, Anderson H, Flavin MT, Pai YH, Mata-Greenwood E, Pengsuparp T, et al. *In vitro* anti-HIV activity of biflavonoids isolated from rhus succedanea and garcinia multiflora. J Nat Prod 1997;60(9):884–8. [Epub 1997/10/10].

[40] Amico KR. Standard of care for antiretroviral therapy adherence and retention in care from the perspective of care providers attending the 5th international conference on HIV treatment adherence. J Int Assoc Physicians AIDS Care (Chic) 2011;10(5):291–6. [Epub 2011/05/12].
[41] Kalichman SC, Cherry C, Amaral C, White D, Kalichman MO, Pope H, et al. Health and treatment implications of food insufficiency among people living with HIV/AIDS, Atlanta, Georgia. J Urban Health 2010;87(4):631–41. [Epub 2010/04/27].
[42] Kalichman SC, Pellowski J, Kalichman MO, Cherry C, Detorio M, Caliendo AM, et al. Food insufficiency and medication adherence among people living with HIV/AIDS in urban and peri-urban settings. Prev Sci 2011;12(3):324–32. [Epub 2011/05/25].
[43] Franke MF, Murray MB, Munoz M, Hernandez-Diaz S, Sebastian JL, Atwood S, et al. Food insufficiency is a risk factor for suboptimal antiretroviral therapy adherence among HIV-infected adults in urban Peru. AIDS Behav 2011;15(7):1483–9. [Epub 2010/08/18].
[44] Kalichman SC, Grebler T, Amaral CM, McKerney M, White D, Kalichman MO, et al. Food insecurity and antiretroviral adherence among HIV positive adults who drink alcohol. J Behav Med 2013. [Epub 2013/09/12].
[45] Hobfoll SE, Jackson AP. Conservation of resources in community intervention. Am J Community Psychol 1991;19(1):111–21. [Epub 1991/02/01].
[46] Hobfoll SE. Conservation of resources and disaster in cultural context: the caravans and passageways for resources. Psychiatry 2012;75(3):227–32. [Epub 2012/08/24].
[47] Alvaro C, Lyons RF, Warner G, Hobfoll SE, Martens PJ, Labonte R, et al. Conservation of resources theory and research use in health systems. Implement Sci 2010;5:79. [Epub 2010/10/22].
[48] Cantrell RA, Sinkala M, Megazinni K, Lawson-Marriott S, Washington S, Chi BH, et al. A pilot study of food supplementation to improve adherence to antiretroviral therapy among food-insecure adults in Lusaka, Zambia. J Acquir Immune Defic Syndr 2008;49(2):190–5. [Epub 2008/09/05].
[49] Martinez H, Palar K, Linnemayr S, Smith A, Derose KP, Ramirez B, et al. Tailored nutrition education and food assistance improve adherence to HIV antiretroviral therapy: evidence from Honduras. AIDS Behav 2014;18(Suppl. 5):566–77. [Epub 2014/05/03].
[50] Ivers L, Chang Y, Jerome G, Freedberg K. Food assistance is associated with improved body mass index, food security, and attendance to clinic in an HIV program in central Haiti: a respective observation study. AIDS Res Ther 2010.
[51] Nyamathi A, Sinha S, Ganguly KK, Ramakrishna P, Suresh P, Carpenter CL. Impact of protein supplementation and care and support on body composition and CD4 count among HIV-infected women living in rural India: results from a randomized pilot clinical trial. AIDS Behav 2013;17(6):2011–21. [Epub 2013/02/02].
[52] de Pee S, Grede N, Mehra D, Bloem MW. The enabling effect of food assistance in improving adherence and/or treatment completion for antiretroviral therapy and tuberculosis treatment: a literature review. AIDS Behav 2014;18(Suppl. 5):531–41. [Epub 2014/03/13].
[53] Kalichman SC, Grebler T. Stress and poverty predictors of treatment adherence among people with low-literacy living with HIV/AIDS. Psychosom Med 2010;72(8):810–6. http://dx.doi.org/doi:10.1097/PSY.0b013e3181f01be3.
[54] Rotheram-Borus MJ, le Roux IM, Tomlinson M, Mbewu N, Comulada WS, le Roux K, et al. Philani plus (+): a mentor mother community health worker home visiting program to improve maternal and infants' outcomes. Prev Sci 2011;12(4):372–88. [Epub 2011/08/19].
[55] Richter L, Rotheram-Borus MJ, Van Heerden A, Stein A, Tomlinson M, Harwood JM, et al. Pregnant women living with HIV (WLH) supported at clinics by peer WLH: a cluster randomized controlled trial. AIDS Behav 2014;18(4):706–15. [Epub 2014/01/29].
[56] Rotheram-Borus MJ, Richter LM, van Heerden A, van Rooyen H, Tomlinson M, Harwood JM, et al. A cluster randomized controlled trial evaluating the efficacy of peer mentors to support South African women living with HIV and their infants. PLoS ONE 2014;9(1):e84867. [Epub 2014/01/28].

CHAPTER

5

Carotid Intima–Media Thickness and Plaque in HIV-Infected Patients on the Mediterranean Diet

Klaudija Višković[1] *and Josip Begovac*[2]

[1]Head of Department of Radiology and Ultrasound, University Hospital for Infectious Diseases, Zagreb, Croatia, [2]University Hospital for Infectious Diseases, The University of Zagreb, School of Medicine, Šalata, Zagreb, Croatia

5.1 INTRODUCTION

The impact of human immunodeficiency virus (HIV) infection and exposure to antiretroviral therapy (ART) on the development of subclinical atherosclerosis is incompletely understood [1]. An HIV-infected patient has a significantly higher risk of developing cardiovascular events during the progression of HIV disease [2]. Atherosclerosis, myocardial infarction, cerebrovascular injury, pulmonary hypertension, and thrombosis are consistently described as major clinical complications in both ART-treated and naive HIV-positive patients [3]. Several factors may contribute to an increased risk of coronary and cerebrovascular artery disease in HIV-infected patients: chronic endothelial or myocardial inflammation due to HIV infection *per se*; lipid changes associated with ART; and the interaction of these with traditional risk factors for cardiovascular disease (CVD) (smoking, hypertension, age, etc.) [1]. The metabolic alterations that precede CVD induce a chain of pathophysiological events that predispose patients to endothelial dysfunction and progressive arterial

Health of HIV Infected People, Volume 2.
DOI: http://dx.doi.org/10.1016/B978-0-12-800767-9.00005-4

stiffness [1]. HIV infection strongly interferes with the biology of several cellular targets such as macrophage and endothelial cells [4]. HIV induces a profound derangement of lipid metabolism and inflammatory cytokine networks that are directly involved in atherogenesis and progressive impairment of the cardiovascular system [5].

High-resolution ultrasound enables vessel wall evaluation and carotid intima–media thickness (CIMT) measurement and, because the thickening of the CIMT is an early marker of atherosclerosis, assessment of risk of coronary and cerebro artery disease [6]. Increased CIMT is associated with an increased risk of global cardiovascular events, including myocardial infarction, stroke, and ischemic stroke [1]. Carotid plaque area is more strongly associated with traditional risk factors and is more predictive of myocardial infarction than of stroke [7].

The Mediterranean diet has long been related to lower CVD risk and there is much evidence suggesting that the Mediterranean diet could serve as an anti-inflammatory dietary pattern that could help fight diseases related to chronic inflammation, including metabolic syndrome [8]. The Mediterranean diet is characterized by high consumption of legumes, fruits, vegetables, grains, and olive oil; moderate consumption of fish; moderate consumption of wine and dairy products; and low consumption of red and processed meat, cream, and pastries [9].

In this chapter, we describe the influence of adherence to the Mediterranean diet on B-mode ultrasound–measured CIMT and the presence of plaques in HIV-infected patients.

5.2 ULTRASOUND MEASUREMENT OF CIMT

The large superficial arteries, particularly the carotid arteries, can be visualized at high resolution with B-mode (or "brightness" mode) ultrasound using linear array transducers for superficial and vascular structures (frequency range, 5–15 MHz) (Figure 5.1). Carotid ultrasonography can measure CIMT and detect focal atheroscleorotic plaque using ultrasound and therefore can provide precise information about atherosclerotic burden (Figures 5.2 and 5.3). The measurement of CIMT has several advantages for monitoring of atherosclerosis. It can be performed with no adverse effects on subjects, it provides better visualization of atherosclerotic changes on the arterial wall than other imaging modalities, and it has been shown to be well-correlated with CIMT measured on microscoping examination [10,11].

The resolution obtained with linear transducers is approximately 0.044 mm axially and 0.25 mm laterally. CIMT measurements can be performed and ultrasound images can be obtained from the near and far walls of the right and left distal common carotid arteries (CCAs), the

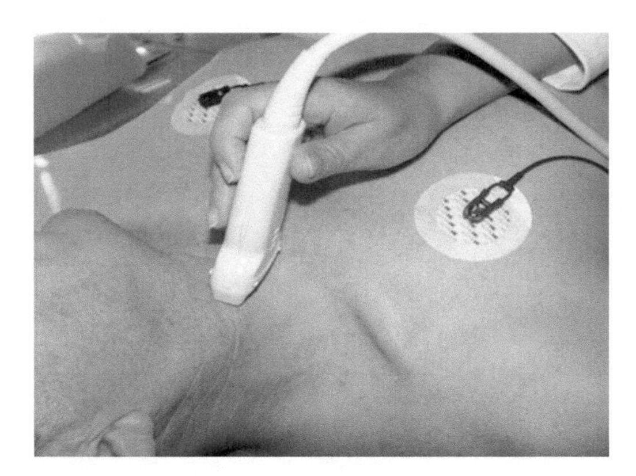

FIGURE 5.1 Patient positioning in B-mode ultrasound measurement of carotid intima–media thickness (CIMT) performed with a linear probe.

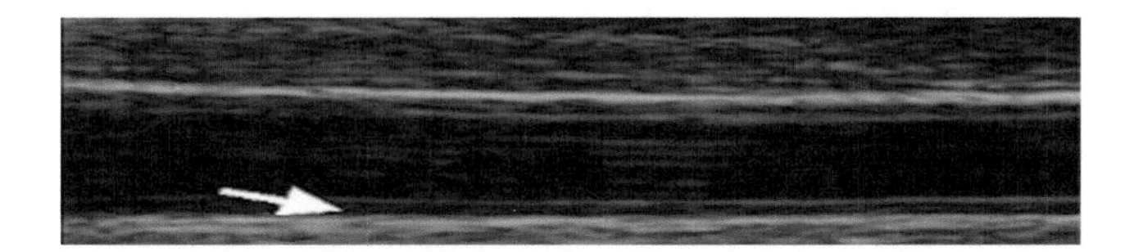

FIGURE 5.2 B-mode ultrasound image of carotid intima–media complex (arrow).

carotid bifurcation, and the proximal internal carotid arterial segments. CIMT in an individual patient is therefore often a composite of intima–media thickness (IMT) measurements of various images of various segments and angles [6].

For CIMT measurements, longitudinal images of the carotid arteries should be obtained in which the leading edges of the lumen–intima and media–adventitia interfaces (the "double-line pattern") of the arterial wall represent intima–media complex [12] (Figure 5.2). Typically, normal common carotid CIMT at age 10 is approximately 0.4–0.5 mm, whereas from the first decade of life onward this progresses to 0.7–0.8 mm or more [13]. Different studies used different protocols for B-mode ultrasound CIMT measurements [4,14–16]. According to our experience, we recommend the following protocol: a circumferential scan should be performed with image acquisition at four predefined angles of the near and far walls of the right and left CCA, carotid bifurcation, and internal carotid artery (ICA) [17–19]. Five-second imaging sequences should be saved in Digital Imaging in Communications in Medicine (DICOM) format and written to optical disk for transfer to reading centers. If different reading centers are included in the same study, then they should use standardized equipment and protocols to process stored images [20].

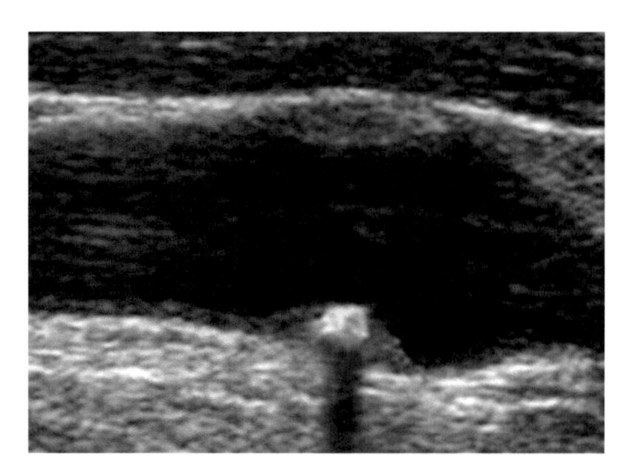

FIGURE 5.3 B-mode ultrasound image of calcified carotid plaque.

Electrocardiographic (ECG) gating to determine the minimum end-diastolic diameter is optimal with either approach because of cyclic variation in CIMT diameter attributable to pulsatile changes in distending pressure. The most preferable site for the measurement of CIMT is the far wall rather than the near wall of the carotid artery because acoustic reflection of the echo-dense intima into the lumen and/or the high gain setting in near wall measurements may lead to overestimation of CIMT [13]. Because the CCA is tubular and can be aligned perpendicular to the transducer beam, reproducibility and yield of CCA IMT are superior to that of IMT of the carotid bifurcation (bulb) or ICA [21]. The small size of the CIMT (usually <1 mm) necessitates computer-assisted measurement using electronic calipers [21]. Semiautomated measurement may be performed for a selected segment (usually 1 cm in length) using an edge detection algorithm [21].

Discrete plaques, commonly defined as focal thickening at least 50% greater than the surrounding wall, can be reliably detected and localized by thorough scanning of the extracranial carotid arteries [22] (Figure 5.3). However, because the overwhelming majority of plaques are nonobstructive and cannot be quantified using Doppler technology, precise quantification of plaque burden is problematic [21]. Although plaque diameter (maximum excursion into the vessel lumen) is readily measurable, the diameter may correlate poorly with plaque size or volume given the variable and complex three-dimensional morphology of plaques. Semiquantitative approaches include averaging of plaque diameters, the number of segments (CCA, bulb, ICA, external carotid artery [ECA]) containing plaque, or plaque number [21].

Semiautomated readings of CIMT should be analyzed with the use of automated measurement software (imaging and data analysis) [23]. From each image sequence, the reader should select one frame in end diastole for measurement of CIMT. The leading edge (far wall) and trailing edge (near wall) of boundaries between the media and adventitia and between the lumen and intima should be traced within the region of interest specified by the reader. Maximum CIMT thickness should be determined from a set of measurement perpendicular to the media–adventitia boundary [21]. The readers should be unaware of study group assignments and a previous CIMT measurement when reading an image. Quality-assurance process should include central training and certification of all sonographers and readers [21].

Despite this continuous relationship between CIMT and risk, an absolute definition of an abnormally high CIMT (measured in the absence of plaque) is problematic due to the strong influence of age on arterial wall thickness in both normotensive and hypertensive individuals [15,21]. Furthermore, hypertension increases CIMT, probably because of medial hypertrophy, independent of typical atherosclerotic changes [24]. Thus, the use of an absolute threshold to define an abnormal CIMT may result in systematic underdetection in younger individuals and overdetection in older individuals [25]. The 34th Bethesda conference suggested establishing normograms or ratios of observed to predicted IMT based on age and other potential covariates depending on the population and application, such as the approximate age-adjusted 75th percentile values for CIMT [10,21]. The Manheim CIMT Consensus defines plaque as a focal structure encroaching into the arterial lumen by at least 0.5 mm or 50% of the surrounding wall or demonstrates a plaque thickness of >1.5 mm [25]. The European Society of Hypertension and European Society of Cardiology have defined either a mean CIMT more than 0.9 mm or the presence of carotid plaque as a marker of target organ damage in hypertension [26]. In our measurements of CIMT in HIV-infected subjects, we defined subclinical atherosclerosis as CIMT ≥0.9 mm and/or the presence of ≥1 carotid plaque [17,27,28].

5.3 CHARACTERISTICS OF MEDITERRANEAN DIET

Adequate nutrition is important for optimal immune and metabolic function in HIV-infected patients [29]. Food insecurity is a recognized risk factor for HIV, and up to 50% of currently infected urban patients may be food-insecure [30]. It is independently associated with increased mortality, decreased ART adherence, and incomplete virologic suppression [30].

Dietary support may therefore improve clinical outcomes in HIV-infected individuals by reducing the incidence of HIV-associated complications, including atherosclerosis and attenuating progression of HIV disease, improving the quality of life and ultimately reducing disease-related mortality [31].

Abnormalities in lipid metabolism have been reported among patients infected with HIV even before the introduction of ART [31]. Elevated levels of triglycerides and decreased total cholesterol and high-density lipoprotein (HDL) cholesterol have been shown to be positively correlated with the progression of HIV infection and have become a common finding in AIDS [32].

The population of the area around the Mediterranean basin adheres to the Mediterranean diet, which is rich in nuts, fruit, vegetables, legumes, whole-wheat bread, fish, and olive oil [9,31]. Alcohol, mostly red wine, is consumed with meals in moderate amounts. The relatively lower occurrence of chronic diseases such as cancer, diabetes, obesity, and CVDs has been linked to these dietary habits [33]. There is no single Mediterranean diet, but rather there are as many Mediterranean eating patterns as there are Mediterranean countries [34]. Olive oil, fish, and red wine have a central position in the culinary habits in this region, despite cultural and religious differences [35]. As an instrument for nutritional assessment, there are validated questionnaires [36–38]. In our studies we used a questionnaire, originally developed by Babio et al. [8], that was suitable for the nutritional habits of the largest number of Croatian people living at the Mediterranean coast.

The phenolic compounds present in olive oil may interact with the inflammatory cascade by their antioxidant action [39,40]. A relatively high concentration of oleic acid, the main monosaturated fatty acid in the membrane of phospholipids, makes the cell susceptible to oxidation by reducing the formation of proinflammatory molecules [40]. These properties may translate into a number of health benefits, including cardiovascular protection.

Red wine contains a variety of phenolic compounds that exert anti-inflammatory, antioxidant, and anti-atherogenic action [41]. Among the phenolic compounds in red wine, resveratrol (3,4,5-trihydroxystilbene) is prominent and has a beneficial effect on low-density lipoprotein (LDL) oxidation, thrombogenicity, ischemia, and vascular tone [42].

Omega-6 and omega-3 polyunsaturated fatty acids (PUFA), also named $n-6$ and $n-3$ PUFAs, from fish cannot be synthesized from scratch by mammalian cells [43]. The presence of these acids is highly dependent on dietary intake. Experiments by Yaqoob and Calder [39] have demonstrated that $n-3$ fatty acid supplementation suppresses inflammation and diminishes oxidative stress. It is believed that the protective effect of the Mediterranean diet is not related to serum concentrations of total LDL or HDL cholesterol, but rather to changes observed in plasma fatty acids [44].

5.4 CIMT IN HIV-INFECTED PATIENTS

Although some studies have shown increased CIMT in the setting of HIV infection, other studies have not confirmed this finding [1,45]. Greater

CIMT than in controls (0.004 mm) has also been associated with HIV infection in a meta-analysis of 13 cross-sectional studies [46,47]. However, a significant difference in CIMT and plaque prevalence between HIV-infected patients and non-HIV-infected participants has not been found [1,48,49]. These differences among studies may be due, in part, to limited sample size in some studies, different patient populations, and the limited ability of anatomic imaging to comprehensively define the cardiovascular risk [50].

Atherosclerotic lesions in HIV-infected patients tend to occur at areas experiencing low endothelial shear stress, which are local wall stresses that are generated by patterns of blood flow, such as the carotid bifurcation region [51]. Low shear stress promotes atherosclerosis by a variety of mechanisms, including impairment of endothelial function by downregulation of endothelial nitric oxide synthase (eNOS), upregulation of endothelin-1, increased endothelial uptake of LDL, promotion of oxidative stress, and increased plaque thrombogenicity.

Low endothelial shear stress also enhances the proatherogenic effect of chronic inflammation, because it allows for the attachment and infiltration of inflammatory cells via activation of NF-κB14,15 and subsequent upregulation of adhesion molecules, chemokines, and proinflammatory cytokines [51]. Low endothelial shear stress has also been implicated in the transition of stable atherosclerotic lesions to vulnerable plaques, resulting in acute coronary syndromes via combination of vascular inflammation, change in the extracellular matrix, and wall remodeling [52].

According to the study by Hsue et al. [4], the rate of CIMT progression in HIV-infected patients has a mean value of 0.074 mm/year (SD, 0.13). This is several-fold higher than the mean value reported in studies of non-HIV-infected subjects [53]. Development of plaque occurred more frequently in the bifurcation and internal carotid regions in HIV-infected individuals as compared with controls, and it was less frequent in the common carotid in both groups [51]. Data from uninfected individuals demonstrate that the carotid bifurcation region is uniquely prone to inflammatory effects as a result of low endothelial shear stress; the findings of Hsue et al. [51] in their study performed in 2012 suggest that the impact of HIV infection on vascular function may be most apparent in branch points due to the effects of inflammation. Previous studies have suggested that there is an association between the use of proteases inhibitors (PI) and increased CIMT in HIV-infected subjects [54,55].

It is still unclear if the rate of CIMT progression is similarly faster in ART-naive, HIV-infected adults as in HIV-infected adults using ART. According to the study by Hileman et al. [56], in ART-naive HIV-infected adults at low risk for HIV disease progression and low cardiovascular risk, CIMT progression rate was similar to that of matched controls. In addition to traditional CVD risk factors, higher levels of soluble tumor necrosis factor-α receptor (sTNFR) I predicted greater bulb CIMT changes

[56]. Independent predictors of CIMT progression in HIV-infected, ART-naive adults were higher systolic blood pressure, total cholesterol, and high sensitivity C-reactive protein [57]. Independent predictors of bulb CIMT progression were higher non-HDL cholesterol and high-sensitivity C-reactive protein. Other inflammation markers were not associated with CIMT progression [57].

5.5 CIMT IN HIV-INFECTED PATIENTS ADHERENT TO MEDITERRANEAN DIET

The higher dietary consumption of olive oil in a typical Mediterranean diet may be associated with lower values of CIMT in non-HIV-infected persons at high cardiovascular risk, as reported by Buil-Cosiales et al. [58].

However, HIV-infected individuals also present with high prevalence of traditional risk factors of CVD that are associated with inflammation, including tobacco use, substance abuse, dyslipidemia, and obesity [30]. Smoking is common in HIV-infected patients and The Data Collection on Adverse Events of Anti-HIV Drugs (DAD) study investigators found that smoking was the most powerful predictor of CVDs [15]. The prevalence of hypertension also appears quite elevated when compared with the general population [15].

To evaluate the influence of adherence to the Mediterranean diet on CIMT and the presence of plaques in HIV-infected patients using ART and non-HIV-infected participants, and to determine if HIV infection contributes independently to subclinical atherosclerosis, we conducted a cross-sectional study of 110 HIV-infected patients using ART and 131 non-HIV-infected participants at the University Hospital for Infectious Diseases in Zagreb, Croatia, from 2009 to 2011 [17].

One-quarter of HIV-infected participants in our study were using PI regimens for at least 12 months [17]. We did not find any difference in surrogate markers of atherosclerosis between these participants and HIV-infected participants using other ART regimens [17]. However, we cannot rule out the possibility that our small sample size is too small.

Our study demonstrated an association of subclinical atherosclerosis with specific and traditional dietary habits, which had been associated with decreased all-cause mortality and improvement in cardiovascular risk factors in prior studies in the general population [17]. We also provided evidence that HIV infection treated with ART was associated with accelerated atherosclerosis in older individuals [17].

In other studies conducted in Croatia, there was no association found between plasma lipid changes during the first year of ART and adherence to the Mediterranean diet [59]. This was similar to results for the non-HIV-infected population, in which adherence to the Mediterranean diet was not correlated well with levels of serum lipids [59].

References

[1] Currier JS, Kendall MA, Zackin R, et al. Carotid artery intima–media thickness and HIV infection: traditional risk factors overshadow impact of protease inhibitor exposure. AIDS 2005;19(9):927–33.
[2] Gibellini D, Borderi M, Clo A, et al. HIV-related mechanisms in atherosclerosis and cardiovascular diseases. J Cardiovasc Med (Hagerstown) 2013;14(11):780–90.
[3] Grunfeld C, Delaney JA, Wanke C, et al. Preclinical atherosclerosis due to HIV infection: carotid intima–medial thickness measurements from the FRAM study. AIDS 2009;23(14):1841–9.
[4] Hsue PY, Lo JC, Franklin A, et al. Progression of atherosclerosis as assessed by carotid intima–media thickness in patients with HIV infection. Circulation 2004;109(13):1603–8.
[5] Anuurad E, Semrad A, Berglund L. Human immunodeficiency virus and highly active antiretroviral therapy-associated metabolic disorders and risk factors for cardiovascular disease. Metab Syndr Relat Disord 2009;7(5):401–10.
[6] Eigenbrodt ML, Evans GW, Rose KM, et al. Bilateral common carotid artery ultrasound for prediction of incident strokes using intima–media thickness and external diameter: an observational study. Cardiovasc Ultrasound 2013;11:22.
[7] Spence JD. Technology insight: ultrasound measurement of carotid plaque—patient management, genetic research, and therapy evaluation. Nat Clin Pract Neurol 2006;2(11):611–9.
[8] Babio N, Bullo M, Salas-Salvado J. Mediterranean diet and metabolic syndrome: the evidence. Public Health Nutr 2009;12(9A):1607–17.
[9] Turcinov D, Stanley C, Rutherford GW, Novotny TE, Begovac J. Adherence to the Mediterranean diet is associated with a lower risk of body-shape changes in Croatian patients treated with combination antiretroviral therapy. Eur J Epidemiol 2009;24(5):267–74.
[10] Lee CJ, Park S. The role of carotid ultrasound for cardiovascular risk stratification beyond traditional risk factors. Yonsei Med J 2014;55(3):551–7.
[11] Pignoli P, Tremoli E, Poli A, Oreste P, Paoletti R. Intimal plus medial thickness of the arterial wall: a direct measurement with ultrasound imaging. Circulation 1986;74(6):1399–406.
[12] Smrzova A, Horak P, Skacelova M, et al. Intima media thickness measurement as a marker of subclinical atherosclerosis in SLE patient. Biomed Pap Med Fac Univ Palacky Olomouc Czech Repub 2013.
[13] Bots ML, Evans GW, Riley WA, Grobbee DE. Carotid intima–media thickness measurements in intervention studies: design options, progression rates, and sample size considerations: a point of view. Stroke 2003;34(12):2985–94.
[14] Perwaiz Khan S, Gul P, Khemani S, Yaqub Z. Determination of site-specific carotid-intima media thickness: common-carotid artery and carotid bifurcation in hypercholesterolemia patients. Pak J Med Sci 2013;29(5):1249–52.
[15] Ho JE, Hsue PY. Cardiovascular manifestations of HIV infection. Heart 2009;95(14):1193–202.
[16] Maggi P, Quirino T, Ricci E, et al. Cardiovascular risk assessment in antiretroviral-naive HIV patients. AIDS Patient Care STDS 2009;23(10):809–13.
[17] Viskovic K, Rutherford GW, Sudario G, Stemberger L, Brnic Z, Begovac J. Ultrasound measurements of carotid intima–media thickness and plaque in HIV-infected patients on the Mediterranean diet. Croat Med J 2013;54(4):330–8.
[18] Ferraioli G, Tinelli C, Maggi P, et al. Arterial stiffness evaluation in HIV-positive patients: a multicenter matched control study. Am J Roentgenol 2011;197(5):1258–62.
[19] Kastelein JJ, van Leuven SI, Burgess L, et al. Effect of torcetrapib on carotid atherosclerosis in familial hypercholesterolemia. N Engl J Med 2007;356(16):1620–30.

[20] de Groot E, Hovingh GK, Wiegman A, et al. Measurement of arterial wall thickness as a surrogate marker for atherosclerosis. Circulation 2004;109(23 Suppl. 1):III33–III38.
[21] Redberg RF, Vogel RA, Criqui MH, Herrington DM, Lima JA, Roman MJ. 34th Bethesda conference: task force #3—What is the spectrum of current and emerging techniques for the noninvasive measurement of atherosclerosis? J Am Coll Cardiol 2003;41(11):1886–98.
[22] Raggi P, Taylor A, Fayad Z, et al. Atherosclerotic plaque imaging: contemporary role in preventive cardiology. Arch Intern Med 2005;165(20):2345–53.
[23] Liang Q, Wendelhag I, Wikstrand J, Gustavsson T. A multiscale dynamic programming procedure for boundary detection in ultrasonic artery images. IEEE Trans Med Imaging 2000;19(2):127–42.
[24] Papita A, Albu A, Fodor D, Itu C, Carstina D. Arterial stiffness and carotid intima–media thickness in HIV infected patients. Med Ultrasound 2011;13(2):127–34.
[25] Touboul PJ, Hennerici MG, Meairs S, et al. Mannheim intima–media thickness consensus. Cerebrovasc Dis 2004;18(4):346–9.
[26] Mancia G, Fagard R, Narkiewicz K, et al. 2013 ESH/ESC practice guidelines for the management of arterial hypertension. Blood Press 2014;23(1):3–16.
[27] Inaba Y, Chen JA, Bergmann SR. Carotid plaque, compared with carotid intima–media thickness, more accurately predicts coronary artery disease events: a meta-analysis. Atherosclerosis 2012;220(1):128–33.
[28] Polak JF, Pencina MJ, Pencina KM, O'Donnell CJ, Wolf PA, D'Agostino Sr. RB. Carotid-wall intima–media thickness and cardiovascular events. N Engl J Med 2011;365(3):213–21.
[29] Raiten DJ, Mulligan K, Papathakis P, Wanke C. Executive summary—nutritional care of HIV-infected adolescents and adults, including pregnant and lactating women: what do we know, what can we do, and where do we go from here? Am J Clin Nutr 2011;94(6):1667S–76S.
[30] Willig AL, Overton ET. Metabolic consequences of HIV: pathogenic insights. Curr HIV/AIDS Rep 2014;11(1):35–44.
[31] Tsiodras S, Poulia KA, Yannakoulia M, et al. Adherence to Mediterranean diet is favorably associated with metabolic parameters in HIV-positive patients with the highly active antiretroviral therapy-induced metabolic syndrome and lipodystrophy. Metabolism 2009;58(6):854–9.
[32] Turcinov D, Begovac J. Predicted coronary heart disease risk in Croatian HIV infected patients treated with combination antiretroviral therapy. Coll Antropol 2011;35(1):115–21.
[33] Pauwels EK. The protective effect of the Mediterranean diet: focus on cancer and cardiovascular risk. Med Princ Pract 2011;20(2):103–11.
[34] Serra-Majem L, Ribas L, Ngo J, et al. Food, youth and the Mediterranean diet in Spain. Development of KIDMED, Mediterranean diet quality index in children and adolescents. Public Health Nutr 2004;7(7):931–5.
[35] Sofi F. The Mediterranean diet revisited: evidence of its effectiveness grows. Curr Opin Cardiol 2009;24(5):442–6.
[36] Babio N, Bullo M, Basora J, et al. Adherence to the Mediterranean diet and risk of metabolic syndrome and its components. Nutr Metab Cardiovasc Dis 2009;19(8):563–70.
[37] di Giuseppe R, Bonanni A, Olivieri M, et al. Adherence to Mediterranean diet and anthropometric and metabolic parameters in an observational study in the "alto molise" region: the MOLI-SAL project. Nutr Metab Cardiovasc Dis 2008;18(6):415–21.
[38] Panagiotakos DB, Pitsavos C, Arvaniti F, Stefanadis C. Adherence to the Mediterranean food pattern predicts the prevalence of hypertension, hypercholesterolemia, diabetes and obesity, among healthy adults; the accuracy of the MedDietScore. Prev Med 2007;44(4):335–40.
[39] Yaqoob P, Calder PC. Fatty acids and immune function: new insights into mechanisms. Br J Nutr 2007;98(Suppl. 1):S41–5.

[40] Owen RW, Haubner R, Wurtele G, Hull E, Spiegelhalder B, Bartsch H. Olives and olive oil in cancer prevention. Eur J Cancer Prev 2004;13(4):319–26.
[41] Booyse FM, Pan W, Grenett HE, et al. Mechanism by which alcohol and wine polyphenols affect coronary heart disease risk. Ann Epidemiol 2007;17(Suppl. 5):S24–31.
[42] Opie LH, Lecour S. The red wine hypothesis: from concepts to protective signalling molecules. Eur Heart J 2007;28(14):1683–93.
[43] Bullo M, Amigo-Correig P, Marquez-Sandoval F, et al. Mediterranean diet and high dietary acid load associated with mixed nuts: effect on bone metabolism in elderly subjects. J Am Geriatr Soc 2009;57(10):1789–98.
[44] Renaud S, de Lorgeril M, Delaye J, et al. Cretan Mediterranean diet for prevention of coronary heart disease. Am J Clin Nutr 1995;61(Suppl. 6):1360S–1367SS.
[45] Kaplan RC, Kingsley LA, Gange SJ, et al. Low CD4+ T-cell count as a major atherosclerosis risk factor in HIV-infected women and men. AIDS 2008;22(13):1615–24.
[46] Longenecker CT, Hoit BD. Imaging atherosclerosis in HIV: carotid intima–media thickness and beyond. Transl Res 2012;159(3):127–39.
[47] Hulten E, Mitchell J, Scally J, Gibbs B, Villines TC. HIV positivity, protease inhibitor exposure and subclinical atherosclerosis: a systematic review and meta-analysis of observational studies. Heart 2009;95(22):1826–35.
[48] Depairon M, Chessex S, Sudre P, et al. Premature atherosclerosis in HIV-infected individuals—focus on protease inhibitor therapy. AIDS 2001;15(3):329–34.
[49] Bongiovanni M, Casana M, Cicconi P, et al. Predictive factors of vascular intima media thickness in HIV-positive subjects. J Antimicrob Chemother 2008;61(1):195–9.
[50] Hsue PY, Scherzer R, Hunt PW, et al. Carotid intima–media thickness progression in HIV-infected adults occurs preferentially at the carotid bifurcation and is predicted by inflammation. J Am Heart Assoc 2012;1(2).
[51] Hsue PY, Ordovas K, Lee T, et al. Carotid intima–media thickness among human immunodeficiency virus-infected patients without coronary calcium. Am J Cardiol 2012;109(5):742–7.
[52] Koskinas KC, Chatzizisis YS, Baker AB, Edelman ER, Stone PH, Feldman CL. The role of low endothelial shear stress in the conversion of atherosclerotic lesions from stable to unstable plaque. Curr Opin Cardiol 2009;24(6):580–90.
[53] de Freitas EV, Brandao AA, Pozzan R, Magalhies ME, Castier M, Brandao AP. Study of the intima–media thickening in carotid arteries of healthy elderly with high blood pressure and elderly with high blood pressure and dyslipidemia. Clin Interv Aging 2008;3(3):525–34.
[54] Delaney JA, Scherzer R, Biggs ML, et al. Associations of antiretroviral drug use and HIV-specific risk factors with carotid intima–media thickness. AIDS 2010;24(14):2201–9.
[55] Lekakis J, Tsiodras S, Ikonomidis I, et al. HIV-positive patients treated with protease inhibitors have vascular changes resembling those observed in atherosclerotic cardiovascular disease. Clin Sci (Lond) 2008;115(6):189–96.
[56] Hileman CO, Carman TL, Longenecker CT, et al. Rate and predictors of carotid artery intima media thickness progression in antiretroviral-naive HIV-infected and uninfected adults: a 48-week matched prospective cohort study. Antivir Ther 2013;18(7):921–9.
[57] Hileman CO, Longenecker CT, Carman TL, McComsey GA. C-reactive protein predicts 96-week carotid intima media thickness progression in HIV-infected adults naive to antiretroviral therapy. J Acquir Immune Defic Syndr 2014;65(3):340–4.
[58] Buil-Cosiales P, Irimia P, Berrade N, et al. Carotid intima–media thickness is inversely associated with olive oil consumption. Atherosclerosis 2008;196(2):742–8.
[59] Turcinov D, Stanley C, Canchola JA, Rutherford GW, Novotny TE, Begovac J. Dyslipidemia and adherence to the Mediterranean diet in Croatian HIV-infected patients during the first year of highly active antiretroviral therapy. Coll Antropol 2009;33(2):423–30.

SECTION II

NUTRITION AND LIFESTYLE

CHAPTER

6

Nutritional Treatment Approach for ART-Naïve HIV-Infected Children

Marianne de Oliveira Falco[1] *and*
Erika Aparecida da Silveira[2]

[1]Department of Nutrition, Society Intensive Care, Goiás, Brazil, Postgraduate Studies Program Ph. D. in Health Sciences, Medical School, Federal University of Goiás, GO, Brazil, [2]Researcher, teacher of Postgraduate Studies Program in Health Sciences, Department of Surgery, Medical School, Federal University of Goiás, GO, Brazil

6.1 INTRODUCTION

There are currently 3.3 million children up to 14 years old living with human immunodeficiency virus/acquired immunodeficiency syndrome (HIV/AIDS) worldwide, with two-thirds in sub-Saharan Africa [1,2]. Sub-Saharan Africa, along with Asian countries, is an area with the second largest occurrence of infected children [1]. Besides the high prevalence of HIV infection, it is also a region of food insecurity [3].

Food insecurity and HIV infection are major triggers of dietary deficiencies and malnutrition [3]. Malnutrition in areas of food insecurity affects 18–47% of children infected with HIV [4,5].

Immune system impairment, anemia, and malnutrition are the top three causes of HIV disease progression [2,6–10]. In HIV-infected children, malnutrition is associated with complications such as opportunistic infections, disabsorptive diseases, fluid and electrolyte disorders, and micronutrient deficiencies, which contribute to a significant increase in mortality, reaching 30% among hospitalized malnourished children [11,12]. These complications impair nutritional status, generating a vicious cycle (Figure 6.1) [13–15].

Health of HIV Infected People, Volume 2.
DOI: http://dx.doi.org/10.1016/B978-0-12-800767-9.00006-6

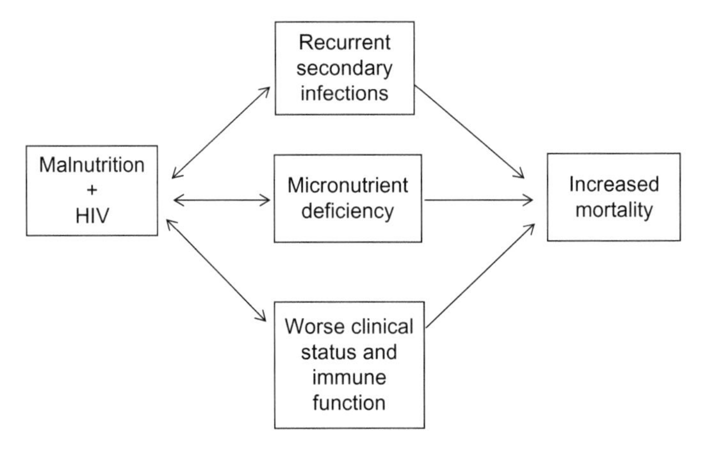

FIGURE 6.1 Vicious cycle of malnutrition, HIV, and morbimortality.

Given this framework, international organizations propose that 50% of HIV treatment is nutritional treatment and 50% is medical care [10,16].

6.1.1 Proposals and Investigations About Nutritional Approach for HIV-Infected Children

Proposals and research on the nutritional approach in HIV-infected children are guided by consolidated actions and often have positive outcomes. For example, supplementation with micronutrients, such as vitamin A, zinc, and iron, along with breastfeeding have provided encouraging evidence of improvement in morbidity and mortality in uninfected malnourished children [17–19]. These recommended approaches, widely disseminated since 2003 by the World Health Organization (WHO), are exposed, compared, and discussed along with other proposals in this chapter [20].

6.2 NUTRITIONAL TREATMENT AND READY-TO-USE FORMULAS

6.2.1 Breastfeeding

Breast milk is the best and most complete food for infants. It helps prevent malnutrition, diarrhea, and recurrent infections. Therefore, it is an important immunomodulatory factor in the presence of HIV [7,16].

Children from 6 to 11 months who are exposed to HIV and who were not breastfed are at increased risk for hospitalization and have higher incidences of fever, diarrhea, and severe malnutrition [21]. In areas where ART is available, such as Brazil, North America, Europe, East Mediterranean region, and the Western Pacific [22], HIV-infected mothers should be strongly encouraged to breastfeed for 12 months or at least for a minimum of 6 months. Where ART is not available, the recommendation is the same because the protective effect of breastfeeding against morbidities arising from HIV infection is greater than the risk of HIV transmission during breastfeeding [16].

Not breastfeeding implies a survival risk for the child, especially in areas where there is food insecurity [22,23]. Its replacement with artificial feeding should only occur when there is an agreement between the mother and the health care professional that it is safe, feasible, affordable, and sustainable [16].

6.2.2 Weaning and Complementary Feeding

The weaning process, with the introduction of new foods, exposes HIV-infected children to the risk of malnutrition and other diseases, especially in areas of food insecurity, low income, and inadequate sanitation [7,16]. Early weaning increases rates of diarrhea and mortality, especially in malnourished children, compared with children who had long-term breastfeeding [7].

For the treatment and control of malnutrition, complementary foods, easy acquisition formulas, or preparation formulas are recommended. For severely malnourished children and HIV-positive children, the same formulas composed of milk, oil, sugar and a mix of vitamins and minerals are indicated [7]. F-75 formula, used as a first early treatment of severe malnutrition, has low osmolarity, avoiding severe metabolic and electrolyte imbalances of the refeeding syndrome. F-100 formula, used in the rehabilitation phase, has a higher caloric density and higher osmolarity.

Health professionals prescribed the formulas according to nutritional status and clinical status to achieve 1.0–1.2 kcal/kg, 13% protein, and approximately 30–40% lipids. For micronutrient deficiencies, depending on the composition and quantity of complementary foods offered to children, supplementation with multivitamins and minerals is required [7,24,25]. The formulas prescribed are low-cost, are composed of local food, and are much more accessible than the industrial formulas. They are distributed by treatment centers or delivered to homes by health workers who actively search out malnourished children, and they can even be commercially acquired [25].

In a detailed analysis conducted by the authors of this chapter, many industrialized formulas have higher protein concentrations than observed in those recommended by the WHO (approximately 14–20% of the nutritional composition). Studies reporting some advantage of industrialized formulas instead of the F-75 and F-100 formulas were not found. Nevertheless, it is known that HIV infection increases energy expenditure and, consequently, protein requirements [26–28]. Besides the aforementioned formulas, there are other variations that are described in this chapter.

Because of the high prevalence of malnutrition and its comorbidities, a study in South Africa has proposed implementing an intensification program to treat malnutrition in the region's hospitals and to assess what ready-to-use formulas are more commonly prescribed. The study included children aged younger than 1 year and those aged between 1 and 5 years. The program involved nutritionists training to better-identify symptoms of malnutrition, such as diarrhea, vomiting, and edema, encouraging breastfeeding and formula prescriptions for children according to malnutrition severity and clinical status. Of the children without diarrhea, 16% used supplemental formula F-75 and the other 84% used industrialized formulas similar to breast milk. Of those with diarrhea, 14% used F-75 and 86% used formulas similar to human milk; the most used formula was soy protein–based, with no lactose. In children without diarrhea, the most commonly used formulas were those acidified with a protein compound based on whey protein, which is similar to breast milk [29]. In this study, the most prescribed formulas for malnutrition in the absence or presence of diarrhea were industrialized. This finding contrasts with the 2013 WHO indication for treating malnutrition in areas of food insecurity (use of F-75 and F-100) [19].

Regarding the use of supplementary food to treat malnutrition, a study conducted with children exposed to HIV in Malawi assessed the acceptability of weaning among mothers, adherence to use of formula, and possible food intolerances in children. The food supplement substitute for breast milk was composed of peanut butter, soy milk powder, sugar, soy oil, soy protein, and a mixture of 22 vitamins and minerals. In each 100 g, there were 15 g of protein and 550 kcal. The food supplement was provided at the beginning of the weaning process, week 24 until week 48, starting with 75 g/day and increasing to 100 g/day. According to mothers' self-report, 91% of children were successfully weaned and 18% had side effects such as diarrhea, vomiting, and constipation at the beginning [30].

In the same perspective, a multicenter cohort study conducted for 8 weeks in the United States, Bahamas, and Brazil evaluated nutritionally complete industrialized formula supplementation in newborn infants exposed to HIV. Children who received formula in calorie and high-protein dilution with 29% more macronutrients and micronutrients showed weight gain, but height was not significantly increased compared with children who received standard formula. No difference was observed regarding adverse effects, tolerance, changes in mortality, or CD4 count in both groups, suggesting that concentrated formulas may be necessary for nutritional status recovery of children exposed to HIV.

The use of industrial formulas in the weaning process is common in regions with lower food insecurity and a lower concentration of children with HIV; however, it is very difficult to extrapolate the results, even if positive for the use of commercial formulas, for most HIV-infected children living in areas of food insecurity.

Formulas using regional foods, like those recommended by the WHO, ensured adequate tolerability and effective weaning in HIV-exposed and malnourished infants [7,19]. Thus, it can be seen that the WHO recommendations are valid. Moreover, high-calorie formula with 29% more micronutrients increased weight in newborns exposed to HIV, although there were no conclusions regarding improvement in immune function.

For children who regained appetite, clinically stabilized, were without infectious complications, or were under home care, the most indicated complementary foods are ready-to-use therapeutic foods (RUTF), which are prepared from basic and typical foods of the region where it is handled, ready to use, have high-caloric density, and are consumed without dilution [25]. RUTF have low moisture, 10–12% protein and 45–60% fat. In nutritional treatment using RUTF, attention should be given to micronutrients requirements, which are often not achieved with only the intake of complementary foods. Therefore, supplementation is needed.

Given the context of severe child malnutrition, particularly in sub-Saharan Africa, other studies analyzed supplementation with complementary formulas in malnourished children. A clinical trial evaluated children of Zulu origin who were between 6 and 36 weeks of age, mostly acutely malnourished, and had prolonged diarrhea (7 or more days) and opportunistic infection but were clinically stable. All children received dietary counseling to reduce diet lactose content and standard care for diarrhea: fluids replenishment with electrolytes and multivitamin supplementation (vitamins A, C, D, thiamine, riboflavin, pyridoxine, nicotinamide, and B12, double the requirements of the recommended daily allowance (RDA), 5 mg of folic acid per day for 7 days, 15 mg of zinc sulfate per day for 14 days, and a single dose of vitamin A 100,000 IU for children between ages 6 and 12 months and 200,000 IU for children older than age 12 months. The formula is lactose-free (trade name AL110) and contains casein, maltodextrin, lipids, vitamins, and essential minerals. The control group received usual formula and standard care for diarrhea (100–110 kcal/kg/day and 2.2 g protein/day). Children in the intervention group received an adaptation of the standard formula to offer 150 kcal/kg/day and 4.0–5.5 g protein/kg per day for 14 weeks. Children in the intervention group showed greater weight gain and fewer days of diarrhea, but improvements in immune function and mortality were not observed [31].

In Malawi, severe malnourished HIV-infected children without ART and between 6 and 60 months of age were followed-up for 4 months after hospital discharge. They were supplemented with F-75 and F-100 formulas for severe malnutrition [20]. At the end of follow-up, HIV-infected children had higher mortality when associated with worse clinical status and lower CD4 count at baseline. Compared with uninfected children who received the same intervention, no difference regarding nutritional status improvement was found [32]. Improvement in diarrhea was observed with administration of supplementary diet with reduced lactose content or F-75/F-100 formulas. Clinical improvement was seen in children who received longer intervention and use of F-75 and F-100 for 4 months or more. It is not possible to state a conclusion about the immune function because the study aims are different and use CD4 as either an outcome [31] or an as explanatory variable [32]. One can see that nutritional status improvement occurred independent of the prescribed formula and that recovery is possible for severely malnourished children, reflecting better quality of life.

6.3 VITAMINS AND MINERALS

Micronutrient deficiency in HIV-positive children is highly prevalent and recurrent in food insecurity areas [14]. Micronutrient supplements are unique or multiple vitamins, minerals, and trace elements formulations [33]. Micronutrients have multiple functions, such as regulation of immune function [34]. In a patient with HIV, micronutrient deficiency is associated with more rapid progression of HIV and higher rates of morbidity (diarrhea, lung infections) and mortality [33].

In endemic areas of micronutrient deficiency or food insecurity, micronutrients must be replenished through fortified foods or multivitamins, regardless of nutritional status, in an attempt to maintain adequate serum levels [35]. Some studies suggest that micronutrient requirements according to the RDA are not always sufficient to maintain stable serum levels [14]. Thus, a recommendation of two standard deviations above the requirement for the general population is indicated for people with HIV/AIDS [34,36].

To correct micronutrient deficiency, it is necessary for the child to undergo viral load suppression and to have overall stability of virus replication, that is, CD4 levels more than 35% in children younger than 11 months, more than 30% in children between 12 and 35 months of age, more than 25% in children between 36 and 59 months of age, or more than 500% in children older than 5 years, according to the WHO classification [34,37].

6.3.1 Iron

Iron is an essential mineral for proper child development and is primordial in the progression and maintenance of motor and cognitive systems. Its deficiency causes anemia [38], which is the second largest hematological change in HIV-infected children, second only to T-cell alterations, especially in areas of food insecurity [3,8]. Additionally, anemia in pregnant women is associated with increased risk of death in children younger than 2 years of age [39]. The prevalence of anemia in HIV-positive children varies between 50% and 91%, higher than in the population of HIV-uninfected children [40]. In Malawi, the prevalence of iron deficiency was 48% in children younger than 24 months and 17.7% in children older than 24 months [41]. Deficiency can be caused by HIV infection itself, opportunistic infections, malnutrition, or the use of antiretroviral medication [33,42]. Iron deficiency is associated with worse outcomes in relation to morbidity, mortality, and progression of HIV disease [40].

A systematic review of children approximately 12 years old and infected with HIV who attended the hospital or outpatient clinic evaluated the safety and efficacy of iron supplementation in clinical and immunological improvement and changes in viral load. The findings showed controversial outcomes and it was not possible to assess the effectiveness. The authors concluded that iron supplementation in anemic children with iron deficiency was able to improve serum iron stores, anemia, and weight gain, although some studies found higher risk of opportunistic infectious diseases and HIV disease progression [42].

HIV-infected children without acute malnutrition between 6 and 59 months of age in Malawi received daily doses of iron 3 mg/day plus multivitamin supplementation (vitamin A, 1,500 IU; vitamin C, 35 mg/mL; and vitamin D, 400 IU/mL) for 3 months. Iron supplementation resulted in better hemoglobin levels and reduced the persistence of anemia at 6-month follow-up when compared with infants who received only multivitamins. The CD4 counts improved in 3 months, although this improvement was not maintained at 6 months. There was also an increased risk of malaria and lower incidence of respiratory infections. Children with iron deficiency who received iron supplementation had significantly slower progression to AIDS in 3 months, but comparing intervention and control groups there was no significant difference. Also, no difference was observed for hospitalizations between groups. In this study, 35% were using ART, but ART had no influence on any of the aforementioned outcomes [41].

For effective correction of iron deficiency, the WHO recommends that in areas of food insecurity with high prevalence of HIV-infected children and anemia, iron supplementation must be the same as for HIV-uninfected children [8,33]. For maintenance of serum levels, the treatment of opportunistic infectious diseases and stabilization of HIV infection stage are relevant [8]. Iron supplementation in HIV-positive children in endemic areas of malaria and tuberculosis should be performed as a preventive measure as soon as the care for the prevention of these diseases is established. Otherwise, there may be an increase in their incidence [41].

There was improvement in anemia and serum iron when supplementation with multivitamins was used. Further investigations are necessary to elucidate the benefits, effectiveness, and efficacy regarding outcomes related to clinical improvement with iron supplementation alone or together with multivitamins,.

6.3.2 Zinc

Adequate serum zinc levels are essential for maintaining the immune function. Its deficiency is related to the decline of the CD4 count and reduced survival [43]. Zinc supplementation in HIV-positive children is recommended as adjuvant treatment for acute or chronic diarrhea and for the reduction of opportunistic infectious diseases, especially in those affected by malnutrition and in food insecurity areas [14,18]. Confirming the aforementioned data, a double-blind randomized clinical trial conducted in South Africa with HIV-positive children between 6 and 60 months of age observed significant reductions in viral load and diarrhea with supplementation of 10g daily zinc for 6 months. This study was a marker of evidence for treatment of diarrhea and the first controlled clinical trial of this type [44].

Currently, concern about the access to treatment for infectious comorbidities such as diarrhea has spread. Diarrhea is a major cause of morbidity and mortality in newborns and children around the world, and HIV-infected children are more likely to suffer from this disorder, both in frequency and severity [18]. Given this concern, a study conducted in western Kenya followed-up children between 2 months and 5 years of age. Their caregivers were asked to provide zinc as adjuvant treatment for diarrhea. Packages of zinc 20mg and two sachets of oral rehydration were left in the houses visited every 2 months. The control group was instructed to seek treatment in a health care clinic. There was no difference in the incidence of diarrhea in the two groups, but the children who had zinc delivered to their residency had an improvement in their diarrhea, with reduced frequency of bowel movements and improved stool consistency compared with the control group. There were no differences in the reduction of infectious morbidity between groups [45]. Families who had zinc provided to their homes used it for treating diarrhea without any difficulties. Zinc is suggested for diarrhea treatment in health centers and pharmacies because there were no observed adverse effects with its supplementation [45].

Health services are crucial for the successful treatment of people living with HIV/AIDS. It is exactly where they will find medical assistance, guidance, and monitoring for HIV infection stabilization as well as medicine, whether antiretroviral therapy or antibiotics for the treatment of infectious comorbidities. It should still be a place for access to nutritional treatment and supplementation guidelines. Nevertheless, as demonstrated by Feikin et al. [45], the low adherence in seeking treatment at health services is characteristic of communities in sub-Saharan Africa because of cultural issues. This problem is already receiving attention from the WHO, which is seeking greater integration of services and expansion of health networks to facilitate access to the most remote communities [46].

6.3.3 Vitamin A

Vitamin A deficiency is a major nutritional issue in developing regions. Vitamin A is essential for the integrity of the epithelium and proper fetal development, because it participates in the cell division process, bone tissue formation, and epithelia integrity maintenance, including that of the intestinal mucosa [47,48].

In endemic areas, hypovitaminosis A can compromise the immune system of up to 40% of HIV-infected children. Vitamin A supplementation is recommended, especially in areas of food insecurity for all children with HIV, regardless of nutritional status, from ages 6 months to 5 years to improve development and child growth and to reduce risk factors associated with diarrhea morbidity [33]. The recommended dose for HIV-infected children is 100,000 IU for babies 6–12 months of age and 200,000 IU for children older than age 12 months [33]. Vitamin A supplementation in children exposed to HIV who are older than age 6 months varies between 50,000 and 200,000 IU [33]. The indicated treatment of diarrhea in HIV-positive children with acute malnutrition is the same concomitant dose administration of zinc [19], with particular attention to clinical status, level of disability and intervals of administration; no randomized studies showed increased morbidity with high-dose vitamin A administration [19,49]. Vitamin A supplementation plus zinc improves immune function, integrity of the intestinal mucosa, and the incidence and severity of diarrhea, in addition to providing improvement in growth in the short term [14,19,34].

In accordance with WHO recommendations [19] and the conclusions reached by studies by Irlam et al. in 2010 and 2013 [14,34] regarding the joint administration of vitamin A and zinc to treat diarrhea, three double-blind clinical trials were developed in South Africa with HIV-infected children and HIV-uninfected children (exposed or not to the virus) 6–24 months of age. The intervention was divided into three different exposures: supplementation with daily doses of vitamin A 1,250 IU; daily supplementation with vitamin A 1,250 IU plus 10 mg of zinc; and daily multivitamin supplementation including zinc and vitamin A. The HIV-positive children had a higher incidence of diarrhea than HIV-negative children. Although different than expected, the HIV-positive children receiving vitamin A plus zinc or micronutrient supplementation had a higher incidence of severe or persistent diarrhea during follow-up than those with only receiving vitamin A. In HIV-uninfected children, vitamin A supplementation plus zinc or micronutrient supplementation reduced the incidence of diarrhea in those with short stature compared with those who received only vitamin A [50]. The highest incidence of diarrhea in HIV-infected children after supplementation with vitamin A plus zinc or micronutrient supplementation can be justified by the small sample size of infected children (32) compared with the sample number of uninfected children (341), thus limiting inferences [50].

Yet another trial evaluating the same population and supplementation to verify the percentage of days of diarrhea per child and the prevalence and incidence of respiratory diseases at the end of follow-up before the three proposed supplementation schemes (vitamin A, vitamin A plus zinc, or supplementation with multivitamins) found no effect on diarrhea or on respiratory diseases in any of the supplemented groups [51]. A major limiting factor in the inferences in this study was a failure to identify the stage of HIV disease progression [51].

Finally, the third test developed by the same group of researchers evaluated the effects of daily doses of vitamin A 1,250 IU plus 10 mg of zinc or doses of vitamin A plus zinc compound with multiple micronutrients. HIV-infected children, children exposed to HIV, and HIV-negative children participated in the study. HIV-negative children showed better growth and reduction of diarrhea when supplemented with zinc plus vitamin A and micronutrients. Children infected with HIV had worse growth; analysis of incidence of diarrhea was not possible because of small sample size and high sample loss. Zinc in combination with vitamin A and micronutrients did not present significant results for diarrhea and respiratory diseases in children exposed to HIV or HIV-positive children [50]. Supplementation with zinc plus vitamin A did not reduce the incidence or prevalence of diarrhea in the studies presented, but it should be considered in the small sample of HIV-infected children.

Research was conducted in Kampala and Uganda for HIV-infected children between 15 and 36 weeks of age receiving 200,000 IU vitamin A supplementation every 3 months. A protective effect against mortality was found in approximately 60% of children who received the supplement [52].

In infected pregnant women living in areas of high prevalence of vitamin A deficiency, the WHO recommends supplementation with a single dose of 200,000 IU soon after birth in an effort to reduce vertical transmission [53]. However, a clinical trial conducted in Africa with 400,000 IU vitamin A supplementation in pregnant women during the postpartum period noted that there was no modification of vertical transmission during breastfeeding. In this same study, the newborns were supplemented with a single dose of 50,000 IU vitamin A after birth. There was a 28% reduction in mortality in HIV-infected neonates during the intrauterine period and in those with negative C-reactive protein (CRP). In infected children who had positive CRP, there was no difference in mortality. In HIV-uninfected children, supplementation with vitamin A doubled the chance of death in 2 years; 40% of children who died had positive CRP, indicating an infectious process. In a more detailed analysis regarding deaths in HIV-negative children, it was found that 61% of the 40% who died were already infected by HIV and were not diagnosed during the cohort. It is hypothesized that the strong interaction between the immune system and vitamin A supplementation could have influenced the worsening of HIV status, increased viral load in mothers, and consequently increased vertical transmission. Apart from that, most of the deaths in children were associated with secondary infectious diseases. These two aspects may indicate that vitamin A may cause side effects and accelerate HIV disease progression [37].

Vitamin A supplementation is beneficial when there is clinical stability in HIV-infected children, but there must be clinical supervision and monitoring because of possible side effects and severity of secondary infectious diseases or HIV disease progression. More evidence is needed to establish whether supplementation provides benefits similar to those found in adults with HIV [54–56]. Vitamin A supplementation associated with zinc had no effect on diarrhea and respiratory diseases.

6.3.4 Vitamin D and Calcium

Vitamin D deficiency is highly prevalent and can reach up to 80% and is associated with increased morbidity and mortality, advancing stage of disease, disturbances in bone metabolism, and immunological changes [57]. Only one trial was found demonstrating efficacy and safety for cholecalciferol supplementation in children older than age 6 years. Cholecalciferol 4,000 or 7,000 IU/day was supplemented; after 12 months, both doses were able to maintain serum concentration less than 32 ng/mL. The dose of 7,000 IU was significantly more effective than 4,000 IU [58].

Regarding clinical outcomes, a double-blind clinical trial was conducted in the United States among HIV-positive individuals with a mean age of 10.6 years who were supplemented with 100,000 IU cholecalciferol every 2 months and 1 g/day of calcium every 12 months. When compared with the placebo group, it was observed that the supplemented dose is safe and effective to maintain 25(OH)D levels $\geq$ 30 ng/mL, but there was no change in the immune function or progression of HIV [59].

Modest results were found for vitamin D supplementation and associated factors among HIV-infected children without ART because, despite being an advent of recent investigations, in most studies it was used in those using ART, and these individuals were not the focus of this chapter [60,61].

Thus, it is not possible to infer conclusions about vitamin D supplementation. Even at doses above the RDA, vitamin D supplementation showed no effect on the clinical and immunological stages of HIV-infected children.

6.3.5 Micronutrients

It is a fact that HIV-infected children have micronutrient deficiencies. A study in Nigeria reported 77.1% zinc deficiency, 71.4% selenium deficiency, and 70.0% vitamin C deficiency in ART-naïve children aged 18 months or older [61]. Therefore, micronutrient supplementation would be the most practical, inexpensive, effective, and possibly easiest way for the health care team to manage the child and the caregiver [3]. The RDA recommendations are not always sufficient to maintain stable blood levels of vitamins, minerals, and trace elements [15,33].

The best combination of micronutrients and individual dosage of each micronutrient, as well as the most adequate moment for supplementation in the face of infectious processes, disease stage, and nutritional status for serum level stability are still the focus of investigations. Among the composition of some multivitamins, some are of substantial importance, such as zinc, selenium, and vitamin C, which showed significant effects on reduction of morbidity and mortality in HIV-positive supplemented children [14].

A study in which 67.1% of the children were in an advanced clinical stage of HIV infection demonstrated that a deficiency of selenium, zinc, and vitamin C was significantly more prevalent during the later stages of HIV and associated with low weight for age and immunological status worsening. Children with adequate micronutrient levels had higher weight for age than children with micronutrient deficiencies [62]. Multiple micronutrient deficiencies were found in this study, reinforcing the importance of this nutritional assessment in HIV-positive children. Thus, it is important to discuss the most appropriate supplementation approach with health care team members.

The micronutrient supplementation in malnourished children of Pretoria, between 6 and 24 months of age, significantly improved appetite. The supplementations were as follows: vitamin A, 300 mg; vitamin B1, 0.6 mg; vitamin B2, 0.6 mg; vitamin B3, 8 mg; vitamin B6, 0.6 mg; vitamin B12, 1 mg; folic acid, 70 mg; vitamin C, 25 mg; vitamin D, 5 mg; vitamin E, 7 mg; copper, 700 mg; iron, 8 mg; selenium, 30 mg; and 8 mg zinc [63]. The improved appetite may consequently improve the nutritional status, reducing susceptibility to opportunistic infections. Future research evaluating results of micronutrient supplementation on these outcomes are relevant.

HIV-infected children between 4 and 24 months age without ART hospitalized with pneumonia or diarrhea and growth restriction received daily supplementation with multivitamins until discharge. The composition of the multivitamin supplement was as follows: 300 mg retinol; 0.6 mg thiamin; riboflavin 0.6 mg; 8 mg niacin; pyridoxine 0.6 mg; 1 mg cobalamin; folic acid 70 mg; 25 mg ascorbic acid; 1,25-dihydrocholecalciferol 5 mg; 7 mg L-α-tocopherol; 700 mg copper; iron 8 mg; 30 mg selenium; and zinc 8 mg. Supplementation reduced days of diarrhea and pneumonia, reflecting a significant reduction in duration of hospitalization, but no results regarding the nutritional status were observed [64].

Multivitamin use was also evaluated in children aged 1–5 years in Uganda to estimate the incidence and prevalence of diarrhea. Supplementation was daily during 6-month follow-up. The control group received micronutrients according to the RDA (vitamins A, B1, B2, niacin, C, and D) and the intervention group received twice the RDA for vitamins A, B1, B2, niacin, B6, B12, C, D, E, folate, selenium, zinc, copper, iron, and iodine. At the end of the study, there was no reduction in diarrhea among groups [65]. Similarly, in Tanzania, daily doses of 150–600% above the RDA requirements for age of vitamins C, E, thiamin, riboflavin, niacin, B6, B12, and folate, were offered to HIV-exposed infants between the sixth week and the seventh month of life. From the seventh month, two daily capsules with 200–400% of the RDA for age was provided. There was a reduction in fever, vomiting, and hospitalization time. For those with low birth weight, there was an increase in risk of fever, vomiting, and lower risk of diarrhea [66].

Children in India, with and without ART, who were 15 years of age or younger were supplemented with 25 mcg copper; 5 mg zinc; 10 mg selenium; 38 μg iodine; and vitamins A, B1, B2, B6, B12, B5, D, and E. At the end of 6 months, there was significant improvement in BMI and clinical and immunological status [67].

As previously described, isolated micronutrient supplements are not necessarily able to improve clinical status, weight gain, or linear growth. Several compositions of various dosages of micronutrients have been proposed for several outcomes. Vitamin A, selenium, and zinc were a part of all presented studies. Positive results in relation to improved appetite, immune function, nutritional status, reduction of diarrhea, pneumonia, and duration of hospitalization were reported. However, it is difficult to make inferences for clinical practice, because the formulas and the outcomes assessed are distinct. The only conclusion from the presented results was that doses of micronutrients according to the requirements of the RDA or higher were able to reduce the length of hospitalization. The improvement seems to be related to the patient's clinical, immunological, and nutritional status at entry and the combination of supplemented micronutrients.

6.4 PROBIOTICS

Probiotics are nonpathogenic live microorganisms that contribute to the improvement of the immune gut barrier, avoiding bacterial translocation at the cost of environment acidification and the consequent destruction of pathogenic bacteria [68,69]. This action provides better health of the host when administered in adequate doses and clinical situations [70].

Faced with this possibility, children 2 to 12 years of age in Porto Alegre, Brazil, were given daily intervention with milk formula plus 14 g *Bifidobacterium bifidum* with *Streptococcus thermophilus* 2.5×10^{10} for

2 months or standard formula without probiotics. The hypothesis that the use of probiotics increases CD4 count and improves stool consistency was raised. There was an increase in CD4 lymphocyte count regardless of ART use in children who received probiotics. Also, an improvement in stool consistency was observed independent of probiotics use [71]. In India, children 15 years of age or younger without ART received probiotics (*Lactobacillus sporogenes*) 2.5×1.01 colony-forming units (CFU) twice daily for 3 months. Those younger than 6 years of age received 10 g and those 6 years of age or older received 20 g. Children showed improvement in the clinical stage of HIV: stage II changed to stage 1 in 30.8% of children. It is important to highlight that the control group showed significant worsening of CD4 count in relation to baseline [67].

Double-blind, randomized, multicenter clinical trial evaluated supplementation with nutritionally complete formulas and *B. lactis* in newborns exposed to HIV for 6 months. No difference in growth and morbidities such as diarrhea and opportunistic infections was observed; however, weight was higher in children who received probiotics compared with those who received standard formulas without the addition of probiotics [72]. Another trial in hospitalized premature infants aged younger than 34 weeks who were HIV-exposed or not exposed (children of HIV-uninfected mothers) in South Africa included daily doses of probiotics (*Lactobacillus rhamnosus* 0.35×10^9 CFU and *B. infantis* 0.35×10 CFU^9) for 28 days along with breast milk. Among those exposed to HIV, there was greater head growth and increased growth on Z score for height. However, when compared with HIV-negative children, there were no differences in growth. Adverse effects in relation to probiotics use were evaluated (food intolerance and abdominal distension), but there was no difference between groups [73].

Probiotic administration improved stage of HIV infection. Newborns who received probiotics along with breast milk or industrialized formula had an improvement in nutritional status. Searches using probiotics as nutritional treatment in children without ART are recent but have demonstrated promising and positive results.

6.5 CONCLUSION

There is great concern regarding facilitating the weaning process in HIV-exposed children to maintain proper immune response, prevent opportunistic diseases, and ensure adequate development even before the evidence of risks in those not breastfeeding.

The use of complementary formulas in the weaning process in HIV-positive children is open for discussion. Investigations occur with different interventions, but it is interesting that formulas recommended by

WHO show good tolerability and their utilization in the weaning process ensured good adhesion in malnourished children. The results with respect to weight gain and height were checked only regarding the use of high-calorie and high-protein formulas. These findings are consistent with studies evaluating increased energy expenditure in HIV-positive children. Reflections on this finding are noteworthy.

Improvements in diarrhea and nutritional status in malnourished children were observed with the use of both industrialized formulas (lactose-free and F-75/F-100). The immune status showed improvement in malnourished children who received longer interventions and who received complementary foods based on regional foods.

When evaluating isolated micronutrient supplementation, zinc stands out for notable efficacy in the treatment of diarrhea and prevention of opportunistic infections. Doses above the RDA are related to improvement in diarrhea in severely malnourished children. Supplementation with vitamin A showed a protective effect on mortality. However, in the presence of immune disorders, it may cause HIV disease progression and increased risk for secondary infectious diseases. Vitamin A administered with zinc showed no significant effect on the incidence or prevalence of diarrhea and growth in HIV-positive children. Supplementation with vitamin D showed no beneficial effect in relation to the immune system and stage evolution of HIV.

Iron supplementation improved hemoglobin levels, reduced persistence of anemia, and promoted weight gain. However, the replenishment of iron deserves attention in HIV-positive children because its use has shown conflicting results regarding the worsening of morbimortality.

Micronutrient deficiency is associated with nutritional status and is highly prevalent among HIV-infected children. Micronutrient supplementation seems to provide better health conditions in ART-naïve children. Positive results in relation to improved appetite, improved nutritional status, immunological markers, reduced prevalence and incidence of diarrhea, and days of hospitalization were perceived in compositions that contained vitamin A, zinc, and selenium. It is possible to question whether the best approach would be to supplement formulas with multiple micronutrients rather than in isolation. Many outcomes of micronutrient supplementation indicated improvement in diarrhea, immune status, and delay in HIV disease progression. Usage as a single intervention or in combination with others, such as formulas, has presented good results regarding physical development and weight gain in malnourished children.

Despite the widespread use of probiotic *Lactobacillus* and *Bifidobacterium* strains in children with good results in the reduction of days of treatment in infectious diseases [74] and acute diarrhea [75] in uninfected children, the studies evaluating benefits in HIV-positive children are scarce and with modest results. HIV disease progression improvement and progress in infectious diseases of the gastrointestinal tract and anthropometric markers have been noted.

Findings show that considerable effort is being undertaken to find the best nutritional approach for HIV-positive children. However, given the scale of abnormalities arising from HIV infection, there is still much to be investigated. Working with skilled staff and expanded access to health care may be relevant in the prevention and treatment of the resulting deficiencies of the evolution of HIV. Way of ensuring the survival of these children can make a big difference in immune development and in the advancement of AIDS.

References

[1] UNAIDS. Report on the global AIDS epidemic. Joint United Nations Programme on HIV/AIDS; Geneva: 2013:1–198.
[2] UNICEF. The state of the world's children 2014 in numbers revealing disparities, advancing children's rights every child counts. United Nations Children's Fund; New York: 2014:1–110.
[3] UNICEF. Improving child nutrition: the achievable imperative for global progress. United Nations Children's Fund; New York: 2013:1–132.
[4] Kimani-Murage EW, Norris SA, Pettifor JM, et al. Nutritional status and HIV in rural South African children. BMC Pediatr 2011;11:23.
[5] Nhampossa T, Sigaúque B, Machevo S, et al. Severe malnutrition among children under the age of 5 years admitted to a rural district hospital in southern Mozambique. Public Health Nutr 2013;16:1565–74.
[6] UNICEF. Prevention of mother-to-child transmission (PMTCT) of HIV. United Nations Children's Fund; New York: 2012:1–39.
[7] WHO Essential nutrition actions: improving maternal, newborn, infant and young child health and nutrition. Geneva, Switzerland: World Health Organization; 2013. pp. 1–146.
[8] McLean E, Cogswell M, Egli I, Wojdyla D, de Benoist B. Worldwide prevalence of anaemia: who vitamin and mineral nutrition information system, 1993–2005. Public Health Nutr 2009;12:444–54.
[9] de Pee S, Semba RD. Role of nutrition in HIV infection: review of evidence for more effective programming in resource-limited settings. Food Nutr Bull 2010;13:S313–44.
[10] UNAIDS WHO. Technical guidance note for global fund HIV proposals: food and nutrition. Joint United Nations Programme on HIV/AIDS; Geneva: 2011:1–10.
[11] Musoke PM, Fergusson P. Severe malnutrition and metabolic complications of HIV-infected children in the antiretroviral era: clinical care and management in resource-limited settings. Am J Clin Nutr 2011;94:1716S–20S.
[12] Fergusson P, Tomkins A. HIV prevalence and mortality among children undergoing treatment for severe acute malnutrition in Sub-Saharan Africa: a systematic review and meta-analysis. Trans R Soc Trop Med Hyg 2009;103:541–8.
[13] Piwoz EG, Preble EA. HIV/AIDS and nutrition: a review of the literature and recommendation for nutrition care and support in sub Saharan African. USAID 2000:1–66.
[14] Irlam JH, Siegfried N, Visser ME, Rollins NC. Micronutrient supplementation for children with HIV infection. Cochrane Database Syst Rev 2013:10. CD010666.
[15] Mankal PK, Kotler DP. From wasting to obesity, changes in nutritional concerns in HIV/AIDS. Endocrinol Metab Clin North Am 2014;43:647–63.
[16] WHO UNAIDS UNFPA UNICEF Guidelines on HIV and infant feeding. Principles and recommendations for infant feeding in the context of HIV and a summary of evidence. Geneva, Switzerland: World Health Organization; 2010. pp. 1–58.

[17] Bhutta ZA, Ahmed T, Black RE, et al. What works? Interventions for maternal and child undernutrition and survival. Lancet 2008;371:417–40.
[18] WHO Recommendations on the management of diarrhoea and pneumonia in HIV-infected infants and children: integrated management of childhood illness (IMCI). Geneva, Switzerland: World Health Organization; 2010. pp. 1–60.
[19] WHO Guideline updates on the management of severe acute malnutrition in infants and children. Geneva, Switzerland: World Health Organization; 2013. pp. 1–123.
[20] WHO Guidelines for the inpatient treatment of severely malnourished children. Geneva, Switzerland: World Health Organization; 2003. pp. 1–50.
[21] Marquez C, Okiring J, Chamie G, et al. Increased morbidity in early childhood among HIV-exposed uninfected children in Uganda is associated with breastfeeding duration. J Trop Pediatr; 2014. pii: fmu045. [Epub ahead of print].
[22] WHO Global update on HIV treatment 2013: results, impact and opportunities: WHO report in partnership with UNICEF and UNAIDS. Geneva, Switzerland: World Health Organization; 2013. pp. 1–30.
[23] Kindra G, Coutsoudis A, Esposito F. Effect of nutritional supplementation of breast-feeding HIV positive mothers on maternal and child health: findings from a randomized controlled clinical trial. BMC Public Health 2011;11:946.
[24] WHO Management of severe malnutrition: a manual for physicians and other senior health workers. Geneva, Switzerland: World Health Organization; 1999. pp. 1–68.
[25] WHO WFP UNSSCN UNICEF Community-based management of severe acute malnutrition. Geneva, Switzerland: World Health Organization; 2007. pp. 1–8.
[26] Grunfeld C, Pang M, Shimizu L, Shigenaga JK, Jensen P, Feingold KR. Resting energy expenditure, caloric intake, and short-term weight change in human immunodeficiency virus infection and the acquired immunodeficiency syndrome. Am J Clin Nutr 1992;55:455–60.
[27] Bell SJ, Chavali S, Baumer J, Forse RA. Resting energy expenditure, caloric intake, and short-term change in HIV infection and AIDS. J Parenter Enteral Nutr 1993;17:392–4.
[28] Batterham MJ. Investigating heterogeneity in studies of resting energy expenditure in persons with HIV/AIDS: a meta-analysis. Am J Clin Nutr 2005;81:702–13.
[29] Biggs C. Clinical dietetic practice in the treatment of severe acute malnutrition in a high HIV setting. J Hum Nutr Diet 2013;26:175–81.
[30] Parker ME, Bentley ME, Chasela C, et al. The acceptance and feasibility of replacement feeding at 6 months as an HIV prevention method in Lilongwe, Malawi: results from the BAN study. AIDS Educ Prev 2011;23:281–95.
[31] Rollins NC, van den Broeck J, Kindra G, Pent M, Kasambira T, Bennish ML. The effect of nutritional support on weight gain of HIV-infected children with prolonged diarrhea. Acta Paediatr 2007;96:62–8.
[32] Fergusson P, Chinkhumba J, Grijalva-Eternod C, Banda T, Mkangama C, Tomkins A. Nutritional recovery in HIV-infected and HIV-uninfected children with severe acute malnutrition. Arch Dis Child 2009;94:512–6.
[33] WHO Nutrient requirements for people leaving with HIV/AIDS: report of a technical consultation. Geneva, Switzerland: World Health Organization; 2003. pp. 1–31.
[34] Irlam JH, Visser MME, Rollins NN, Siegfried N. Micronutrient supplementation in children and adults with HIV infection. Cochrane Database Syst Rev 2010:12. CD003650.
[35] Sabery N, Duggan C. The American society for parenteral and enteral nutrition (ASPEN) clinical guidelines: nutrition support of children human immunodeficiency virus infection. JPEN J Parenter Enteral Nut 2009;33:588–606.
[36] King JC, Vorster HH, Tome DG. Nutrient intake values (NIVs): a recommended terminology and framework for the derivation of values. Food Nutr Bull 2007;28:S16–26.
[37] Humphrey JH, Lliff PJ, Marinda ET, et al. Effects of a single large dose of vitamin A, given during the postpartum period to HIV-positive women and their infants, on child HIV infection, HIV-free survival, and mortality. J Infect Dis 2006;193:860–71.

[38] UNICEF. The micronutrient initiative. Investing in the future: a united call to action on vitamin and mineral deficiencies global report. United Nations Children's Fund. New York: 2009:1–52.

[39] Isanaka S, Spiegelman D, Aboud S, et al. Post-natal anaemia and iron deficiency in HIV-infected women and the health and survival of their children. Matern Child Nutr 2012;8:287–98.

[40] Calis JC, van Hensbroek MB, de Haan RJ, Moons P, Brabin BJ, Bates I. HIV-associated anemia in children: a systematic review from a global perspective. AIDS 2008;22:1099–112.

[41] Esan MO, van Hensbroek MB, Nkhoma E, et al. Iron supplementation in HIV-infected Malawian children with anemia: a double-blind, randomized, controlled trial. Clin Infect Dis 2013;57:1626–34.

[42] Adetifa I, Okomo U. Iron supplementation for reducing morbidity and mortality in children with HIV. Cochrane Database Syst Rev 2009:1. CD006736.

[43] Zeng L, Zang L. Efficacy and safety of zinc supplementation for adults, children and pregnant women with HIV infection: systematic review. Trop Med Int Health 2011;16:474–82.

[44] Bobat R, Coovadia H, Stephen C, Naidoo KL, McKerrow N, Black RE. Safety and efficacy of zinc supplementation for children with HIV-1 infection in South Africa: a randomised double-blind placebo-controlled trial. Lancet 2005;366:1862–7.

[45] Feikin DR, Bigogo G, Audi A, et al. Village-randomized clinical trial of home distribution of zinc for treatment of childhood diarrhea in rural western Kenya. PLoS One 2014;9:e94436.

[46] WHO Consolidated guidelines on HIV prevention, diagnosis, treatment and care for key populations. Geneva, Switzerland: World Health Organization; 2014. pp. 1–184.

[47] Villamor E, Fawzi WW. Effects of vitamin a supplementation on immune responses and correlation with clinical outcomes. Clin Microbiol Rev 2005;18:446–64.

[48] WHO Guideline: vitamin A supplementation in pregnancy for reducing the risk of mother-to-child transmission of HIV. Geneva, Switzerland: World Health Organization; 2011. pp. 1–25.

[49] Allen LH, Haskell M. Estimating the potential for vitamin A toxicity in women and young children. J Nutr 2002;132:2907S–2919SS.

[50] Chhagan MK, Van den Broeck J, Luabeya KA, Mpontshane N, Tomkins A, Bennish ML. Effect on longitudinal growth and anemia of zinc or multiple micronutrients added to vitamin A: a randomized controlled trial in children aged 6–24 months. BMC Public Health 2010;10:145.

[51] Luabeya KK, Mpontshane N, Mackay M, et al. Zinc or multiple micronutrient supplementation to reduce diarrhea and respiratory disease in South African children: a randomized controlled trial. PLoS One 2007;2:e541.

[52] Semba RD, Ndugwa C, Perry RT, et al. Effect of periodic vitamin A supplementation on mortality and morbidity of human immunodeficiency virus-infected children in Uganda: a controlled clinical trial. Nutrition 2005;21:25–31.

[53] WHO. Safe vitamin A dosage during pregnancy and lactation. Recommendations and report of a consultation. Geneva, Switzerland: World Health Organization; 1998. pp. 1–46.

[54] Baum MK, Shor-Posner G, Lu Y, et al. Micronutrients and HIV-1 disease progression. AIDS 1995;9:1051–6.

[55] Mehendale SM, Shepherd ME, Brookmeyer RS, et al. Low carotenoid concentration and the risk of HIV seroconversion in Pune, India. J Acquir Immune Defic Syndr 2001;26:352–9.

[56] Stephensen CB. Vitamin A, beta-carotene, and mother-to-child transmission of HIV. Nutr Rev 2003;61:280–4.

[57] EACS. Guidelines version 7.01, November 2013. European AIDS Clinical Society; Zurich: 2013:1–81.

[58] Dougherty KA, Schall JI, Zemel BS, et al. Safety and efficacy of high-dose daily vitamin D3 supplementation in children and young adults infected with human immunodeficiency virus. J Pediatr Infect Dis 2014;27:1–10.
[59] Arpadi SM, McMahon D, Abrams EJ, et al. Effect of bimonthly supplementation with oral cholecalciferol on serum 25-hydroxyvitamin D concentrations in HIV-infected children and adolescents. Pediatrics 2009;123:e121–6.
[60] Chun RF, Liu NQ, Lee T, Schall JI, Denburg MR, Rutstein RM. Vitamin D supplementation and antibacterial immune responses in adolescents and young adults with HIV/AIDS. J Steroid Biochem Mol Biol 2014;S0960-0760(14):00144–47.
[61] Foissac F, Meyzer C, Frange P, et al. Determination of optimal vitamin D3 dosing regimens in HIV-infected paediatric patients using a population pharmacokinetic approach. Br J Clin Pharmacol 2014;78:1113–21.
[62] Anyabolu HC, Adejuyigbe EA, Adeodu OO. Serum micronutrient status of HAART-naïve, HIV infected children in Southwestern Nigeria: a case controlled study. AIDS Res Treat 2014 2014:351043.
[63] Mda S, van Raaij JM, Macintyre UE, de Villiers FP, Kok FJ. Improved appetite after multi-micronutrient supplementation for six months in HIV-infected South African children. Appetite 2010;54:150–5.
[64] Mda S, van Raaij JM, de Villiers FP, MacIntyre UE, Kok FJ. Short-term micronutrient supplementation reduces the duration of pneumonia and diarrheal episodes in HIV-infected children. J Nutr 2010;140:969–74.
[65] Ndeezi G, Thorkild T, Ndugwa CM, James TK. Multiple micronutrient supplementation does not reduce diarrhoea morbidity in Ugandan HIV-infected children: a randomized controlled trial. Paediatr Int Child Health 2012;32:14–21.
[66] Duggan C, Manji KP, Kupka R, et al. Multiple micronutrient supplementation in Tanzanian infants born to HIV-infected mothers: a randomized, double-blind, placebo-controlled clinical trial. Am J Clin Nutr 2012;96:1437–47.
[67] Gautam N, Dayal R, Agarwal D, et al. Role of multivitamins, micronutrients and probiotics supplementation in management of HIV infected children. Indian J Pediatr 2014;14 1407-1406.
[68] Vanderhoof JA. Probiotics: future directions. Am J Clin Nutr 2001;73:1152S–55S.
[69] Brenchley JM, Douek DC. HIV infection and the gastrointestinal immune system. Mucosal Immunol 2008;1:23–30.
[70] FAO Health and nutritional properties of probiotics in food including powder milk with live lactic acid bacteria. Rome, Italy: Food and Agriculture Organization; 2001. pp. 1–56.
[71] Trois L, Cardoso EM, Miura E. Use of probiotics in HIV-infected children: a randomized double-blind controlled study. J Trop Pediatr 2008;54:19–24.
[72] Velaphi SC, Cooper PA, Bolton KD, et al. Growth and metabolism of infants born to women infected with human immunodeficiency virus and fed acidified whey-adapted starter formulas. Nutrition 2008;24:203–11.
[73] Niekerk EV, Kirsten GF, Nel DG. Probiotics, feeding tolerance, and growth: a comparison between HIV-exposed and unexposed very low birth weight infants. Nutrition 2014;30:645–53.
[74] King S, Glanville J, Sanders ME, Fitzgerald A, Varley D. Effectiveness of probiotics on the duration of illness in healthy children and adults who develop common acute respiratory infectious conditions: a systematic review and meta-analysis. Br J Nutr 2014;112:41–54.
[75] Applegate JA, Fischer Walker CL, Ambikapathi R, Black RE. Systematic review of probiotics for the treatment of community-acquired acute diarrhea in children. BMC Public Health 2013;13:S16.

CHAPTER

7

Nutrition Therapy for HAART-Naïve HIV-Infected Patients

Marianne de Oliveira Falco[1] *and Erika Aparecida da Silveira*[2]

[1]Department of Nutrition, Society Intensive Care, Goiás, Brazil, Postgraduate Studies Program Ph. D. in Health Sciences, Medical School, Federal University of Goiás, Brazil, [2]Researcher, teacher of Postgraduate Studies Program in Health Sciences, Department of Surgery, Medical School, Federal University of Goiás, Brazil

7.1 INTRODUCTION

What to do about acquired immunodeficiency syndrome (AIDS)? This pandemic affects millions of people, especially in sub-Saharan Africa, which is a region of food insecurity [1]. Researchers in this area and various institutions around the world constantly seek, through research, resolutions to address and improve the quality of life of millions of people living with human immunodeficiency virus (HIV)/AIDS (PLWHA), malnutrition, and exposure to chronic diseases arising from the HIV inflammatory process [2]. Nutrition therapy plays an important role in this population, reducing complications associated with HIV and providing consequent improvement in quality of life and morbimortality of PLWHA [3,4]. This chapter addresses some suggestions in this context.

Despite the advent of ART, thousands of people worldwide do not have access to this treatment, mainly in sub-Saharan Africa and resource-limited settings [5]. In many endemic countries, the population looks for health care only when opportunistic infections attributable to HIV have deteriorated the clinical and nutritional status of these patients [6]. In such cases, the start of ART is not a priority. The primary concern is to stabilize the clinical and nutritional status of the patient, and then to resort

Health of HIV Infected People, Volume 2.
DOI: http://dx.doi.org/10.1016/B978-0-12-800767-9.00007-8

to controlling HIV infection with HAART thereafter [6,7]. In this context, this chapter discusses some evidence of nutritional treatment for patients who are not using HAART.

7.2 MALNUTRITION AND DIARRHEA

The countries with the highest rates of HIV infection also have a high prevalence of malnutrition because they are often regions with lack of access to adequate food (in quality and quantity) to meet all macronutrients and micronutrients requirements [8,9]. Malnutrition and the consequent micronutrient deficiency feeds a vicious cycle of immunodeficiency, susceptibility to opportunistic infections, and progression of HIV infection [10]. Malnutrition is the result of macronutrient (protein and energy) and micronutrient deficiency, resulting in weight loss and loss of muscular tissue. Three factors contribute to malnutrition in HIV/AIDS: inadequate food intake, disabsortive disorders, and increased energy expenditure [11].

Among opportunistic infections, most affect the gastrointestinal tract and can affect 50–90% of PLWHA. Diarrhea in its acute or chronic form is associated with increased morbidity and mortality, weight loss, and malnutrition [12,13]. In sub-Saharan Africa, there is a worrisome scenario of malnutrition. A study of 11 countries in that region estimated 10.3% of adult HIV-infected women with malnutrition were associated with lower levels of education, agricultural work, rural residence, and highest poverty rates [14].

In PLWHA, gut permeability is altered by the disease itself. Hence, the intestinal mucosa should be the focus of attention and care to avoid bouts of infection [15]. In this perspective, along with nutritional therapy, home water treatment has been successful in the prevention and reduction of diarrhea in countries where there is food insecurity and precarious sanitation [16], and this is a recommendation of the World Health Organization (WHO) [17]. A meta-analysis confirmed the effectiveness of this recommendation [18]. A recent study showed efficacy in reducing diarrhea by the treatment of household water with clay filters manufactured with the addition of silver solution [19].

However, diarrhea is not an exclusive problem of countries with some degree of food insecurity and poor sanitation. It also affects HIV-infected patients in developed countries when it is inter-related with HIV/AIDS immune dysfunction. Aiming new nutritional approaches for diarrhea treatment to HIV-infected patients, a product based on colostrum was designed that is rich in immunoglobulins and antibacterial peptides and that has high nutritional value. This product comprised 32% bovine colostrum powder, 30% rice flakes, 12% banana flakes, 20% maltodextrin, and 4% sugar. A clinical trial was developed in northern Uganda to assess its effect in adults. Patients were supplemented for 28 days with 50 g of this product twice per day in addition to receiving regular care for diarrhea, which included fluid replacement with electrolyte fluid, use of antidiarrheal medication and antibiotics in appropriate doses, and nutritional counseling. The control group received routine care for diarrhea. After 9 weeks, there was a reduction in the frequency of diarrhea and muscle fatigue, increase in body weight (7.3 kg per patient), and increased CD4+ count [20]. This product is currently commercially available and seems to be a good option for the treatment of diarrhea and weight gain in HIV patients.

Given the impact of arising comorbidities related to HIV infection in public health and their interdependence with mortality, the WHO states that 50% of care toward PLWHA must be nutritional care [21]. For nutritional assessment and counseling, it is worth mentioning that resting energy expenditure is increased in PLWHA [22]. Energy requirements are increased by 10% in asymptomatic adults and by 20–30% in symptomatic adults [22]. In the nutrition therapy process, it is important to consider the body mass index (BMI) and unintentional weight loss, which are classified in relation to the usual weight (7.5% in 6 months or 10% in 1 year). The assessment of weight loss is essential for determining the nutritional risk to guarantee that the treatment can meet the nutritional needs of the patient and contribute to a better quality of life [23].

A meta-analysis evaluated seven studies on food with macronutrient and micronutrient supplementation and nutritional counseling for PLWHA. An increase in weight and lean mass was observed, but these results in relation to CD4+ count, viral load, and mortality were not statistically significant. However, the researchers pointed out methodological heterogeneity and poor quality of the studies [24].

Some dietary supplements are already well-established for the treatment of malnutrition through food adequacy. Ready-to-use therapeutic food (RUTF) is the most indicated and used for adults. RUTF can be used as a supplement or as a single food source and has high caloric density. In 100 g, this product has 520 kcal, 10–12% protein (of which at least half is from milk and vegetable protein isolates), 45–60% fat (canola or soybean oil), and 24 vitamins and minerals [9].

A study involving HIV-infected breastfeeding women with a BMI less than 24.5 kg/m^2 concluded that they had less muscle loss than the control group after supplementation with a daily dose of 50 g of fortified soymilk with peanuts, totaling 280 kcal and 8 g protein, for 9 months of lactation [25].

Protein deficiency is closely related to low-calorie intake. Regarding adequate supply of protein for recovery of nutritional status, it is still unclear whether the recovery is better with higher protein intake or protein of high biological value. Protein deficiency is strongly associated with morbimortality, but the supplementation of proteins requires caution.

Oversupply, especially in patients with inflammatory processes, can lead to fat accumulation and refeeding syndrome in cases of severely malnourished patients [11].

The refeeding syndrome is defined by changes in fluids and electrolytes that cause metabolic and hormonal changes, which can result in a higher proportion of deaths. The excess of protein and calorie supply is among its causes, usually from artificial formulas offered to severely malnourished individuals. To prevent refeeding syndrome, it is necessary to identify the patient at risk who may have some characteristics such as more than 10 days without eating, change in food absorption process, increased energy expenditure, and severe malnutrition. These patients should start with 20–50% of the total caloric intake required, which should be calculated in relation to the current body weight. Until the feeding process stabilizes, cardiac and metabolic functions and electrolytes should be monitored continuously [26].

A clinical trial involving adults in Botswana evaluated supplementation of fortified sorghum meal by 12 months. Sorghum was fortified with a mix of vitamins and minerals containing 250 g dry product (vitamin A, 250 RE; vitamin B1, 0.35 mg; vitamin B2, 0.50 mg; vitamin B3, 4.50 mg; vitamin B6, 0.50 mg; folate, 0.06 mg; and iron, 2.80 mg). The intervention did not affect CD4 count and viral load. The authors concluded that the intervention could be more efficient in malnourished individuals with impaired immune status once the patients in the study were eutrophic and had a stable CD4 count [27]. Supplementation with fortified foods needs further investigations to observe its effects in relation to the nutritional status of patients at baseline and HIV disease progression.

7.3 MINERALS

It is known that HIV promotes several deficiencies usually associated with malnutrition, infectious processes, and evolution stage of HIV infection. To verify the presence of some mineral deficiencies, a cross-sectional study conducted in Nigeria in adults showed that HIV-positive individuals have significantly more deficiencies of selenium, zinc, and magnesium than uninfected individuals [28]. Therefore, guided supplementation and appropriate dosages may be much more than just knowing the proper dosage. Beyond anything, it would promote nutritional status recovery and, consequently, the conditions of morbidity and mortality.

Why recover nutritional deficiencies if there are absorption disorders, malnutrition, and infectious processes? Several studies evaluating these and other outcomes were proposed in this context. Some micronutrients such as selenium and zinc were most widely investigated because of their immunomodulatory capacity. Others such as iron and folate are less investigated, but agreement regarding disability in patients reinforces their relevance as recommended for adults not infected with HIV [29]. In 2003, the WHO established some criteria regarding mineral deficiencies and proper supplementation. Some proposals regarding the supplementation of minerals and their possible relationships with best health status in PLWHA are described here.

7.3.1 Iron

Anemia is a public health problem that affects developing and developed countries at all stages of the life cycle, most predominantly in children and pregnant women. Iron deficiency is responsible for almost 50% of cases, but other risk factors for anemia include iron malabsorption, parasitic infections, acute and chronic infections such as HIV, and deficiencies of vitamins A and B12, folic acid, and riboflavin [29].

The WHO recommends supplementation of iron and folic acid during prenatal care for pregnant women living with HIV/AIDS to prevent anemia [30]. In pregnant women, the nutritional requirements of iron and folic acid are increased [31]. For pregnant women with HIV, the recommended amount of folic acid is 0.4 or 4 mg/day for those who have had children with malformations of the neural tube [32]. The recommendation of iron does not exceed the recommended daily allowance (RDA) for pregnant women. In regions where the prevalence of anemia in pregnant women is less than 40%, the recommendation is 60 mg iron plus 0.4 μg folic acid daily for 6 months. In regions where the prevalence is higher than 40%, the recommendation is the same except that 3 additional months of supplementation postpartum are required [31].

7.3.2 Zinc

Zinc deficiency is present in 30–51% of HIV-infected individuals [33]. Zinc is an essential mineral that plays a role in the immune system and protein synthesis [34]. Because of their fundamental role in the human body, the need for zinc supplementation in HIV-infected individuals is well-established, mainly because of its role in the immune system. However, there is still no consensus regarding the dose or when the supplementation should occur (at which stage of disease and during which nutritional status) because it can cause adverse effects in HIV-infected individuals [33]. As observed by Siegfried et al. [10], supplementation with 25 mg zinc in the prenatal period inhibited iron absorption in malnourished pregnant women living with HIV, which is an unfavorable outcome of zinc supplementation.

Zinc deficiency can have negative effects as observed (for 6 months) in cohort of adults living in Miami. During the follow-up, those who presented with and continued to have zinc deficiency exhibited more rapid progression of HIV infection stage and lower survival regardless of whether they initiated antiretroviral therapy during follow-up. Thus, zinc deficiency was a predictor of early disease progression and mortality [35]. Positive effects of long-term supplementation of 12 mg elemental zinc in women and 15 mg in men were observed for the control and prevention of diarrhea and delayed immunological failure [36].

In this context, the safe supplementation would be based on the RDA. However, it is important to assess the level of vitamin and mineral depletion of each patient. In malnourished individuals, or in areas of known food insecurity, supplementation should be beyond the levels of the RDA to correct the deficiencies, given that lower doses may not have the desired effect. In a study in which 55% of the sample had severe zinc deficiency at baseline, supplementation of 50 mg of zinc twice daily for 14 days in adults did not reduce diarrhea when compared with the control group [37].

Regarding HIV-infected pregnant women without antiretroviral treatment, a double-blind clinical trial evaluated zinc supplementation 25 mg/day up to 6 months after delivery, which is greater than the RDA dose of 11 mg/day. Besides zinc, all patients received prenatal supplements of 400 mg iron sulfate, 20 mg thiamine, 20 mg riboflavin, 25 mg B6, 100 mg niacin, 50 g vitamin B12, 0.8 mg folic acid, 500 mg vitamin C, and 30 mg vitamin E. Zinc supplementation did not reduce preterm births, mortality in neonates, or mortality in pregnant women, and it had no effect on birth weight, CD4 count, or viral load. The authors concluded that zinc supplementation in antenatal care in an attempt to achieve better outcomes in pregnant women with HIV is not pertinent [38].

Micronutrient supplementation is still inconclusive with respect to significant improvement in diarrhea and intestinal barriers [39], but it is possible to affirm that zinc has an important role [40].

7.3.3 Selenium

Selenium is correlated with complex enzymatic and metabolic functions, an important antioxidant and essential nutrient, therefore demanding that food intake allows for adequate serum levels [41].

Selenium seems to have a significant role in the prevention of viral replication, but the mechanisms are not well-elucidated [42]. A recent study evaluating supplementation with 200 μg of selenium for 24 months in the early phase of HIV did not find effects at the end of follow-up related to viral replication or CD4 count, and the stage of disease progression did not change over time [43].

A double-blind clinical trial conducted in HIV-infected hospitalized adults evaluated 200 mg/day selenium supplementation for 12 months. At the end of follow-up, there was a reduction in hospitalization and hospital cost of 58% in the supplemented group [44].

Research conducted in Tanzania evaluated supplementation with 200 μg selenium in HIV-infected pregnant women during and after pregnancy for 6 months. There was a reduction in maternal diarrhea, especially in its acute form, and an improvement in child survival. However, the results are limited because of the low prevalence of selenium deficiency in the study population [45].

The RDA recommendations for individuals not infected with HIV is 55 μg/day for those aged older than 18 years, 60 μg/day for pregnant women, and 70 μg/day for infants [46]. In the studies described, supplementation was more than twice that of the selenium RDA (200 μg). According to findings, supplementation with selenium reduces hospitalization and improves the immune system, but the same dosage in outpatients was not able to reduce the stage of evolution of HIV infection and did not affect the immune system. In pregnant women, the effect was only significant in relation to the improvement of diarrhea. Because of the diversity of populations studied, it can be inferred that selenium may improve levels of CD4 and viral load in immunosuppressed HIV-positive patients. However, the outcome in those with clinical stability and without selenium deficiency with supplementation, even at high doses, did not affect the progression of the disease and the immune system.

7.3.4 Calcium

Calcium plays an important role in bone resorption, nerve impulse transmission, and muscle contraction [47]. Calcium has been investigated in past decades in the context of cardiovascular disease and hypertension because of its role in lipid metabolism. The current hypothesis is that low calcium intake and low serum calcium act by inhibiting lipolysis and reducing lipid oxidation [48]. HIV/AIDS patients also have metabolic disorders, but its etiology remains unclear [47].

In this context, a study of 100 adult patients with HIV/AIDS was developed in Rio de Janeiro to assess food consumption and calcium intake. This research found that the lowest calcium intake doubles the chances of metabolic syndrome and hypertension. Also, consuming two or more servings of dairy food was significantly associated with lower BMI and smaller waist circumference, and calcium intake more than 700 mg/day was associated with increased consumption of fruits and fruit juice, fiber, and saturated fat [49].

Thus, calcium appears to have a significant role in preventing metabolic disorders in PLWHA, although more studies are required to strengthen this hypothesis. It is noteworthy that higher calcium intake was associated with a pattern of a healthier diet. Perhaps the benefits are linked to the dietary profile as a whole rather than calcium alone. The recommendation for calcium intake in PLWHA is 1–1.2 g/day, which is not different from the recommendation for the general population [47].

7.4 VITAMINS

7.4.1 Vitamin D

Vitamin D is essential for maintaining the mineral balance in the body, especially in the regulation of calcium, phosphorus, and magnesium. Some evidence indicates the action of vitamin D in other cells such as hematopoietic cells, lymphocytes, epidermal cells, pancreatic islets, muscles, and neurons. It also works as a mediator in inflammatory and autoimmune processes, blood pressure control, cardiovascular diseases, diabetes, and cancer [50,51].

Vitamin D deficiency is prevalent in HIV and is related to skin color, seasonality, sun exposure, polymorphisms in the vitamin D receptor, inadequate food intake, and use of antiretroviral medication [51,52]. The European AIDS Clinical Society classifies vitamin D deficiency levels as less than 10 ng/mL or less than 25 nmol/L, insufficiency levels as less than 20 ng/mL or less than 50 nmol/L, and adequate levels as ≥30 ng/mL [47].

Research on vitamin D supplementation in people with HIV/AIDS is relatively recent, but some results are encouraging. Adequate levels of vitamin D were associated with reduced complications related to HIV and disease progression, with consequent delay starting ART, mortality reduction, maintenance of body weight, and reduced incidence of infections in the gastrointestinal tract and bone disease [47,53,54].

Supplementation with 4,000 or 7,000 IU was effective in improving immune response in ART-naïve young adult response, although it was necessary to supplement for 52 weeks [55]. Another study, also involving young adults, used a supplemental dose of 100,000 IU every 3 months during a follow-up period of 12 months, which successfully increased serum 25 (OH)D, but it was not significant for immune response improvement [56].

There is much to research in this area, particularly regarding the appropriate dose, dosing interval, and associated interfering factors (such as weight, CD4 count, and serum 25 (OH)D at the start of supplementation), among others. So far, daily intake of 800–2,000 IU vitamin D is recommended to maintain serum 25 (OH)D ≥30 ng/mL [47]. However, a recent clinical trial assures that the ingestion of high daily doses of vitamin D, that is, 7,000 IU, are safe and effective in maintaining 25 (OH)D serum levels ≥30 ng/mL [57].

7.4.2 Vitamin A

Vitamin A acts as an inflammatory marker and its deficiency is associated with more rapid progression of HIV and worsening infectious condition [58,59]. Currently, vitamin A supplementation is considered safe. Reaffirming its role as an inflammatory marker, a clinical trial was conducted in Kenya with women supplemented with 10,000 IU/day of vitamin A for 6 months. The acute phase of the disease was observed among those who remained vitamin A deficient at the end of follow-up, that is, levels of C-reactive protein (CRP) $\geq$10 mg/dL [60].

Some evidence indicated positive results with vitamin A supplementation during pregnancy [61,62]. Nevertheless, research in Africa involving pregnant women showed that postpartum vitamin A (400,000 IU) supplementation had no effect on the vertical transmission of HIV, suggesting that vitamin A supplementation only during the postpartum period can be ineffective for improving the immune system to reduce vertical transmission during breastfeeding [63].

In areas of food insecurity, the prevalence of vitamin A deficiency in pregnant women is high. The pregnancy itself and HIV infection can aggravate the deficiency. For proper development of the fetus and maternal health maintenance, vitamin A is essential because its deficiency is associated with increased risk of vertical transmission [64]. In areas of endemic vitamin A deficiency, mainly Africa and Southeast Asia, where it is considered a public health problem, the WHO recommends a single dose of vitamin A (200,000 IU) to be administered to HIV-infected pregnant women after delivery as soon as possible to prevent vertical transmission of HIV in breastfeeding [64]. If not possible, then the vitamin A dose should be administered no later than 6 weeks after delivery. In nonendemic areas, the recommendation is the RDA during pregnancy and lactation [30].

Defining appropriate doses to achieve outstanding results with respect to nonvertical transmission is still controversial. Despite positive effects on the immune system, vitamin A supplementation is not part of the public health recommendation for preventing vertical transmission. The recommendation for adequacy of vitamin A consists of only a healthy and balanced diet [65]. However, how is it possible to eat a healthy diet to the extent of ensuring adequate levels of vitamin A when the higher prevalence of hypovitaminosis occurs in an area of food insecurity? Therefore, there may be no other choice for health professionals but to supplement.

It is important to highlight that vitamin A supplementation is affordable [65]. Given the findings regarding the relevance of vitamin A on the immune system and the inflammatory process, why not supplement all HIV-infected pregnant women with vitamin A during primary antenatal care, or at least HIV-infected pregnant women living in areas of food insecurity?

7.5 MULTIVITAMINS

According to WHO, the best way to ensure proper support of micronutrients is through a balanced diet [30]. In the areas of food insecurity, this action is quite limited. Besides the food shortage in these regions, ensuring adequate food supply requires government strategic planning to better access to health networks and nutritionists, that is, it involves costs often unavailable in nutritional risk areas [31,66].

Deficiencies of vitamins A, B6, B12, C, D, E, β-carotene, selenium, copper, zinc, magnesium, and iron have been evidenced among HIV individuals, particularly in areas of food insecurity, once micronutrient requirements are increased in this population [67]. HIV-infected individuals in areas of food insecurity often have malnutrition, which leads to worsening of immunological status and higher prevalence of infectious diseases. Thus, because of the stress caused by infectious processes and the presence of disabsortive disorders such as acute or chronic diarrhea, micronutrient absorption is impaired [59].

In this context, particular attention should be given to pregnant women. The problem of micronutrient deficiency may be even greater in this population, considering the higher nutritional requirements for maternal health and adequate fetal growth and development [10].

Since the beginning of the HIV, there have been reports that micronutrient deficiency is directly related to immune system worsening even before the development of disease [68], contributing to the advancement of the stage of HIV infection and increased mortality [69]. From these findings, various research emerged to expand knowledge about the effects of multivitamin supplementation in nutrition therapy for HIV [58,70].

In 1998, Fawzi et al. [71] conducted a double-blind clinical trial with pregnant women in Tanzania to assess an intervention with multiple doses of vitamins 22-times higher than the recommended RDA for adults. One of the intervention arms comprised multivitamin supplementation containing 20 mg thiamine, 20 mg riboflavin, 25 mg vitamin B6, 100 mg niacin, 50 μg vitamin B12, 0.8 mg folate, 500 mg vitamin C, and 30 mg vitamin E. By the end of follow-up, a decrease in preterm birth and low birth weight was observed. Also, multivitamin supplementation improved the immune system, delayed disease progression, and delayed initiation of antiretroviral therapy.

Another study in pregnant women in Tanzania evaluated multivitamin supplementation (vitamin B complex, vitamin C, and vitamin E) ten-times the RDA recommendation. Unlike the aforementioned study, there was no reduction in premature births, low birth weight, and fetal death. The immunological status was not investigated [45].

The recommendations of vitamins and minerals for pregnant women and infants with HIV are equivalent to the RDA for adults without HIV [30]. The American Society for Parenteral and Enteral Nutrition (ASPEN) recommends that pregnant women and infants should be supplemented, although more clinical trials to verify the dose–response and its associated factors in an attempt to maintain nutritional security and best health status for this specific group are needed [72].

To try to understand the effect of a multiple micronutrient supplementation in HIV patients without ART, a placebo-controlled trial was performed in Thailand. There was a significant reduction in mortality in the micronutrient group supplemented with a multivitamin tablet twice daily for 48 weeks [69]. Another clinical trial conducted in Zambia assessed multivitamin supplementation for 9 months, showing a reduction in episodes of diarrhea and mortality in HIV-infected patients. However, the results of both studies are controversial because the deaths were not related to micronutrient deficiencies, but rather to digestive hemorrhage and heart failure [73].

A clinical trial conducted in Botswana, sub-Saharan Africa, assessed supplementation of selenium and multivitamins for 24 months in ART-naïve HIV-infected adults with CD4 counts more than 350/μL and BMI higher than 18 kg/m². There were three intervention groups: supplementation with 20 μg/day selenium plus multivitamins (20 mg thiamine, 20 mg riboflavin, 100 mg niacin, 25 mg vitamin B6, 50 μg vitamin B12, 800 μg folic acid, 500 mg vitamin C, and 30 mg vitamin E); only multivitamin supplement; and selenium alone. In the selenium plus multivitamins group, progression of HIV disease decreased at the end of follow-up and onset of ART was delayed for up to 2 years. The other groups of intervention did not show significant change in any of the outcomes related to HIV progression (CD4 count or viral replication) [43].

Micronutrient supplementation is an affordable alternative, especially when considering many morbidities resulting from deficiencies [31] and the high cost of treatment, which will postpone progression of HIV disease, antiretroviral treatment, antibiotic therapy, hospitalization, and, perhaps the greatest of all costs, the loss of human life [30].

The knowledge of micronutrient supplementation at this time seems to indicate its positive and safe effects, yet much remains necessary to evaluate. Issues regarding which micronutrients need to be supplemented and in what dosage require more evidence for their elucidation. Research methodologies involve different profiles of supplementation, as well as different contexts with respect to nutritional status, coexistence of pregnancy, micronutrient profile, and stage of HIV infection, making it difficult to make a conclusive statement.

7.6 PROBIOTICS

The integrity of the intestinal mucosa is an important factor that deserves attention in the health care of HIV-infected patients because of their susceptibility to recurrent diarrhea regardless of nutritional status [15]. In this context, the use of probiotics has been investigated in several studies. Probiotics are live microorganisms that confer a health benefit of the host when administered in adequate amounts and can be used in food products such as yogurts and industrialized supplements. *Lactobacillus* and *Bifidobacterium* are the most widely used probiotic strains [74].

Nevertheless, the effects are strain-specific and dependent on the amount of probiotic bacteria used. Next, two studies without significant results regarding diarrhea and other outcomes and a study with positive results are presented.

A clinical trial conducted in Tanzania with 65 women evaluated oral intake of capsules containing *Lactobacillus rhamnosus* GR-1 and *Lactobacillus reuteri* RC-14 at 2×10^9 CFU/day twice daily, for 25 weeks. There was no difference between control and intervention groups regarding the duration of diarrhea and stool consistency, the probability of stomach pain, bloating, nausea, and other gastrointestinal symptoms, IFNγ, IL-10, IgG, and IgE [75]. Another clinical trial, also in Tanzania used a supplement of 125 mL of yogurt containing *L. rhamnosus* GR-1 at 1.23×10^9 CFU/mL plus 1,500 IU vitamin A, vitamin E 5.7 IU, niacin 3.8 mg, vitamin B1 0.3 mg, 0.6 µg vitamin B12, vitamin B6 0.3 mg, 21 mg vitamin C, iron 3.3 mg, 13 µg selenium, 2.4 mg zinc, omega 3 (DHA) 13 mg, and omega 3 (EPA) 19 mg. No differences were observed between the intervention and control groups, which received only micronutrients, in relation to BMI, anemia, and CD4 count [76].

However, in another clinical trial involving women, rapid resolution in gastrointestinal symptoms (nausea, flatulence, and diarrhea) compared with baseline and significant improvement in CD4 count compared with the control group after 30 days of follow-up were observed. The control group received 100 mL of yogurt fermented with *Lactobacillus bulgaricus* and *Streptococcus thermophilus delbrueckii*. The intervention group received the same fermented yogurt supplemented with *L. rhamnosus* GR-1 and *L. reuteri* RC-14 [77].

There is evidence of positive outcomes regarding the use of probiotics in acute and hospitalized patients in relation to reducing the use of antibiotics, such as improvement of diarrhea and improvement of the immune system. These positive effects are related to some properties of strains, such as production of substances that prevent infection and growth of pathogenic bacteria in the gut that contribute to the maintenance of the intestinal barrier, preventing bacterial translocation [78,79]. Great efforts have been put forth by scientists regarding probiotics and the possibility of outcomes and comorbidities arising from HIV disease progression prevention, such as deterioration of the immune system, acute and chronic diarrhea, and disabsortive syndrome, among others.

These results underlie interesting proposals for those with HIV/AIDS, even with some inconclusive results presented in the aforementioned research. There is a great perspective regarding the wide use of probiotics for infectious bouts.

7.7 CONCLUSION

Nutritional therapy is essential for patients with HIV because it promotes improvement in nutritional status and in the response of the immune system, prevents and treats malnutrition, and improves diarrhea.

Overall, the results indicate that supplementation can reduce the frequency and incidence of other opportunistic infections and recover the intestinal barrier to prevent new cases of diarrhea that majorly contribute to disabsorptive processes. Considering the relevance of proper absorption of micronutrients for the correction of comorbidities resulting from HIV infection, it is crucial to think about the treatment of diarrhea as a focus of primary care and not only as a prophylactic treatment, as indicated by these studies.

Therefore, supplementation appears to promote a better health state, better quality of life, and increased survival of patients. Because it can delay the start of ART, it directly implies a smaller burden to the public health system. However, multivitamin supplementation should be further investigated in relation to its dose–response and real benefits for PLWHA because many studies use different combinations and dosages.

Regarding a higher intake of macronutrients, it would be of great value to estimate energy requirements using specific formulas for patients with HIV through advanced proposals such as indirect calorimetry so that details regarding when to start supplementation, adequate volumes, and proper caloric density can be determined [80].

Specific studies on ART-naïve PLWHA need to be further explored with more robust statistical approaches that differentiate outcomes for individuals with and without antiretroviral therapy; studies including both types of individuals may bring distinct biases in the results. In this chapter, the benefits of nutritional treatment with a focus on macronutrients and micronutrients were discussed according to the evidence available in the literature. Thus, the aim was to contribute to the work of various professionals and researchers engaged in this area whose objective is to improve treatment for PLWHA, considering that the nutritional approach has great relevance in the context of ART-naïve patients. It is believed that future research in the area of possible nutritional treatments for significant advances in health and quality of life will occur, as will lower costs for public health associated with HIV/AIDS.

References

[1] UNAIDS. Report on the global AIDS epidemic. Joint United Nations Programme on HIV/AIDS; Geneva: 2013. pp. 1–198.

[2] Raiten DJ, Mulligan K, Papathakis P, Wanke C. Executive summary—nutritional care of HIV-infected adolescents and adults, including pregnant and lactating women:

What do we know, what can we do, and where do we go from here? Am J Clin Nutr 2011;94(Suppl.):1667S–76S.
[3] Fields-Gardner C, Campa A. American dietetics association. Position of the American dietetic association: nutrition intervention and human immunodeficiency virus infection. J Am Diet Assoc 2010;110:1105–19.
[4] Grobler L, Siegfried N, Visser ME, Mahlungulu SSN, Volmink J. Nutritional interventions for reducing morbidity and mortality in people with HIV. Cochrane Database Syst Rev 2013;2 CD004536.
[5] WHO Global update on HIV treatment 2013: results, impact and opportunities: WHO report in partnership with UNICEF and UNAIDS. Geneva, Switzerland: World Health Organization; 2013. pp. 1–126.
[6] WHO Guidelines for the clinical management of HIV infection in adults and adolescents. National AIDS-STD control programme. Department of Health, Ministry of Health Myanmar: World Health Organization; Geneva, 2007. pp. 1–92.
[7] Isanaka S, Mugusi F, Hawkins C, et al. Effect of high-dose vs standard-dose multivitamin supplementation at the initiation of HAART on HIV disease progression and mortality in Tanzania: a randomized controlled trial. JAMA 2012;308:1535–44.
[8] de Pee S, Semba RD. Role of nutrition in HIV infection: review of evidence for more effective programming in resource-limited settings. Food Nutr Bull 2010;31:S313–44.
[9] Manary MJ. Local production and provision of ready-to-use therapeutic food (RUTF) spread for the treatment of severe childhood malnutrition. Food Nutr Bull 2006;27(Suppl.):S83–9.
[10] Siegfried N, Irlam JH, Visser ME, Rollins NN. Micronutrient supplementation in pregnant women with HIV infection. Cochrane Database Syst Rev 2012;3 [CD009755].
[11] Hsu JWC, Pencharz PB, Macallan D, Tomkins A. Macronutrients and HIV/AIDS: a review of current evidence a review of current evidence. Durban: World Health Organization; 2005. pp. 1–36.
[12] Fekadu S, Taye K, Teshome W, Asnake S. Prevalence of parasitic infections in HIV-positive patients in Southern Ethiopia: a cross-sectional study. J Infect Dev Ctries 2013;7:868–72.
[13] WHO Consolidated guidelines on HIV prevention, diagnosis, treatment and care for key populations. Geneva, Switzerland: World Health Organization; 2014. pp. 1–184.
[14] Uthman OA. Prevalence and pattern of HIV-related malnutrition among women in sub-Saharan Africa: a meta-analysis of demographic health surveys. BMC Public Health 2008;8:226.
[15] Brenchley JM, Douek DC. HIV infection and the gastrointestinal immune system. Mucosal Immunol 2008;1:23–30.
[16] Lule JR, Mermin J, Ekwaru JP, et al. Effect of home-based water chlorination and safe storage on diarrhea among persons with human immunodeficiency virus in Uganda. Am J Trop Med Hyg 2005;73:926–33.
[17] Hutton G, Haller L. Evaluation of the costs and benefits of water and sanitation improvements at the global level. Geneva: World Health Organization; 2004. pp. 1–87.
[18] Clasen T, Schmidt WP, Rabie T, Roberts I, Cairncross S. Interventions to improve water quality for preventing diarrhoea: systematic review and meta-analysis. BMJ 2007;334:782.
[19] Abebe LS, Smith JA, Narkiewicz S, et al. Ceramic water filters impregnated with silver nanoparticles as a point-of-use water-treatment intervention for HIV-positive individuals in Limpopo Province, South Africa: a pilot study of technological performance and human health benefits. J Water Health 2014;12:288–300.
[20] Kaducu FO, Okia SA, Upenytho G, Florén CH. Effect of bovine colostrum-based food supplement in the treatment of HIV-associated diarrhea in Northern Uganda: a randomized controlled trial. Indian J Gastroenterol 2011;30:270–6.

[21] UNAIDS Technical guidance note for global fund HIV proposals: food and nutrition. Geneva, Switzerland: World Health Organization; 2011. pp. 1–9.
[22] Mittelsteadt AL, Hileman CO, Harris SR, Payne KM, Gripshover BM, McComsey GA. Effects of HIV and antiretroviral therapy on resting energy expenditure in adult HIV-infected women—a matched, prospective, cross-sectional study. J Acad Nutr Diet 2013;113:1037–43.
[23] Integrated Treatment Centre. Special preventive programmes. Department of Health, Hong Kong. Manual HIV 2001. Int Treat Cen 2002; 1–342.
[24] Mahlungulu SSN, Grobler L, Visser MME, Volmink J. Nutritional interventions for reducing morbidity and mortality in people with HIV. Cochrane Database Syst Rev 2007;3 [CD004536].
[25] Kindra G, Coutsoudis A, Esposito F. Effect of nutritional supplementation of breast-feeding HIV positive mothers on maternal and child health: findings from a randomized controlled clinical trial. BMC Public Health 2011;11:946.
[26] Mehanna HM, Moledina J, Travis J. Refeeding syndrome: what it is, and how to prevent and treat it. BMJ 2008;336:1495–8.
[27] Motswagole BS, Mongwaketse TC, Mokotedi M, Kobue-Lekalake RI, Bulawayo BT, Thomas TS, et al. The efficacy of micronutrient-fortified sorghum meal in improving the immune status of HIV-positive adults. Ann Nutr Metab 2013;62:323–30.
[28] Okwara EC, Meludu SC, Okwara JE, et al. Selenium, zinc and magnesium status of HIV positive adults presenting at a university teaching hospital in Orlu-eastern Nigeria. Niger J Med 2012;21:165–8.
[29] WHO Worldwide prevalence of anaemia 1993–2005: WHO global database on anaemia. Geneva, Switzerland: World Health Organization; 2008. pp. 1–40.
[30] WHO Nutrient requirement for people leaving with HIV/AIDS: report of a technical consultation. Geneva, Switzerland: World Health Organization; 2003. pp. 1–27.
[31] WHO/BASICS/UNICEF Nutrition essentials: a guide for health managers. Geneva, Switzerland: World Health Organization; 1999. pp. 1–264.
[32] CDC. Panel on opportunistic infections in HIV-infected adults and adolescents. Guidelines for prevention and treatment of opportunistic infections in HIV-infected adults and adolescents. Center for Disease Control and Prevention; 2009. pp. 1–416.
[33] Zeng L, Zang L. Efficacy and safety of zinc supplementation for adults, children and pregnant women with HIV infection: systematic review. Trop Med Int Health 2011;16:474–82.
[34] Coovadia HM, Bobat R. Zinc deficiency and supplementation in HIV/AIDS. Nutr Res 2002;22:179–91.
[35] Baum MK, Campa A, Lai S, Lai H, Page JB. Zinc status in human immunodeficiency virus type 1 infection and illicit drug use. Clin Infect Dis 2003;37(Suppl.):S117–23.
[36] Baum MK, Lai S, Sales S, Page JB, Campa A. Randomized controlled clinical trial of zinc supplementation to prevent immunological failure in HIV-positive adults. Clin Infect Dis 2010;50:1653–60.
[37] Cárcamo C, Hooton T, Weiss NS, Gilman R, Wener MH, Chavez V, et al. Randomized controlled trial of zinc supplementation for persistent diarrhea in adults with HIV-1 infection. J Acquir Immune Defic Syndr 2006;43:197–201.
[38] Fawzi WW, Msamanga GI, Spiegelman D, et al. A randomized trial of multivitamin supplements and HIV disease progression and mortality. N Engl J Med 2004;351:23–32.
[39] Kelly P, Shawa T, Mwanamakondo S, Soko R, Smith G, Barclay GR, et al. Gastric intestinal barrier impairment in tropical enteropathy and HIV: limited impact of micronutrient supplementation during a randomised controlled trial. BMC Gastroenterol 2010;10:72.
[40] Kelly P, Feakins R, Domizio P, et al. Paneth cell granule depletion in the human small intestine under infective and nutritional stress. Clin Exp Immunol 2004;135:303–9.

[41] Rayman MP. The importance of selenium to human health. Lancet 2000;356:233–41.
[42] Hurwitz BE, Klaus JR, Llabre MM, et al. Suppression of human immunodeficiency virus type 1 viral load with selenium supplementation: a randomized controlled trial. Arch Intern Med 2007;167:148–54.
[43] Baum MK, Campa A, Lai S, et al. Effect of micronutrient supplementation on disease progression in asymptomatic, antiretroviral-naive, HIV-infected adults in Botswana: a randomized clinical trial. JAMA 2013;310:2154–63.
[44] Burbano X, Miguez-Burbano MJ, McCollister K, et al. Impact of a selenium chemoprevention clinical trial on hospital admissions of HIV-infected participants. HIV Clin Trials 2002;3:483–91.
[45] Kawai K, Kupka R, Mugusi F, et al. A randomized trial to determine the optimal dosage of multivitamin supplements to reduce adverse pregnancy outcomes among HIV-infected women in Tanzania. Am J Clin Nutr 2010;91:391–7.
[46] IOM Food and nutrition board. Dietary reference intakes for vitamins C, vitamin E, selenium and carotenoids. Washington, DC: The National Academies Press; Zurich: 2000. pp. 1–506.
[47] EACS. Guidelines version 7.01, November 2013. Zurich: European AIDS Clinical Society; 2013. pp. 1–81.
[48] Astrup A. The role of calcium in energy balance and obesity: the research for mechanisms. Am J Clin Nutr 2008;88:873–4.
[49] Leite LHM, Sampaio ABMM. Dietary calcium, dairy food intake and metabolic abnormalities in HIV-infected individuals. J Hum Nutr Diet 2010;23:535–43.
[50] Hayes CE, Nashold FE, Spach KM, Pedersen LB. The immunological functions of the vitamin D endocrine system. Cell Mol Biol 2003;49:277–300.
[51] Holick MF. Vitamin D deficiency. N Engl J Med 2007;357:266–81.
[52] Hewison M. An update on vitamin D and human immunity. Clin Endocrinol (Oxf) 2012;76:315–25.
[53] Mehta S, Mugusi FM, Spiegelman D, et al. Vitamin D status and its association with morbidity including wasting and opportunistic illnesses in HIV-infected women in Tanzania. AIDS Patient Care STDS 2011;25:579–85.
[54] Eckard AR, McComsey GA. Vitamin D deficiency and altered bone mineral metabolism in HIV-infected individuals. Curr HIV/AIDS Rep 2014;11:263–70.
[55] Chun RF, Liu NQ, Lee T, Schall JI, et al. Vitamin D supplementation and antibacterial immune responses in adolescents and young adults with HIV/AIDS. J Steroid Biochem Mol Biol 2014;S0960-0760(14):00144–00147. [Epub ahead of print].
[56] Giacomet V, Vigano A, Manfredini V, Cerini C, Bedogni G, Mora S, et al. Cholecalciferol supplementation in HIV-infected youth with vitamin D insufficiency: effects on vitamin D status and T-cell phenotype: a randomized controlled trial. HIV Clin Trials 2013;14:51–60.
[57] Dougherty KA, Schall JI, Zemel BS, et al. Safety and efficacy of high dose daily vitamin D3 supplementation in children and young adults infected with HIV. J Pediatr Infect Dis Soc 2014. [Epub ahead of print].
[58] Irlam JH, Visser MME, Rollins NN, Siegfried N. Micronutrient supplementation in children and adults with HIV infection. Cochrane Database Syst Rev 2010;12 CD003650.
[59] Villamor E, Fawzi WW. Effects of vitamin A supplementation on immune responses and correlation with clinical outcomes. Clin Microbiol Rev 2005;18:446–64.
[60] Baeten JM, McClelland RS, Richardson BA, Bankson DD, Lavreys L, Wener MH, et al. Vitamin A deficiency and the acute phase response among HIV-1-infected and -uninfected women in Kenya. J Acquir Immune Defic Syndr 2002;31:243–9.
[61] Semba RD. The role of vitamin A and related carotenoids in immune function. Nutr Rev 1998;56:S38–48.
[62] Fawzi WW. Nutritional factors and vertical transmission of HIV-1. Epidemiology and potential mechanisms. Ann N Y Acad Sci 2000;918:99–114.

[63] Humphrey JH, Iliff PJ, Marinda ET, et al. Effects of a single large dose of vitamin A, given during the postpartum period to HIV-positive women and their infants, on child HIV infection, HIV-free survival, and mortality. J Infect Dis 2006;193:860–71.
[64] WHO Safe vitamin A dosage during pregnancy and lactation. Recommendations and report of a consultation. Geneva: World Health Organization; 1998. pp. 1–34.
[65] WHO Guideline: vitamin A supplementation in pregnancy for reducing the risk of mother-to-child transmission of HIV. Geneva, Switzerland: World Health Organization; 2011. pp. 1–20.
[66] Koethe JR, Marseille E, Giganti MJ, Chi BH, Heimburger D, Stringer JS. Estimating the cost-effectiveness of nutrition supplementation for malnourished, HIV-infected adults starting antiretroviral therapy in a resource-constrained setting. Cost Eff Resour Alloc 2014;12:10.
[67] Academy of Science of South Africa. HIV/AIDS, TB and nutrition: scientific inquiry into the nutritional influences on human immunity with special reference to HIV infection and active TB in South Africa. Academy of Science of South Africa; 2007. pp. 1–283.
[68] Baum MK, Shor-Posner G, Lu Y, et al. Micronutrients and HIV-1 disease progression. AIDS 1995;9:1051–6.
[69] Jiamton S, Pepin J, Suttent R, et al. A randomized trial of the impact of multiple micronutrient supplementation on mortality among HIV-infected individuals living in Bangkok. AIDS 2003;17:2461–9.
[70] Irlam JH, Siegfried N, Visser ME, Rollins NC. Micronutrient supplementation for children with HIV infection. Cochrane Database Syst Rev 2013;10 [CD010666].
[71] Fawzi WW, Msamanga GI, Spiegelman D, et al. Randomised trial of effects of vitamin supplements on pregnancy outcomes and T cell counts in HIV-1-infected women in Tanzania. Lancet 1998;351:1477–82.
[72] Sabery N, Duggan C. The American Society for Parenteral and Enteral Nutrition (ASPEN) clinical guidelines: nutrition support of children human immunodeficiency virus infection. J Parenter Enteral Nut 2009;33:588–606.
[73] Kelly P, Katubulushi M, Todd J, et al. Micronutrient supplementation has limited effects on intestinal infectious disease and mortality in a Zambian population of mixed HIV status: a cluster randomized trial. Am J Clin Nutr 2008;88:1010–7.
[74] Guarner F, Khan AG, Eliankim J. World Gastroenterology Organisation Global Guidelines: probiotics and prebiotics, October 2011. J Clin Gastroenterol 2012;46:468–81.
[75] Hummelen R, Changala J, Butamaya NL, et al. Effect of 25 weeks probiotic supplementation on immune function of HIV patients. Gut Microbes 2011;2:80–5.
[76] Hummelen R, Hemsworth J, Changalucha J, et al. Effect of micronutrient and probiotic fortified yogurt on immune-function of anti-retroviral therapy naïve HIV patients. Nutrients 2011;3:897–909.
[77] Anukam KC, Osazuwa EO, Osadolor HB, Bruce AW, Reid G. Yogurt containing probiotic *Lactobacillus rhamnosus* GR-1 and *L. reuteri* RC-14 helps resolve moderate diarrhea and increases CD4 count in HIV/AIDS patients. J Clin Gastroenterol 2008;42:239–43.
[78] Schultz MJ, Haas LE. Antibiotics or probiotics as preventive measures against ventilator-associated pneumonia: a literature review. Crit Care 2011;15:R18.
[79] Salari P, Nikfar S, Abdollahi M. A meta-analysis and systematic review on the effect of probiotics in acute diarrhea. Inflamm Allergy Drug Targets 2012;11:3–14.
[80] Ziegler TR, McComsey GA, Frediani JK, Millson EC, Tangpricha V, Eckard AR. Habitual nutrient intake in HIV-infected youth and associations with HIV-related factors. AIDS Res Hum Retroviruses 2014;30:888–95.

CHAPTER

8

The Role of Nutrition Training for Health Workers in Addressing Poor Feeding Practices and Undernutrition Among HIV-Positive Children

Bruno F. Sunguya[1], David P. Urassa[2], Junko Yasuoka[1] and Masamine Jimba[1]

[1]Department of Community and Global Health, Graduate School of Medicine, The University of Tokyo, Hongo, Bunkyo-ku, Tokyo, Japan, [2]School of Public Health and Social Sciences, Muhimbili University of Health and Allied Sciences, Dar es Salaam, Tanzania

8.1 INTRODUCTION

The human immunodeficiency virus (HIV) epidemic has had a variable course over the past three decades. After years of rapid escalation of new cases of infections, the epidemic is now stable and even showing signs of decline in some parts of the world [1]. The rate of new infections is decreasing in some age groups; however, transmission rates are still escalating in children and adolescents [2]. Approximately 700 newborns and young children are infected every day; as a result, 3.3 million children are currently infected with HIV. These children are vulnerable to a number of adverse health outcomes, including undernutrition, short life expectancy, and ill health caused by unprecedented opportunistic infections.

HIV contributes to 3% of child mortality, and undernutrition is an underlying cause of more than one-third of total child deaths [3]. The mortality rate is high among children because of this dual burden of

Health of HIV Infected People, Volume 2.
DOI: http://dx.doi.org/10.1016/B978-0-12-800767-9.00008-X

immune-debilitating conditions [4]. In addition, opportunistic infections increase the demand for energy and further drive HIV-positive children into undernutrition. A lack of adequate nutrition and energy may also jeopardize the efficacy of antiretroviral therapy (ART) [5]. Moreover, adherence to ART is low among children who are undernourished [5], making it difficult to achieve viral suppression [5,6].

Undernutrition may have short- and long-term effects on HIV-positive children. The short-term effects include impaired immunity, increased risk of opportunistic infections, morbidity, and mortality. The long-term effects include poor cognitive functioning, poor achievement of developmental milestones, and poor levels of education [7–10]. As a result, even when HIV-positive children survive with ART, if they are undernourished they may not be able to function like their HIV-negative counterparts who received adequate nutrition during childhood [2]. They may suffer from chronic diseases as they grow up, or they may die young [11]. Early nutritional deficits are also linked to noncommunicable diseases in adulthood such as diabetes, dyslipidemia, hypertensive heart disease, stroke, and hypercholesterolemia [12].

To address child undernutrition among HIV-positive children, it is imperative to focus on interventions that can target its causes. This calls for proper nutrition and feeding counseling by trained health workers who routinely care for such children. Through training, health workers can acquire the skills to integrate nutrition care into the existing care and treatment system.

The aim of this chapter is to describe nutrition training for health workers and to discuss how they can address undernutrition among HIV-positive children. First, we identify the nutritional needs of HIV-positive children with or without ART at various stages of the disease. Second, we explain the need to apply tailor-made nutrition interventions within the local context. Third, we explain the role of health worker nutrition training in addressing feeding practices and undernutrition. In addition, we use the example of one intervention in Tanga, Tanzania, and extrapolate from this to training interventions for health workers who care for HIV-positive children. Fourth, we identify the challenges that health workers should expect and highlight successful, sustainable models of nutrition training.

8.2 HIV-POSITIVE CHILDREN: NUTRITIONAL NEEDS AND THE NEED FOR TAILORED INTERVENTIONS

8.2.1 Nutritional Needs of HIV-Positive Children

HIV-positive children have special nutritional needs at various disease stages [13]. The World Health Organization (WHO) recommends increasing nutrition intake depending on children's clinical disease stage, opportunistic infection, and nutritional status. HIV-positive children with no symptoms may have the same energy expenditure as other healthy children of the same age; however, their food consumption should be altered when the need arises because of the risk posed by the disease [13]. For example, newly infected HIV-positive children who are 6 months of age or older and have mild symptoms require 10% more energy than that needed to sustain an HIV-negative or otherwise healthy child of the same weight [13]. Additional energy and nutrients may be obtained through normal diets that are otherwise provided to the household if these are of adequate diversity, quality, and frequency.

HIV-positive children who have acute respiratory tract infections tend to lose energy [13]. Malignant conditions also require high energy. Moreover, energy is continually lost when a child has chronic diarrhea. To cope with infections and to replenish nutritional loss, HIV-positive children need an additional 20–30% of energy [13].

Children with advanced HIV experience severe undernutrition. To help with their recovery, such children need at least 50–100% more energy [13]. They can obtain such high levels of energy from ready-to-use therapeutic food until they have recovered their weight loss [13,14]. If not yet initiated, then ART should also be administered to them to prevent opportunistic infections [13].

Chronic infections at any stage of the disease cause loss of appetite, vomiting, and lethargy. Oral thrush and esophageal candidiasis also cause painful swallowing, leading to poor feeding and possibly undernutrition [13]. Appropriate medical interventions are important to treat such conditions. It is also important to provide children with small and appropriate meals that are easy to swallow.

8.2.2 Need for Tailor-Made Nutrition Interventions for HIV-Positive Children

When caregivers are well-informed about child nutrition, they can improve their feeding practices and ultimately the nutritional status of HIV-positive children. Nutrition knowledge can help to counter misconceptions, myths, and restrictive traditional beliefs about nutritious food and good feeding behaviors. Even in food-insecure regions, such knowledge can help caregivers to use the limited food available and preserve the rest for dry seasons. In food-rich regions, well-informed caregivers can use available food resources to bring about desired feeding practices. Improved nutrition knowledge can also help to improve food preparation hygiene, preventing diseases such as diarrhea [13] (Box 8.1).

Health workers need to provide nutrition counseling to improve the nutrition knowledge of the caregivers [13]. However, health workers often do not have the knowledge and skills to provide such important care in

BOX 8.1

POOR FEEDING PRACTICES DUE TO POOR NUTRITION KNOWLEDGE OF CAREGIVERS

Caregivers' nutrition knowledge affects the way they feed their children. Even where food is available, adequate knowledge is necessary to achieve the appropriate amount, type, and frequency of feeding. Lack of such knowledge may cause caregivers to follow community norms in feeding practices, which may be related to misconceptions.

In Tanga, Tanzania, a high proportion of caregivers of HIV-positive children did not know how to feed their children with the right amount, frequency, and types of foods. This was one of the most important determinants of undernutrition. One of them reported the following:

> *Even under normal circumstances, she knows that the normal feeding frequency is 2. Now, today she is HIV-positive, and she is supposed to get 5 meals a day...she does not know this and budget-wise, she finds that the 5 meals are too much...so she cooks 'bada porridge'...this is cassava-made porridge in the morning and the child will eat again in the afternoon (evening), and that is it... (A 43-year-old HIV-positive home-based care worker and a mother of 3 children, one of whom is HIV-positive)*

Nutrition counseling may help to resolve misunderstandings of caregivers if performed by trained health workers using common examples. If caregivers understand the need to properly feed their children, then they may find ways to improve existing practices using the available resources, even under financial hardship.

most settings [15] or to prevent HIV-positive children from suffering from acute or chronic undernutrition [16]. Recurrent undernutrition is common if local determinants are not considered and if it is managed using only traditional methods [17].

Lack of practical nutrition training in professional schools is a major cause of health workers' poor knowledge of undernutrition prevention [18]. Most medical and nursing schools worldwide lack adequate clinical nutrition training [19]. As a result, health workers graduate without gaining sufficient knowledge and skills to treat undernutrition. Although guidelines to manage undernutrition exist [20,21], they focus on its treatment as a disease and do not emphasize prevention of undernutrition or address its underlying causes. Patients therefore suffer repeated episodes of undernutrition on returning to the environment in which it developed. The guidelines have also failed to address child undernutrition in the context of HIV [20,21].

It is essential to provide in-service nutrition training that is tailored to local needs to improve the knowledge, skills, and competence of health workers [15]. Such needs include the awareness of local determinants of undernutrition. Nutrition training can help health workers to address local restrictive beliefs and myths against proper feeding practices, and to be aware of their own misconceptions. In addition, training can boost skills in providing care, including nutrition counseling [15].

Knowledgeable health workers can provide tailored nutrition counseling to caregivers of HIV-positive children. Caregivers can easily follow such advice if it focuses on solving the problem and uses existing resources (e.g., improving feeding practices using foods similar to those available to caregivers) [22]. They are more likely to change old behaviors if provided with options that are affordable and simple to prepare. In addition, if counseling is repeated frequently and made part of existing routine care, it can make more enduring effects. Nutrition training of health workers and subsequent counseling with monitoring are effective interventions to improve caregivers' knowledge of feeding practices [23].

8.3 NUTRITION TRAINING FOR HEALTH WORKERS PROVIDING CARE TO HIV-POSITIVE CHILDREN

8.3.1 Shortage of Health Workers: Turning a Crisis into an Opportunity

Countries with a high burden of HIV [1] also lack sufficient numbers of health workers [24]. Because a limited number of health workers must care for a large number of patients, tasks are obliged to shift to less qualified health workers or mid-level providers [25]. Such a shift can ameliorate both the health workforce crisis and child undernutrition. To achieve this, nutrition training must be designed to match workers' levels of understanding.

Nutrition training for health workers has been effective in improving knowledge and practices among physicians, nurses, and specialized health workers, such as nutritionists and dieticians [23,26–29]. It has also been effective in improving the knowledge and feeding practices of lay health workers who treat children [30–32]. However, mid-level providers have not yet been targeted for this type of training, and so there is little evidence of its effectiveness.

Evidence is also lacking regarding both efficacy and effectiveness of nutrition training for feeding practices and management of undernutrition in HIV-positive children. Although WHO has released guidelines for vulnerable groups [13], field testing has not been documented. The guidelines need to be adapted to suit the local epidemiology, food availability, practices, and health worker cadres. They also need to be integrated into the country's nutrition policy for routine implementation.

8.3.2 Local Adaptation of Nutrition Training

Local and national adaptation is important for nutrition training [13], because the causes of undernutrition are multifaceted and vary from region to region among HIV-positive children. For example, undernutrition may result from food insecurity and hunger in drought regions, but from different causes in food-rich areas. Geographical variation may also account for epidemiological differences in opportunistic infections that play a role in undernutrition among HIV-positive children. For example, diarrhea may be more common in wet areas with poor hygienic conditions than in drier areas.

Knowledge of seasonal variations can help to predict the epidemiology of diseases that are responsible for child undernutrition. In regions where a great deal of fruit grows (such as Tanga, Tanzania), the incidence of diarrhea generally increases when the fruits (e.g., mango) are ripe. During wet seasons, flies multiply and become vectors for diarrheal diseases. During the harvesting season, food is more available at affordable prices, so acute forms of undernutrition are proportionally low.

8.3.3 Local Determinants of Undernutrition to Be Examined Prior to Nutrition Training

Household food security is an important determinant of undernutrition [5]. WHO defines it as access to sufficient, safe, and nutritious food to maintain a healthy and active life for all people at all times [33]. It comprises three important pillars [34]. These are food availability, food access, and food use. Household food insecurity is measured using the validated Household Food Insecurity Access Scale [34], although several other scales exist.

It is also important to measure local feeding practices [13], such as feeding frequency (Box 8.2). This is measured as the number of times a child was fed the previous day. WHO recommends a feeding frequency of at least 5 times per day [13]. Another feeding practice of interest is dietary diversity score, measured as the number of food types consumed the previous day. WHO recommends providing HIV-positive children with a variety of foods to improve absorption, provide adequate nutrients, and increase appetite [13]. The quality of the diet is measured by assessing types of nutrition in the previous day's diet and the quantity of food in grams, which allows calculation of the recommended daily allowance (Box 8.3).

BOX 8.2

POOR FEEDING PRACTICES AMONG HIV-POSITIVE CHILDREN IN TANGA, TANZANIA

In Tanga, Tanzania, HIV-positive children had poor feeding practices. More than 88% of such children were fed at a lower than recommended frequency, and this was associated with undernutrition [16]. In the focus group discussion, caregivers mentioned the likely causes of low feeding frequency. For dietary diversity, most caregivers did not know what foods to provide, and in what combination, to yield adequate nutritional diversity. This was related to poor knowledge, food insecurity, and poverty. For some caregivers, the health status of HIV-positive children improved when they were provided with a variety of foods that were within their reach [16].

BOX 8.3

IDENTIFYING LOCAL CAUSES OF POOR FEEDING PRACTICES IS IMPORTANT IN DESIGNING EFFECTIVE NUTRITION TRAINING

Each region has a different set of determinants of undernutrition for HIV-positive children. The commonest risk factors are food insecurity and poverty. In Tanga, Tanzania, food is available in abundance, but poor feeding practices are unprecedented and result from risk factors other than those commonly recognized. Households of HIV-positive children succumb to selective food insecurity, caregivers who are unemployed, people who are too weak to engage in farm work, orphanhood, and single parents who may not adequately provide children with necessary nutritional foods,

In Tanga, our children do not have jobs, so no income, not enough money for buying food. He can only afford to buy a small amount of cheap food, which is not enough to feed all 7 grandchildren. (A 70-year-old grandmother of 6 orphans)

I am a single mother, my baby's father died, I remarried again and the second husband divorced me, so I am alone. All expenses are on me. I do not have much help from anyone else. My income is 1.25 USD per day. This is for family food and medicines. It is not enough. So whatever I can, I will do, the food that I can afford is what we can eat. Just enough to pass the day, and I know she is not satisfied with food. Her nutrition status is poor. (A 40-year-old widow with 4 children, one of whom is HIV positive)

continued

BOX 8.3 (*cont'd*)

Knowing local determinants may further streamline counseling and tailor it to suit each individual. A blanket approach to all caregivers may not bring about changes in feeding practices even in a homogenous community. This is because of the diversity of determinants of poor feeding practices and other local factors. It is therefore important to investigate such factors and frequently monitor changes due to time, season, and disease stages.

Child undernutrition is also associated with a number of sociodemographic characteristics [13], such as the number and age of children, orphan status, and caregivers' education level, income, and occupation.

Restrictive feeding behaviors may also affect child undernutrition. These behaviors include taboos regarding feeding children and pregnant women specific nutritious foods such as eggs, liver, and vegetables, among others. It is important to determine the reasons for not eating a particular type of available food [16]. In addition, myths about poor feeding practices should be examined to improve the counseling of caregivers. It is possible to explore such factors in focus group discussions (Box 8.4).

8.4 CONDUCTING NUTRITION TRAINING

8.4.1 Necessary Preparations for Nutrition Training

Successful nutrition training of health workers (especially mid-level providers) requires adequate preparations. These include identifying the targeted health workers, deciding the training venue, preparing patients for practical sessions, assembling training materials, and evaluating nutrition knowledge before training.

8.4.1.1 Identifying the Targeted Health Workers

Nutrition training should target health workers who treat HIV-positive children. They should be trained for integrated nutrition care in the existing HIV care and treatment system [13]. Integrated care can provide better links between services and save time, particularly if there are limited health workers to complete tasks. In most developing countries, health workers are clinicians, registered nurses, adherence nurse counselors,

BOX 8.4

LOCAL RESTRICTIVE BEHAVIORS AND TRADITIONAL BELIEFS SHOULD BE STUDIED AND INCLUDED IN NUTRITION TRAINING

Some of the caregivers in Tanga perceived that eating vegetables downgrades one's social status. In their communities, households that consume meat are considered of high income, whereas those consuming vegetables are perceived as poor. This is because meat is more expensive compared with vegetables, which are diverse and widely available. Therefore, even poor households do not consume vegetables when they can afford meat.

I eat other foods but not green vegetables. Good food includes meat (red or white meat), beef, or chicken. Vegetables are not considered good food here. In our normal diet, we do not eat vegetables even when they are available. (A 25-year-old mother of 2 HIV-positive children)

People do not want to cultivate vegetables; it is not their tradition. Young women are not made to make such gardens...it is not a matter of lack of energy. Even HIV-positive people do not have such tradition. A woman is a person who does not work, only men do that in Tanga. (A 35-year-old businesswoman and a mother of one HIV-positive child)

Such restrictive behaviors are inherited from one generation to another, creating generations of poor feeding practices and micronutrient deficiency. The lack of necessary nutrients for HIV-positive children further damages their ability to fight opportunistic infections, driving them to more advanced stages of the disease and increased risk of morbidity, undernutrition, and mortality. Knowledge of such local restrictive behaviors can help to streamline feeding counseling if health workers also have adequate nutrition counseling skills.

nutritionists, and laboratory technicians. In human resource–constrained areas, mid-level providers commonly serve in these facilities.

8.4.1.2 *Deciding on the Training Venue*

Training may be more effective if it uses existing health facilities. If the training venue is close to the facilities, then the trainees can easily move to and from various practical sessions. Because nutrition training usually takes more than 1 working day, health workers from distant facilities will need to travel to participate. Therefore, choosing training venues close to health facilities saves both time and money.

8.4.1.3 Gaining Cooperation from Patients for Practical Sessions

The inclusion of patients typical of the local context in practical sessions can help health workers learn practical knowledge and skills. However, it is important to include patients with varied characteristics, too. For example, if wasting patients are selected in a region where wasting rate is high, then the training will be more meaningful. Additionally, the inclusion of positive deviant HIV-positive children can promote understanding of survival despite common difficult conditions. For example, if a child is not experiencing wasting, despite experiencing the same difficult conditions as other children, he or she might be considered a positive deviant.

8.4.1.4 Assembling Training Materials

The WHO guidelines for nutrition training follow the Integrated Approach to Nutritional Care of HIV-Infected Children (6 months–14 years). According to these guidelines [13], prospective trainees need pre-training materials about basic nutrition knowledge before undergoing training. It is useful for participants to prepare common cases and discuss how they manage them. In this way, trainers can establish the needs of health workers before nutrition training. Learning materials will also help participants refresh their understanding of the link between undernutrition and HIV infection. Health workers will therefore acquire some basic knowledge before the nutrition training. Because there are differences in basic knowledge among health workers, it is important to prepare training materials and methods based on their level of understanding.

8.4.1.5 Assessment of Nutrition Knowledge Before Training

Prior to nutrition training, health workers' baseline knowledge level should be assessed. After the training, a similar knowledge test will help determine how much participants have learned. Knowledge decay can be also evaluated at a later stage. The training materials based on WHO guidelines contain questions that can assess knowledge levels [13]; these include different aspects of nutrition knowledge, such as food preparation hygiene, counseling knowledge and skills, feeding practices, and opportunistic infections.

8.4.2 An Example of Nutrition Training in Tanga, Tanzania

Nutrition training was conducted among health workers caring for HIV-positive children at care and treatment centers in Tanga, Tanzania [35]. It targeted mid-level providers, or a majority of health workers in Tanzania, who serve populations in rural and semi-urban areas [25] (Figure 8.1).

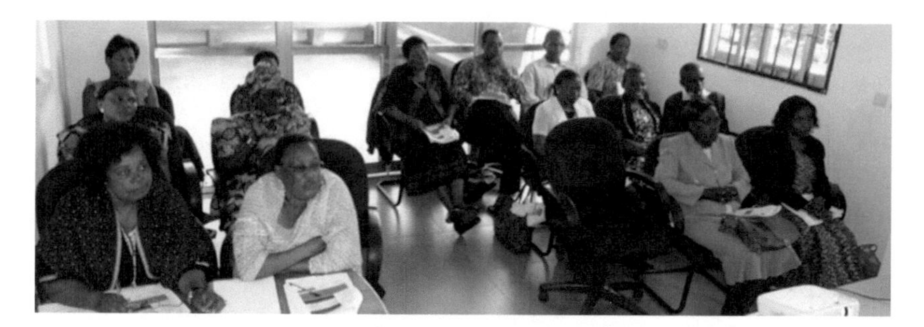

FIGURE 8.1 Participants of the nutrition training in Tanga, Tanzania.

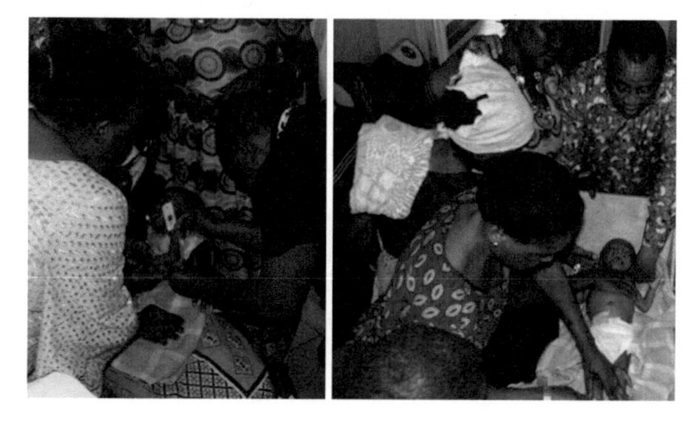

FIGURE 8.2 Participants of the nutrition training in a practical anthropometric session.

The Tanga nutrition training followed the steps recommended by WHO (Figure 8.2). These included formative research to examine the magnitude of undernutrition and poor feeding practices [16]. This research examined and addressed specific determinants of undernutrition (Figure 8.2). It used a mixed methods design consisting of cross-sectional quantitative and qualitative studies. The triangulated results identified the specific factors and feeding practices associated with undernutrition among HIV-positive children.

In total, 16 midlevel providers participated in the nutrition training [35]. The 2-day training occurred at an HIV care and treatment facility and included 18 theoretical and practical sessions. The training emphasized pertinent characteristics previously identified in the formative research. It also emphasized local food availability, norms, and myths of feeding in Tanga and in potential areas of improvement. Before the training, the trainees' baseline nutrition knowledge and skills were assessed using a standard questionnaire.

8.4.2.1 Contents of Nutrition Training

The integrated nutrition training consisted of 10 steps (Table 8.1) that aimed to teach the health workers how to assess, classify, and choose a nutrition care plan. They also aimed to teach health workers about how to implement the nutrition care plan, to manage special cases, and to consider other factors in the care of HIV-positive children [13]. A knowledge

TABLE 8.1 Ten steps of nutrition training in Tanga, Tanzania

ASSESSMENT AND PLANNING	
Step 1	• How to assess and classify child growth • How to take anthropometric measurements and assess nutritional status • How to plot growth curve and monitor growth • Clinical practice on wards in how to assess growth and nutritional status
Step 2	• How to assess child's nutritional needs • How to determine additional nutritional needs • Practical session on how to assess nutritional needs of HIV-positive children
Step 3	• How to classify nutritional needs in terms of a nutrition care plan based on individual characteristics, taught in step 2 • Each nutrition care plan explained, examples given of local foods to cater for each plan • How to move from one care plan to another
IMPLEMENTING CARE PLAN	
Step 4	• How to explore what the child eats and drinks • How to evaluate feeding practices: feeding frequency and dietary diversity • How to examine the child's ability to eat, and monitor associated problems
Step 5	• Who feeds the child and how the child receives food
Step 6	• How to examine the household's food security and socioeconomic status
Step 7	• Discuss local determinants of undernutrition and how to avoid them • Role-play and group discussion on local determinants of undernutrition • Discuss infection control, food preparation hygiene, and opportunistic infections
Step 8	• Make a decision to refer • Discuss conditions that warrant referral • How to prepare patients before referral, based on the local protocol
DEALING WITH SPECIAL NEEDS	
Step 9	• Discuss HIV-positive children with special needs • How to feed the child recovering from illness, who is vomiting, who has severe undernutrition, and who has mouth sores
Step 10	• Discuss HIV-positive children on ART • What to do if the child is not gaining weight on ART, if the child has nausea or vomiting while on ART, and side effects of ART

assessment was conducted before the training was completed, and a question-and-answer session was held to clarify any misconceptions, myths, and beliefs that restrict feeding practices.

8.5 CHALLENGES OF IMPLEMENTING NUTRITION TRAINING

8.5.1 Fragmented Efforts in HIV Programs

In Tanzania, vertical HIV programs are implemented by development partners other than the government. In Tanga, two nongovernmental organizations provide care and treatment in public health facilities. Each organization operates using its own protocol and hires its own health workers in care and treatment centers. The government also provides care for hospitalized patients or those who seek treatment for other conditions. Within this context, it is difficult to plan and implement nutrition training for all health workers who care for HIV-positive children. None of the organizations accept responsibility for developing the existing human resources. In addition, the government lacks funds to train all of its health workers, including those working for other implementing partners. This kind of fragmentation is common in many developing countries.

8.5.2 Health Worker Shortage

A limited number of health workers work in Tanzania, and they provide care and treatment for a large number of HIV-positive patients in routine clinics. For example, on a typical clinic day in Tanga, up to 80 children may visit a care and treatment facility in which only four or fewer mid-level providers work. If health workers have to spend more time on individualized nutrition care and detailed counseling, then they may not be able to complete other tasks. Therefore, even if they acquire a high level of nutrition knowledge from training, they will only be able to provide a general approach to nutrition care. Many sub-Saharan African countries suffer from a shortage of health workers and share these common problems.

8.5.3 Knowledge Decay—Retraining Needs and Costs

Trained health workers experience knowledge decay; therefore, training should not be a one-time investment. Health workers may gradually forget their knowledge unless nutrition training is provided frequently as continuing education. For this case, the training was privately funded for research purposes and may not be sustainable or able to be scaled up. Nutrition training should be institutionalized, and the overall running costs of HIV programs should be used to make it sustainable.

8.6 USE OF SUCCESSFUL MODELS TO IMPLEMENT NUTRITION TRAINING AND PROGRAMS

The effectiveness of nutrition training and subsequent counseling for health workers may be increased by following other successful models and programs. Such successful models include the ART-adherence model, active case finding by directly observed treatment programs (DOTS) in tuberculosis, and the positive deviance approach model.

8.6.1 ART-Adherence Model

Despite numerous challenges, the ART-adherence model in Tanzania has been successful even among children. The adherence counseling is integrated into routine care. In this model, health workers in care and treatment facilities receive frequent ART-adherence counseling training. This helps to sharpen their skills, knowledge, and methods of monitoring adherence. Patients are given simple tools to remember how to use ART on time, including a fixed timetable based on their most routine activities and peer reminder methods. Such local innovations during training are useful and practical. By repeating the training, health workers realize how important adherence counseling is for routine care.

Patients bring their remaining pills or a medicine diary and show their health workers how they use their ART. From this, health workers can know the level of adherence over the previous month and identify reasons for missing doses when pills remain. The health workers and patients are then responsible for moving toward adherence. Health facilities maintain high levels of ART adherence by continuing routine follow-up through pill counting whenever a patient visits there.

Nutrition care may adapt such an innovative and tailor-made ART-adherence model by frequently training health workers. In addition, nutrition care can be integrated into routine HIV care and treatment and can be made a mandatory intervention. In this model, health workers may provide feeding diaries to caregivers of HIV-positive children. It helps health workers and caregivers to plan together using individual feeding patterns, and it helps assist in monitoring progress. Peer reminders may be used in nutrition interventions through nutrition groups as in adherence interventions. In such groups, caregivers can encourage each other and remind themselves of the best feeding practices. A care and treatment center can also ask community health workers and home-based care to extend care and follow-up at home.

8.6.2 Active Case Finding and Supervision by DOTS

The DOTS program is one of the most successful interventions to combat tuberculosis. The DOTS strategy includes five elements: political commitment to ensure adoption of policy and strategies and, to ensure financial sustainability, early and active case detection; standard and effective treatment and patient supervision; effective drugs and supplies; and monitoring and evaluation.

Nutrition interventions that adopt this model may yield better results. For example, the nutritional status of all children, including HIV-positive children, could be improved by strengthening nutrition governance through the adoption of updated nutrition guidelines [36], which recommend integrating nutrition care for HIV-positive children into national policies. Active identification of the early stages of undernutrition will help health workers identify such cases through constant monitoring to determine trends in growth. If health workers receive adequate training to sharpen their skills, then nutrition counseling for feeding practices will improve [22]. Monitoring and evaluation of health workers' nutrition knowledge and skills will help maintain the quality of health care and ensure that HIV-positive patients receive routine and standard care [23].

8.6.3 Positive Deviance Approach

Positive deviants are people who show extraordinarily positive results despite the normal trend in a population [37]. For example, in communities where undernutrition is common, children who have better nutritional status are considered positive deviants. Their caregivers might have taken a different approach toward feeding that may be considered abnormal in such a population. The use of such cases as examples of how nutritional status may improve, regardless of normal trends, can be helpful in changing patterns of undernutrition and poor feeding [38]. This approach has proved useful in Vietnam [37] and other regions with a high prevalence of child undernutrition [38].

A positive deviant approach may also be useful among HIV-positive children in areas where food is available but where caregivers have restrictive feeding practices, similar to those for HIV-negative children [38]. Collecting examples of how others feed their children well can help change the beliefs underlying poor feeding practices, and evidence of children with improved nutritional status can lead to sustainable results. In addition, the identification of centers that conducted successful counseling may help to stimulate other facilities into integrating such interventions, thereby helping to improve nutritional status through feeding practices.

8.7 CONCLUSION

The growing number of HIV-positive children will continue to exacerbate child undernutrition rates unless it is addressed. Both AIDS and undernutrition are preventable if locally available resources are appropriately used. In some countries like Tanzania, food is available but not effectively used.

Nutrition training can benefit health workers of various cadres. Training of qualified health workers and community workers can benefit the general population. If the necessary resources are available, then they have the potential to improve feeding practices and undernutrition among HIV-positive children.

For nutrition training of health workers to be more effective, it is critical to identify specific and local risk factors for undernutrition and poor feeding practices. It is then important to institutionalize the training program to make it sustainable at a country level. In this way, HIV-positive children can live and enjoy their adulthood like other members of society without depending too much on donor agencies.

References

[1] UNAIDS Global report: UNAIDS report on the global AIDS epidemic 2013. Geneva: Joint United Nations Programme on HIV/AIDS (UNAIDS); 2013.
[2] UNICEF Towards an AIDS-free generation—children and AIDS: sixth stocktaking report. New York, NY: United Nations Children's Fund; 2013.
[3] Black RE, Allen LH, Bhutta ZA, Caulfield LE, de Onis M, Ezzati M, et al. Maternal and child undernutrition: global and regional exposures and health consequences. Lancet 2008;371(9608):243–60.
[4] Villamor E, Misegades L, Fataki MR, Mbise RL, Fawzi WW. Child mortality in relation to HIV infection, nutritional status, and socio-economic background. Int J Epidemiol 2005;34(1):61–8.
[5] Weiser SD, Young SL, Cohen CR, Kushel MB, Tsai AC, Tien PC, et al. Conceptual framework for understanding the bidirectional links between food insecurity and HIV/AIDS. Am J Clin Nutr 2011;94(6):1729S–39S.
[6] Weiser SD, Frongillo EA, Ragland K, Hogg RS, Riley ED, Bangsberg DR. Food insecurity is associated with incomplete HIV RNA suppression among homeless and marginally housed HIV-infected individuals in San Francisco. J Gen Intern Med 2009;24(1):14–20.
[7] McDonald CM, Manji KP, Kupka R, Bellinger DC, Spiegelman D, Kisenge R, et al. Stunting and wasting are associated with poorer psychomotor and mental development in HIV-exposed Tanzanian infants. J Nutr 2013;143(2):204–14.
[8] Lowick S, Sawry S, Meyers T. Neurodevelopmental delay among HIV-infected preschool children receiving antiretroviral therapy and healthy preschool children in Soweto, South Africa. Psychol Health Med 2012;17(5):599–610.
[9] Sherr L, Mueller J, Varrall R. A systematic review of cognitive development and child human immunodeficiency virus infection. Psychol Health Med 2009;14(4):387–404.
[10] Kandawasvika GQ, Kuona P, Chandiwana P, Masanganise M, Gumbo FZ, Mapingure MP, et al. The burden and predictors of cognitive impairment among 6- to 8-year-old children infected and uninfected with HIV from Harare, Zimbabwe: a cross-sectional study. Child Neuropsychol 2015;21(1):106–20.
[11] Unicef Improving child nutrition: the achievable imparatives for global progress. New York, NY: United Nations Children's Fund; 2013.
[12] Barker DJ. Fetal origins of coronary heart disease. BMJ 1995;311(6998):171–4.

[13] WHO Guidelines for an integrated approach to the nutritional care of HIV-infected children (6 months to 14 years). Geneva, Switzerland: World Health Organization; 2009.
[14] Sunguya BF, Poudel KC, Mlunde LB, Otsuka K, Yasuoka J, Urassa DP, et al. Ready to use therapeutic foods (RUTF) improves undernutrition among ART-treated, HIV-positive children in Dar es Salaam, Tanzania. Nutr J 2012;11:60.
[15] Sunguya BF, Poudel KC, Mlunde LB, Urassa DP, Yasuoka J, Jimba M. Nutrition training improves health workers' nutrition knowledge and competence to manage child undernutrition: a systematic review. Front Public Health 2013;1:37.
[16] Sunguya BF, Poudel KC, Mlunde LB, Urassa DP, Yasuoka J, Jimba M. Poor nutrition status and associated feeding practices among HIV-positive children in a food secure region in Tanzania: a call for tailored nutrition training. PLoS One 2014;9(5):e98308.
[17] Sunguya BF, Poudel KC, Otsuka K, Yasuoka J, Mlunde LB, Urassa DP, et al. Undernutrition among HIV-positive children in Dar es Salaam, Tanzania: antiretroviral therapy alone is not enough. BMC Public Health 2011;11:869.
[18] Mowe M, Bosaeus I, Rasmussen H, Kondrup J, Unosson M, Rothenberg E, et al. Insufficient nutritional knowledge among health care workers? Clin Nutr 2008;27(2):196–202.
[19] Adams K, Lindell K, Kohlmeier M, Zeisel S. Status of nutrition education in medical schools. Am J Clin Nutr 2006;83(4):941S–4S.
[20] Ashworth A, Jackson A, Khanum S, Schofield C. Ten steps to recovery. Child Health Dialogue 1996(3–4):10–12.
[21] Collins S, Dent N, Binns P, Bahwere P, Sadler K, Hallam A. Management of severe acute malnutrition in children. Lancet 2006;368(9551):1992–2000.
[22] Sunguya BF, Poudel KC, Mlunde LB, Shakya P, Urassa DP, Jimba M, et al. Effectiveness of nutrition training of health workers toward improving caregivers' feeding practices for children aged six months to two years: a systematic review. Nutr J 2013;12:66.
[23] Pelto GH, Santos I, Gonçalves H, Victora C, Martines J, Habicht JP. Nutrition counseling training changes physician behavior and improves caregiver knowledge acquisition. J Nutr 2004;134(2):357–62.
[24] World Health Organization The world health report 2006: working together for health. Geneva, Switzerland: WHO; 2006.
[25] Alliance GHW. Mid-level health providers a promising resource to achieve the health millennium development goals global health workforce alliance, report. Geneva, Switzerland: 2010.
[26] Bhandari N, Mazumder S, Bahl R, Martines J, Black RE, Bhan MK, et al. An educational intervention to promote appropriate complementary feeding practices and physical growth in infants and young children in rural Haryana, India. J Nutr 2004;134(9):2342–8.
[27] Santos I, Victora CG, Martines J, Gonçalves H, Gigante DP, Valle NJ, et al. Nutrition counseling increases weight gain among Brazilian children. J Nutr 2001;131(11):2866–73.
[28] Bhandari N, Bahl R, Nayyar B, Khokhar P, Rohde JE, Bhan MK. Food supplementation with encouragement to feed it to infants from 4 to 12 months of age has a small impact on weight gain. J Nutr 2001;131(7):1946–51.
[29] Roy SK, Fuchs GJ, Mahmud Z, Ara G, Islam S, Shafique S, et al. Intensive nutrition education with or without supplementary feeding improves the nutritional status of moderately-malnourished children in Bangladesh. J Health Popul Nutr 2005;23(4):320–30.
[30] Zaman S, Ashraf RN, Martines J. Training in complementary feeding counselling of healthcare workers and its influence on maternal behaviours and child growth: a cluster-randomized controlled trial in Lahore, Pakistan. J Health Popul Nutr 2008;26(2):210–22.
[31] Vazir S, Engle P, Balakrishna N, Griffiths PL, Johnson SL, Creed-Kanashiro H, et al. Cluster-randomized trial on complementary and responsive feeding education to caregivers found improved dietary intake, growth and development among rural Indian toddlers. Matern Child Nutr 2012;9(1):99–117.

[32] Pachón H, Schroeder DG, Marsh DR, Dearden KA, Ha TT, Lang TT. Effect of an integrated child nutrition intervention on the complementary food intake of young children in rural north Viet Nam. Food Nutr Bull 2002;23(Suppl. 4):62–9.
[33] FAO State of food insecurity in the world. Rome, Italy: Food and Agriculture Organization; 2010.
[34] Coates J, Swindale A, Bilinsky P. Household food insecurity access scale (HFIAS) for measurement of household food access: indicator guide (v. 3). Washington, DC: Food and Nutrition Technical Assistance Project, Academy for Educational Development; 2007.
[35] Sunguya BF, Poudel KC, Mlunde LB, Urassa DP, Jimba M, Yasuoka J. Efficacy of in-service nutrition training for mid-level providers to improve feeding practices among HIV-positive children in Tanga, Tanzania: study protocol for a cluster randomized controlled trial. Trials 2013;14(1):352.
[36] Sunguya BF, Ong KI, Dhakal S, Mlunde LB, Shibanuma A, Yasuoka J, et al. Strong nutrition governance is a key to addressing nutrition transition in low and middle-income countries: review of countries' nutrition policies. Nutr J 2014;13(1):65.
[37] Marsh DR, Schroeder DG, Dearden KA, Sternin J, Sternin M. The power of positive deviance. BMJ 2004;329(7475):1177–9.
[38] Bisits Bullen PA. The positive deviance/hearth approach to reducing child malnutrition: systematic review. Trop Med Int Health 2011;16(11):1354–66.

CHAPTER

9

Nutrition and Food in AIDS Patients

Beata Całyniuk[1], Teresa Kokot[2], Ewa Nowakowska-Zajdel[2], Elżbieta Grochowska-Niedworok[1] and Małgorzata Muc-Wierzgoń[2]

[1]**Department of Human Nutrition, Silesian Medical University, Zabrze, Poland,** [2]**Department of Internal Diseases, Silesian Medical University, Bytom, Poland**

9.1 INTRODUCTION

Infection with human immunodeficiency virus (HIV) from the retrovirus family leads to the loss of the organism's immunity. Moreover, infections that cause mild symptoms in healthy individuals develop into severe forms complicated with high mortality in HIV-positive patients [1].

Full-blown immunodeficiency syndrome is a significant challenge for public health care worldwide and certainly requires multidirectional actions. Acquired immunodeficiency syndrome (AIDS) is a new threat among communicable diseases and primarily requires prophylaxis, early diagnosis, antiviral treatment, and supportive management, including a well-balanced diet.

The classification of HIV infections is based on the criteria developed by the Center for Disease Control and primarily involves the count of CD4 cells per μL and concomitant symptoms associated with AIDS. Causal/antiretroviral treatment is indicated in the case of full-blown AIDS, but also in each infection irrespective of the stage of the disease. The opinions of experts concerning the time when treatment should be implemented vary because the course of the disease is unpredictable and antiviral treatment results in numerous adverse reactions.

Health of HIV Infected People, Volume 2.
DOI: http://dx.doi.org/10.1016/B978-0-12-800767-9.00009-1

In Europe, it is assumed that AIDS is diagnosed based on symptoms irrespective of CD4 cell count, whereas in the United States AIDS is diagnosed in asymptomatic patients in whom the CD4 count is less than 200/μL. Despite the fact that the UNAIDS (The Joint United Nations Programme on HIV and AIDS) reported more than 50% reduction in HIV infection incidence in 25 countries with low and average income in 2012, the number of HIV-positive individuals worldwide was still high in 2011, amounting to 34 million. In 2011, approximately 2.5 million newly diagnosed cases were recorded, which shows a considerable reduction when compared with 2001 (3.2 million cases). Moreover, less deaths have been reported: approximately 1.7 million versus up to 1.9 million in 2001. Insufficient access to antiretroviral therapy (ART) is still observable. Such treatment is not available to approximately 7 million qualified patients worldwide [2]. Today, AIDS is no longer considered a fatal disease, but rather a chronic one; a person with AIDS can live as long as 40 years [3].

According to the WHO report of 2003, proper nutrition may prevent diseases, cure health conditions when combined with other means, help in the recovery processes, or help control diseases [4,5]. The WHO recommends that nutrition intervention should be part of all HIV/AIDS control and therapy programs because it can improve ART effectiveness and metabolic abnormalities caused by the therapy [4]. Diet in AIDS patients is not of primary significance, but it is of considerable importance at each stage. When planning ART, one should also consider interactions of food with drugs [6,7]. The aim of nutrition in HIV-positive patients is to maintain fat-free body mass. Dietary management is the same as in patients with chronic infections and depends on the clinical condition, nutritional status, biochemical disorders, concomitant diseases, and complications in the form of opportunistic infections, neoplasms (Kaposi's sarcoma, lymphatic and reticular neoplasms), or neurological disorders. In patients manifesting only immunological disorders without full-blown syndrome, the diet should aim at maintaining adequate body mass and function of the immune system. When diet is planned in patients with full-blown syndrome, the following must be considered: individual requirements; the degree of damage to the organism; secondary malnutrition; and the presence of opportunistic infections.

Monitoring the nutritional status of HIV-positive patients is, in addition to assessment of immunological status, a significant element of prognosis concerning progression of the infection and risk of death [8,9]. Nutrition plays a significant role in multidisciplinary care of HIV-positive patients; as a type of supportive management, it improves the general condition and contributes to a better quality of life [6,7].

9.1.1 Energy and Food

The condition that makes all life processes run properly is systematic energy intake, the only source of which is chemical energy from food. The energy requirement of an individual depends on sex, body mass index (BMI), age, physiological condition, composition of the body mass, and physical activity [10].

Chandrasekhar and Gupta [11] claim that the effects of nutrition in HIV-positive and AIDS patients should be studied because of the diversity of patients in the population, dosage, and proportions of nutrients, initial levels of deficit, and final effects. The diet should be planned individually as far as its quantitative and qualitative composition is concerned, including individual needs of the organism and patients' preferences. The diet should conform to the principles of reasonable nutrition because, apart from the quantitative composition of nutrients, other factors such as proper selection of products, meals, fluids, and distribution of meals during the day are of vital importance [6]. Meals should not be large in volume, but rather consumed regularly four to six times per day [12] (Table 9.1).

If a full-blown disease has not yet developed in AIDS patients, then energy requirement is the same as in a healthy individual [12], and thus there are no grounds for increasing energy content in a diet. Resting energy expenditure increases by approximately 10%, but total energy expenditure remains unaltered. Delivering an increased number of calories at this time rapidly leads to an increase in the body weight and all its consequences. It is therefore recommended to continuously monitor the nutritional status.

Restrictive diets, which result in rapid weight loss (e.g., cabbage, vegetable, yogurt diets, or "powder" diet), are contraindicated for HIV-positive patients. They lead to protein and vitamin deficiencies as well

TABLE 9.1 Percentage Distribution of Diet in Meals [6,13]

Meal	4 Meals a day	5 Meals a day	6 Meals a day
First breakfast	30%	25%	20%
Second breakfast	15%	10%	10%
Dinner	30%	30%	30%
Afternoon tea	–	10%	10%
Supper	25%	25%	20%
Meal before bedtime	–	–	10%

as metabolism disorders and negatively affect immune processes [13,14]. Concomitant use of antiretroviral drugs may impair absorption and elimination of medicines, and thus render the treatment and selection of a drug-resistant strain ineffective.

The nutritional status is assessed with the use of one of the anthropometric methods, such as measurements of the body weight, height, and waist circumference [15]. These measurements are used to calculate the BMI, observe body weight over time, and assess distribution of the fat tissue.

The basic principle in nutrition for HIV-positive/AIDS patients is maintaining proper fat-free body mass. This means that if the body mass increases, then energy intake must be reduced by limiting the amount of fat and simple carbohydrates with unaltered protein delivery. It is recommended to eliminate sweets and alcohol, reduce the amount of bread, fatty meat, and fried and stewed dishes, to replace butter with low-fat margarine, and to satisfy hunger with vegetables and fruit [13,16]. In the course of HIV infection/AIDS, the immune system is gradually weakened and the nutritional status deteriorates by limiting the possibilities in which the organism can use nutrients, with simultaneous increase in metabolic requirement [17]. That is why losing weight is a frequently observed phenomenon in HIV-positive and AIDS patients.

Unintended loss of more than 5% of the body weight in 3 months or a decrease of BMI to less than 18.5 kg/m^2 indicates that it may be necessary to consider changing the diet and implement dietary supplements [14,18]. Undernutrition may intensify the activity of HIV, thus increasing susceptibility to AIDS-related diseases [19]. Minimal energy intake in people who maintain low physical activity is 1,800–2,200 kcal daily [17]. Such energy intake is also needed by hospitalized patients [20]. Regarding nutrition of malnourished patients, for the purposes of clinical nutrition, it is assumed that daily energy requirement of an adult patient is 25–35 kcal/kg, but it is 5 kcal/kg lower in women due to increased amount of adipose tissue [20]. The guidelines of the National Institutes of Health state that the energy requirement in HIV-positive/AIDS patients is at least 17–20 kcal/kg of the body mass as long as the body weight is stable. In the case of weight loss, the number of calories should be increased to at least 25 kcal/kg [19].

There are several principles that must be followed when preparing meals for HIV-positive/AIDS patients [21,22]:

- high-quality and fresh products should be used
- food in small, single, and hermetically sealed packages is recommended
- foods should be consumed directly after preparation
- when foods are warmed, they should be brought to a boil
- food should be boiled, steamed, or baked in foil

- meals should be small and consumed four to six times daily
- food should be prepared in an aesthetic way
- one should not eat meals that are too hot or too cold

Nutrition should be based on the principles of a light diet. The selection of recommended and contraindicated foods (Table 9.2) is determined by the influence of individual components of the genotype of the pathogen, virulence, mechanism of phagocytosis, cellular resistance, activity of the complement system, and synthesis of antibodies and cytokines [26] (Table 9.2).

9.1.2 Protein

The basic protein requirement of a healthy adult is 0.75–0.90 g/kg of standard body weight. In AIDS patients, it increases to 2.2–1.5 g/kg of standard body weight, which should constitute 10–15% of daily energy intake [13,20]. In the case of chronic infections, which frequently accompany AIDS, protein requirement may increase up to 20% due to increased catabolism [14].

Particular attention should be given to animal protein due to the content of exogenous amino acids (tryptophan, isoleucine, or methionine). The recommended sources of these components are oily fish (mackerel, herring) containing omega-3 fatty acids and lean meats (Table 9.2). Vegetable products are also a good source of protein. Vegetable products of high biological value include soy beans, legumes, and nuts. To ensure an adequate amount of all amino acids, they should be combined with milk products, particularly in the case of vegan diets.

Including fermented milk products (without lactose) is also recommended because they are a source of protein, calcium, and a range of other minerals. When the CD4 level is more than 200 cells/μL, fermented products are indicated; however, when the number of cells decreases, replacing them with gently pasteurized products is recommended. In such products the bacterial flora is inactive and therefore not harmful to an immunodeficient organism [27–29]. If diarrhea is present, then milk should be excluded from the diet.

9.1.3 Fats

Fats should constitute 15–30% of energy in a diet [13,30]. These recommendations are also valid in HIV-positive patients [13,30]. However, particular attention should be given to the proportions of n-3 and n-6 fatty acids. The recommended intake of n-3 fatty acids is 0.5–2% of total energy intake with food, whereas n-6 fatty acids should constitute 5–8% of daily energy intake [13,31]. According to other authors, proper proportions between these acids should be 1:1–2:1, but due to difficulties in observing

TABLE 9.2 Recommended and Contraindicated Products in the Diet of Patients with AIDS [23–25]

Recommended	Contraindicated
CEREAL PRODUCTS	
Wheat bread, graham bread, sponge cake, confectionery bread, groats, rice, noodles, light pasta	Fresh rye bread, whole-wheat bread, rye crisp bread, bran bread
MILK AND MILK PRODUCTS	
Milk with the fat content of 2% or lower, milk and fruit or milk and vegetable drinks, light cottage cheese, cream cheese, yoghurt, kefir, buttermilk (fermented products can be consumed only if CD4 level is normal)	Full-fat ripening-cheese, blue cheese
EGGS	
Boiled eggs, steamed scrambled eggs	Hard-boiled eggs, raw eggs
MEAT, COLD CUTS, POULTRY, FISH	
Boiled meat, lean cold cuts, ham, poultry sirloin, lean veal, baby beef, rabbit, chicken, turkey, fish	Fat cold cuts, canned meat, liver sausage, mutton, pork, goose, duck
FATS	
Butter in limited amounts, margarine with reduced fat content, vegetable oils	Lard, pork fat, tallow, hard margarine, palm oil, cream
VEGETABLES	
Boiled potatoes, carrots, pumpkin, courgette, parsley, pattypan squash, celery, peeled tomatoes, lettuce	Fried potatoes, cabbage vegetables, onion, garlic, leek, cucumbers, rutabaga, radish, turnip, marinated and salted vegetables, dry legume seeds
FRUIT	
Berries, grapes without seeds, rose hips, peaches, apricots, bananas, apples	Citruses, marinated fruits
SUGAR AND SWEETS	
Fruit-flavored starch jelly, pudding, fruit jellies, mousses, meringues, soufflés	Fatty cakes, layer cakes, desserts with stimulants, chocolate, candy bars, ice cream

TABLE 9.3 Sources of Fatty Acids [32,33]

Fatty acids	Sources
Saturated fatty acids	Lard, tallow, fat meat, palm oil, coconut oil full-fat milk products (butter, cheese, cream, milk)
Monounsaturated fatty acids	Olive oil, rapeseed oil margarine, almonds, hazelnuts, tuna, sardine
Polyunsaturated fatty acids—omega 6	Corn oil, soybean oil, sunflower seed oil walnuts, margarine
Polyunsaturated fatty acids—omega 3	Fish oils (cod, mackerel, salmon, sardine) crustaceans, tofu linseed oil, rapeseed oil, soybean oil

such proportions the recommended *n*-6:*n*-3 ratio should not be greater than 5:1 [32]. Food sources of fatty acids are presented in Table 9.3. Fish, particularly sea fish, are the main and direct sources of beneficial omega-3 acids. A considerably high amount of omega-3 acids can be found in salmon, sardines, and crustaceans. Numerous studies indicate that the amount of omega-3 acids in a diet should be increased by consuming fish and seafood [33] (Table 9.3).

Carter et al. [34] presented the effects of supplementation with omega-3 on dyslipidemia in HIV/AIDS patients during ART. Omega-3 fatty acids can promote a reduction in plasma triglycerides by decreasing hepatic synthesis of VLDL cholesterol in the general population, but its effect on HIV/AIDS patients with hypertriglyceridemia is unknown. No significant reduction in total cholesterol has been observed in some studies [34,35], but significant reduction has been shown in others [36,37].

There is no evidence to indicate that any treatment has significantly reduced total cholesterol and LDL cholesterol and increased HDL cholesterol. The intervention group of most of the randomized, controlled study was too small.

Lipid disorders are caused not only by pharmacological therapies but also, and even more frequently, by improper lifestyle—diet that is not well-balanced, alcohol use, tobacco smoking, lack of physical activity, or nonhygienic lifestyle. High concentrations of LDL and low levels of HDL are proven factors of cardiovascular diseases, and a high triglyceride concentration may lead to pancreatitis [23].

The latest findings indicate that the Mediterranean diet, or hypolipidemic diet, may be beneficial for HIV-positive patients [23,38,39]. This diet emphasizes high intake of vegetable products as well as monounsaturated and polyunsaturated fatty acids and low consumption of saturated acids. Docosahexaenoic acid (DHA) and eicosapentaenoic acid (EPA) decrease the level of triglycerides in HIV-positive patients to a considerable degree [38,39].

In individuals infected with HIV virus, lipodystrophy is observed frequently [40–43]. Lipoatrophy develops in approximately 13–34% of HIV-positive patients who receive antiviral treatment [44]. People at particular risk include women, elderly patients, as well as those with low CD4 cell counts and low BMI [45]. Lipoatrophy affects the face and extremities. Moreover, excessive accumulation of the adipose tissue (lipohypertrophy) is also observed in HIV-positive patients [46]. Deposition of the fat tissue is seen in the abdominal region, dorsal aspect of the neck, and breasts [43,47]. It seems that these are two separate pathophysiological processes.

The pathogenesis of lipodystrophy is highly complex. It is determined by the course of HIV infection and antiviral drugs used; however, individual genetic conditions are also significant [44]. The mechanisms responsible for lipodystrophy include mitochondrial toxicity, disorder of adipose tissue gene expression, and insulin resistance [47]. It is suspected that activity of peroxisome proliferator-activated receptors (PPAR) is inhibited in the course of infection, which favors an increase in a triglyceride level [48]. While using reverse-transcriptase inhibitors (drugs that belong to the class of nucleotide analogues), the mitochondrial DNA polymerase is blocked, thereby disturbing mitochondrial function and cellular oxidation processes. Inhibitors of proteases of sterol response element binding proteins lead to impairment of intracellular fatty acid and glucose metabolism and affect adipocyte differentiation [49]. Such changes are accompanied by lipid metabolism disorders (high LDL level, low HDL, sometimes high triglyceride concentrations) [40–43]. These changes are found in certain HIV-positive patients treated with antiretroviral drugs, particularly those who are older. One basic type of nonpharmacological management is following a diet (hypocalorific one) and increasing physical activity [50]. Diet may restore proper cholesterol and triglyceride levels but does not make lipodystrophy symptoms subside. Lazzaretti [30] conducted clinical trials in which adult participants limited their fat consumption (from 31% to 21% of daily energy intake). This resulted in a decrease in plasma triglyceride concentrations.

HIV-infected patients with lipodystrophy were subjects in studies on metformin, glitazones (PPAR activators), and recombinant leptin. It was observed that treatment with metformin or glitazone lowered triglyceride concentrations and free fatty acid levels, improved glucose tolerance, and caused a slight gain of the subcutaneous adipose tissue [45,51]. Recombinant leptin reduced appetite, lowered blood glucose levels, and improved the lipid profile. It needs to be stressed that neither dietary management (except for patients with nutrition disorders) nor medicines used produce desirable therapeutic effects [45,46,51].

9.1.4 Carbohydrates

Carbohydrates cover most of the energy requirements of the organism, that is, 55–75% of daily energy intake. These recommendations are valid for healthy individuals and HIV-positive patients [13].

Carbohydrates should be selected with caution and should include whole-wheat cereal products, vegetables, and fruit [23,43]. The main sources of monosaccharides in a standard diet are sugar, honey, sweets, syrups, and juices [13]. Their intake should be reduced (less than 10% of daily energy intake) [13]. The diet should include complex carbohydrates, which are a source of dietary fiber, such as steel-cut oats, brown rice, whole-meal cereals, bread, pasta, and vegetables such as potatoes.

Dietary fiber is an important element of the diet but should be introduced gradually. Daily intake of 30–40g should be divided carefully into several small meals to prevent gastrointestinal disorders. In this case, we observe an improvement of lipid parameters in the blood because of the influence on decreased absorption of triglycerides and cholesterol [52–54]. An abrupt increase in fiber intake may cause flatulence, constipation, and diarrhea [55].

9.1.5 Vitamins and Minerals

Vitamins and minerals are very important dietary components in immune mechanisms. Immunostimulating properties of vitamins, particularly vitamins B, A, E, and C, as well as microelements—selenium, zinc, and iron—were confirmed in clinical trials and it was demonstrated that their intake reduces the risk of developing full-blown AIDS [56]. The recommendations of vitamin intake for infected patients are considerably higher than for healthy individuals. As of today, however, few studies concerning macroelement supplementation have been conducted.

A normal well-balanced diet contains everything that is essential and there is no need for additional administration of vitamins and minerals. However, if the diet contains too few vegetables and fruit, then some deficiencies—usually temporary and slight—may occur. This concerns certain B vitamins (B1, B2, and B6), magnesium, potassium, and sometimes (although rarely) calcium [47,48]. Deficiencies of other vitamins and minerals are rather impossible unless an individual follows a restrictive diet to lose weight or a vegetarian or vegan diets.

When a diet is well-balanced, the general vitamin requirement does not increase. Some patients use large doses of certain vitamins and microelements because they believe that they reinforce their immune systems. However, a lot of studies prove that large doses of certain vitamins may be harmful [57] and, despite numerous attempts undertaken in developed countries, the influence of vitamin and mineral salt supplementation on the course of HIV infection has not been confirmed [58].

A vitamin B complex, which includes vitamin B1 (thiamine), vitamin B2 (riboflavin), vitamin B6 (pyridoxine), vitamin B12 (cobalamin), niacin, pantothenic acid, biotin, and folate, plays an important role in energy metabolism as well as proper function of the nervous and immune systems. Vitamins B1, B6, and B12 deficiencies were not observed in all patients, particularly in those without clinical symptoms of HIV infection. The trials conducted in a group of 2,100 HIV-positive African subjects revealed that vitamin B complex supplementation prolongs survival [59]. Using the vitamin B complex containing 50 mg of vitamins B1, B2, B6, and B12 is safe.

Vitamin B1 (thiamine) is a water-soluble vitamin. It plays a crucial role in tissue respiration processes and, particularly, in carbohydrate metabolism. It is a component of carboxylase coenzyme (thiamine pyrophosphate). It supports the function of acetylcholine, inhibits cholinesterase, shows synergy with thyroxine and insulin, and stimulates secretion of gonadotrophic hormones. Thiamine accelerates wound healing and has analgesic properties. It is essential for proper functioning of the nervous system. Its daily requirement for a healthy individual is 1.5–3.0 mg. The recommended requirement for HIV-positive people is 2.6 mg [60] or, according to another source, even 20 mg daily [61]. It was also observed that HIV-positive patients with low thiamine concentrations develop full-blown AIDS more frequently [61].

The daily requirement of vitamin B2 is 1.5 mg. The recommended requirement for AIDS patients is approximately the same as for the healthy population. Deepika and Seema [62] showed that nutritional profile for HIV/AIDS patients in India needed interventions to improve nutrient intakes. The intake for riboflavin was well below the recommendation, and during ART (nucleotide analogues) lactic acidosis as a rare and fatal complication was often observed. The signs of mitochondrial toxicity demonstrated by diffuse myopathy and pancreatitis were connected with riboflavin level deficiency. Clinical manifestation improved after treatment with a 50-mg daily dose of riboflavin [63]. This vitamin takes part in amino acid and lipid metabolism, which is of considerable importance in the course of AIDS.

The daily requirement of vitamin B6 is 2 mg. The recommended requirement for HIV-positive patients is 3.00–25.00 mg daily [8]. To support the immune system, vitamin B6 is probably the most important B vitamin in terms of immune support [64]. B6 deficiency is observed in 12–52% of HIV-positive patients [8,64,65] and contributes to disorders of cellular and humoral responses. The deficiency impairs proliferation of lymphocytes and synthesis of interleukin-2, which is responsible for growth and maturation of lymphocytes. This might lead to inhibition of DNA and protein synthesis essential in the process of forming proper immune responses.

The recommended intake of vitamin B12 in healthy adults ranges from 1.5 to 3.0 μg daily. The preferred requirement for HIV-positive patients ranges from 5.00 to 12.00 μg daily [60] or, according to another source, even up to 50 μg daily [64]. As early as in the 1980s, several studies have shown low levels of vitamin B12 in HIV-positive people [66,67].

It is unclear whether low vitamin B12 levels affect HIV disease progression, or whether they are merely a consequence of disease progression. An 18-month study of HIV-positive individuals found that the onset of low serum vitamin B12 levels was associated with CD4 cell count decline, and that normalization of vitamin B12 levels was associated with an improvement in CD4 cell count [68].

Another study that followed-up 310 men for 9 years found that low serum vitamin B12 levels at entry to the study were associated with an 89% increased risk of progression of AIDS after controlling for disease stage, ART, alcohol intake, and age [69]. In the majority of HIV-positive people in every stage of infection, vitamin B12 deficiency manifests itself with pernicious anemia and weakened response of T cells and B cells to antigens, and is associated with nervous system dysfunction.

The recommended daily dose of folate is 400 μg [68]. In AIDS patients, who frequently manifest deficiency, the recommended intake increases to 800–1,000 μg [60,61].

The daily requirement of vitamin PP (niacin, vitamin B3) is 14–35 mg daily in healthy people [70]. For HIV-positive/AIDS patients, a recent study confirmed that 3 g/day could be well-tolerated [71]. Abrams et al. reported that higher nicotinamide intake was associated with higher CD4 cell counts [72]. Tang et al. [73], using the Multicenter AIDS Cohort Study, observed that a daily niacin intake more than three- to four-times the recommended value was an independent factor for slower progression and improved survival. Whether the benefits could be the result of repletion of intracellular NAD concentration in uninfected non-T-lymphocytes rather than direct antiviral effects depends on the metabolic abnormalities. Supplementation with chromium nicotinate 400 mg/day significantly reduced triglyceride levels in HIV/AIDS patients. Chromium nicotinate enhances insulin action and influences glucose and lipid metabolism [74,75].

Research reveals that administering 3–4.5 g niacin to infected people with increased cholesterol levels compared with 40–80 mg of lovastatin daily resulted in a decline in LDL cholesterol level, but to a lesser degree [70].

The daily requirement of vitamin A is 800 μg in healthy people and 1,000 μg for HIV-positive individuals. Numerous studies report reduced B-cell function and antibody production that accompany HIV infection [9,15], which is also associated with vitamin A and beta-carotene deficiencies. Vitamin A should not be taken in doses more than 1,200 IU (i.e., approximately 360 μg of retinol) because of increased risk of neoplasms. Artificial preparations that contain "animal-type" vitamin A, that is, retinol acetate and palmitate, may also be harmful for the organism.

The daily requirement of vitamin E for healthy individuals is 10 mg daily; for infected people it is 30–267 mg [60,61]. Using doses more than 800 mg daily is not recommended. It was observed that chronic use of high doses of this vitamin may be associated with shorter survival. The mechanism of such a phenomenon has not been explained [61]. Moreover, it must be emphasized that preparations containing vitamin E impair absorption of certain drugs.

The preferred doses of vitamin D for healthy people range from 5,000 to 10,000 IU. Doses that exceed 0.7 mg for males and 0.6 mg for females may be harmful. A low concentration of this vitamin is frequently seen in AIDS patients and in the general population [76–78]. Vitamin D deficiency may influence the immune system and exacerbate HIV complications such as opportunistic infections, disease progression, and death, and may have a negative impact on bone, metabolic, cardiovascular, and neurocognitive functions as well. Levels of the vitamin less than 10 ng/mL are widely accepted as showing deficiency [77,78]. A target vitamin D level should be more than 30 ng/mL.

It was observed, that there is an association between vitamin D level and ART. Non-nucleoside reverse-transcriptase inhibitor was associated with a high risk of vitamin D deficiency, but nucleoside reverse-transcriptase inhibitor did not appear to be associated with its deficiency [77,78].

Investigators from Europe, Argentina, and Israel found a strong relationship between low levels of the vitamin, an increased risk of all-cause mortality, and the development of an AIDS-defining condition.

Vitamin C is recommended in a dose of 60–100 mg daily due to its antiviral and antioxidant properties. The preferred requirement for infected people is 200–500 mg daily. The dosage should not exceed 1,000 mg daily because such a dose may be harmful due to delayed elimination of other drugs. There is no convincing evidence indicating that using vitamin C is in any way beneficial for patients. The use of 500 mg at bedtime may result in urinary acidification, which prevents urinary tract infections (particularly in women) [8].

Excessive intake of vitamins A, D, and E is discouraged and even harmful because they interact with antiviral drugs used in AIDS therapies [61].

Some clinical reports indicate that HIV infection and AIDS progression were decelerated in Africans who received multivitamins. However, this effect is nonspecific and is a consequence of considerable vitamin deficiencies in the African population. In developed countries, such intense deficiencies are not encountered and, therefore, the efficacy of vitamin therapies was not proven [79]. Furthermore, studies on megadose vitamin therapies have not demonstrated any beneficial effects—only those resulting from an overdose [79].

In addition to proper nutrition, temporary implementation of dietary supplements is indicated if undernutrition, emaciation, or cachexia is diagnosed. A physician should be consulted regarding implementation of dietary supplements because they may alter the effects of antiretroviral drugs. The results of studies concerning the usage of microelements in pathogenesis of HIV infection frequently deliver contradictory information. Despite the fact that a beneficial effect of vitamins and minerals on defense mechanisms is scientifically confirmed and commonly established, this issue still requires further research.

9.2 NUTRITION AND ART

The past decade has seen substantial advances in the development of ART medications used in combination to reduce the replication of HIV virus and to treat HIV-infected persons. Because of these medications, many HIV-infected persons are able to reduce levels of virus in the bloodstream to undetectable levels. Antiretroviral treatment is an important in the lives of AIDS patients because it should be continued for the rest of their lives, even a few decades.

Combination antiretroviral therapy (cART), which is currently recommended, is based on six groups of antiretroviral drugs. It has a risk of various adverse effects. The following effects are observed in infected patients: metabolism changes such as elevated triglyceride, total cholesterol, and LDL levels; HDL concentration decline; insulin resistance of tissues and glucose tolerance disorders; elevated lactate level; osteopenia and osteoporosis; cardiovascular diseases; hematological abnormalities; gastric symptoms; nephropathies; and skin lesions. Lipodystrophy or lipid metabolism disorders are observed within 3–12 months of the therapy in approximately 40% of patients. Carbohydrate metabolism disorders affect approximately 60% of patients [80]. Nephropathies are associated with both HIV infection and nephrotoxic effects of antiretroviral drugs [81]. The development of such disorders may be delayed by an appropriate diet.

Due to drug-to-drug interactions, the usage of hypolipidemic agents—statins—is limited because of increased probability of myopathy. In this context, a diet with controlled fat intake becomes significant in supportive management [80,82].

Unfavorable interactions of protease inhibitors with proton pump and H2 receptor inhibitors (decreased absorption of, e.g., atazanavir) restrict their usage in treating gastric disorders [81,82]. The diet that reduces acidity of the gastric juice is clinically significant. Moreover, it is recommended to eliminate alcohol during ART. Regular consumption of even slight amounts of alcohol leads to addiction and reacts with medicines [80]. Furthermore, citrus fruits, particularly grapefruits and all grapefruit-containing products, are contraindicated because they impair the mechanism of action of antiretroviral drugs by blocking cytochrome P450 3A4 enzyme.

Prior to initiating therapy, we interview each patient, perform a complete physical examination, conduct a thorough nutritional assessment, evaluate the gut function, and calculate the daily caloric and protein requirements. The selection of appropriate oral, enteral, and parenteral diets is crucial in the successful management of these patients. Because all AIDS patients using ART differ in their nutritional requirements, diet tolerance, and degree of intestinal dysfunction, there is no single nutritional therapy regimen that can be utilized in the treatment of all these patients. Therefore, we recommend special individualized oral diets combined with food supplements and enteral and parenteral diets in the treatment of AIDS patients using ART [78].

In any case, individuals should follow the dietary recommendations that are associated with therapy and consumer a rational, healthy diet without excess calories, sugars, and animal fats and that is rich in vegetables and protein. The diet should be consumed in the form of four to six meals per day.

9.3 SUMMARY

From the very beginning of the HIV and AIDS epidemics, diet has been considered an important factor in the course of infection. The relationship between the nutritional status and ability to generate immune responses has been raising the interest of scientists for many years; still, much new and sometimes surprising information is reported. The influence of nutrients on HIV infection or interaction between food and antiretroviral drugs is being studied all around the world. A nutritionist should therefore be a part of a therapeutic team treating HIV-positive patients.

The diet for AIDS patients should be planned individually by taking into account the phase of the disease, concomitant symptoms, and nutritional status. An adequately prepared diet may have a beneficial effect on the general health status, course of the disease, and quality of life. Nutrition for those with HIV infection and AIDS is even more significant in the course of opportunistic infections. Individual nutrients may affect the genotype of pathogens and their virulence, as well as impair cellular resistance, mechanism of phagocytosis, complement system function, antibody production, and cytokine synthesis [26].

Patients with AIDS are advised to follow a light diet that is rich in protein and that includes products that are a source of whole protein and supply the organism with nutrients in amounts conforming to the requirements [13]. Foods that cause gastrointestinal disorders should be excluded from the diet. Moreover, delivering adequate amounts of vitamins and minerals (in amounts not less than 0.5 kg daily) found in vegetables and fruit is also important. Meals should be smaller in volume and eaten four to six times per day [13,24,25]. The diet needs modification in the cases of body weight changes, symptoms of lipodystrophy, elevated blood LDL and triglyceride concentrations, diagnosis of prediabetes or diabetes, metabolic syndrome, hepatic or renal impairment, arterial hypertension, gastrointestinal symptoms (diarrhea, constipation), and implementation of ART [83]. In addition to proper nutrition, temporary implementation of dietary supplements is indicated if undernutrition, emaciation, or cachexia is diagnosed.

Although huge progress has been made in exploring and treating HIV infection and AIDS within the past 30 years, most of it only refers to prophylaxis. Implementation of ART with the use of new medicines is more and more effective, but still insufficient. Moreover, the progress that has been made in this context refers mainly to developed countries [4].

A global increase in food prices that has occurred in the 21st century that has exceeded expected values, poorer crop yield in some regions of the world, the need for biofuels, unfavorable weather conditions, and restrictions in land cultivation indicate that access to food has become reduced, which might have an unfavorable influence on the nutritional status, course of the disease, and nutritional hazards for ill people. Increasing prices of food and decreased food intake are of particular importance in HIV infection, especially in poor countries [56,61].

Much research has drawn attention to the fact that reducing AIDS epidemics requires HIV screening tests among people from poor countries and treating HIV-positive people according to the current standards. Moreover, spreading knowledge and education concerning risk factors is equivalent to counteracting the disease [58,83]. The productivity of farmers, nutritional safety, nutritional counseling, concomitant diseases including hospitalizations, and patient quality of life are of particular significance [56,61].

Nutritional care and support promote well-being, self-esteem, and a positive attitude for people and their families living with HIV/AIDS.

Healthy and balanced nutrition should be one of the goals of counseling and care for people at all stages of HIV infection. An effective program of nutritional care and support will improve the quality of life of people living with HIV/AIDS by:

- maintaining body weight and strength
- replacing lost vitamins and minerals
- improving the function of the immune system and the body's ability to fight infection
- extending the period from infection to the development of AIDS
- improving response to treatment

- reducing time and money spent on health care
- keeping HIV-infected people active, allowing them to take care of themselves, their family, and their children
- keeping HIV-infected people productive, able to work, able to grow food, and able to contribute to the income of their families [83].

References

[1] Halota W, Juszczyk J. HIV/AIDS: manual for physicians and students. Termedia Poznań; 2006.
[2] <http://www.unaids.org/en/resources/publications/2012/name.76121.en.asp>
[3] Sepkowitz KA. AIDS—the first 20 years. NEJM 2001;344:1764–70.
[4] WHO. Nutrient requirements for people living with HIV/AIDS. Reports of a technical consultation. Geneva, Switzerland; 2003.
[5] Kłosiewicz-Latoszek L, Szostak WB, Podolec P, Kopeć G, Pajak A, Kozek E, et al. Polish forum for prevention guidelines on diet. Kardiol Pol 2008;66:812–4.
[6] Kosmiski L. Energy expenditure in HIV infection. Am J Clin Nutr 2011;94:1677–82.
[7] Koethe JR, Chi BH, Megazzini KM, Heimburger DC, Stringer JS. Macronutrient supplementation for malnourished HIV infected adults: a review of the evidence in resource-adequate and resource-constrained settings. Clin Infect Dis 2009;49:787–98.
[8] Lebiedzińska A, Bierżyńska N, Lemańska M, Jankowska M, Trocha H, Smiatacz T, et al. Witaminy w diecie osób dorosłych HIV-pozytywnych. Bromat Chem Toksykol 2009;62:672–7.
[9] Hughes S, Kelly P. Interactions of malnutrition and immune impairment, with specific reference to immunity against parasites. Parasite Immunol 2006;28:577–88.
[10] Vaz M, Karaolis N, Draper A, Shetty P. A compilation of energy costs of physical activities. PHN 2005;8:1153–83.
[11] Chandrasekhar A, Gupta A. Nutrition and disease progression pre-highly active antiretroviral therapy (HAART) and post-HAART: can good nutrition delay time to HAART and affect response to HAART? Am J Clin Nutr 2011;94:1703–15.
[12] Arbeitman LOBR, Somarriba G, O'Brien R, Ludwig D, Messiah S, Neri D, et al. Prevalence of obesity in HIV-infected children in a Miami cohort. Pediatric Academic Societies Annual Meeting, Boston, MA; 2012; Abstract number 1518.310.
[13] WHO. Diet, nutrition and the prevention of chronic diseases: report of a joint WHO/FAO expert consultation. WHO Technical Report Series 916, Geneva, Switzerland; 2013.
[14] Argemi X, Dara S, You S, Mattei JF, Courpotin C, Simon B, et al. Impact of malnutrition and social determinants on survival of HIV-infected adults starting antiretroviral therapy in resource-limited settings. AIDS 2012;26:1161–6.
[15] Andrade CS, Jesus RP, Andrade TB, Oliveira NS, Nabity SA, Ribeiro GS. Prevalence and characteristics associated with malnutrition at hospitalization among patients with acquired immunodeficiency syndrome in Brazil. PLoS One 2012;7:e. 48717. [Published online November 7, 2012. doi:10.1371/journal.pone.0048717].
[16] Weiss SM, Tobin JN, Antoni M, Ironson G, Ishii M, Vaughn A, et al. Enhancing the health of women living with HIV: the SMART/EST women's project. Int J Womens Health 2011;3:63–77.
[17] Ahoua L, Umutoni C, Huerga H, Minetti A, Szumilin E, Balkan S, et al. Nutrition outcomes of HIV-infected malnourished adults treated with ready-to-use therapeutic food in sub-Saharan Africa: a longitudinal study. J Int AIDS Soc 2011;14:2.
[18] Moh R, Danel C, Messou E, Ouassa T, Gabillard D, Anzian A, et al. Incidence and determinants of mortality and morbidity following early antiretroviral therapy initiation in HIV-infected adults in West Africa. AIDS 2007;21:2483–91.

[19] Mahlungulu S, Grobler LA, Visser ME, Volmink J. Nutritional interventions for reducing morbidity and mortality in people with HIV. Cochrane Database Syst Rev 2007:3. [CD004536].

[20] Lochs H, Valentini L, Schütz T, Allison SP, Howard P, Pichard C, et al. ESPEN guidelines on enteral nutrition. Clin Nutr 2006;25:177–360.

[21] Fields-Gardner C, Campa A. American dietetics a position of the American dietetic association: nutrition intervention and human immunodeficiency virus infection. J Am Diet Assoc 2010;110:1105–19.

[22] Ivers LC, Cullen KA. Food insecurity: special considerations for women. Am J Clin Nutr 2011;94:1740S–44S.

[23] Panagiotakos DB, Pitsavos C, Arvaniti F, Stefanadis C. Adherence to the Mediterranean food pattern predicts the prevalence of hypertension, hypercholesterolemia, diabetes and obesity, among healthy adults; the accuracy of the med diet score. Prev Med 2007;44:335–40.

[24] Itsiopoulos C, Hodge A, Kaimakamis M. Can the Mediterranean diet prevent prostate cancer. Mol Nutr Food Res 2009;53:227–39.

[25] Dilis V, Trichopoulou A. Antioxidant intakes and food sources in Greek adults. J Nutr 2010;140:1274–9.

[26] Chandra RK. Nutrition and immunology: from the clinic to cellular biology and back again. Proc Nutr Soc 1999;58:681–3.

[27] Hummelen R, Hemsworth J, Changalucha J, Butamanya NL, Hekmat S, Habbema JD, et al. Effect of micronutrient and probiotic fortified yogurt on immune-function of anti-retroviral therapy naive HIV patients. Nutrients 2011;3:897–909.

[28] Hummelen R, Changalucha J, Butamanya NL, Koyama TE, Cook A, Habbema JD, et al. Effect of 25 weeks probiotic supplementation on immune function of HIV patients. Gut Microbes 2011;2:80–5.

[29] Irvine SL, Hummelen R, Hekmat S. Probiotic yogurt consumption may improve gastrointestinal symptoms, productivity, and nutritional intake of people living with human immunodeficiency virus in Mwanza, Tanzania. Nutr Res 2011;31:875–81.

[30] Lazzaretti RK, Kuhmmer K, Sprinz E, Polanczyk CA, Ribeiro JP. Dietary intervention prevents dyslipidemia associated with highly active antiretroviral therapy in human immunodeficiency virus type 1-infected individuals: a randomized trial. J Am Coll Cardiol 2012;13:979–88.

[31] Bresson JL, Flynn A, Heinonen M, Hulshof K, Korhonen H, Lagiou P, et al. Labelling reference intake values for *n*-3 and *n*-6 polyunsaturated fatty acid. EFSA J 2009;1176:1–11.

[32] Rustichelli C, Avallone R, Campioli E, Braghiroli D, Baraldi M. Polyunsaturated fatty acid levels in rat tissues after chronic treatment with dietetic oils. J Sci Food Agric 2012;92:239–45.

[33] Lavie CJ, Milani RV, Mehra MR, Ventura HO. Omega-3 polyunsaturated fatty acids and cardiovascular diseases. J Am Coll Cardiol 2009;54:585–94.

[34] Carter VM, Woolley I, Jolley D, Nyulasi JCI, Mijch A, Dart A. A randomised controlled trial of omega-3 fatty acid supplementation for the treatment of hypertriglyceridemia in HIV-infected males on highly active antiretroviral therapy. Sex Health 2006;3:287–90.

[35] Wohl DA, Tien HC, Busby N, Cunningham C, MacIntosh B, Napravnik S, et al. Randomized study of the safety and efficacy of fish oil (omega-3 fatty acid) supplementation with dietary and exercise counseling for the treatment of antiretroviral therapy-associated hypertriglyceridemia. Clin Infect Dis 2005;41:1498–504.

[36] Baril JG, Kovacs CM, Trottier S, Roederer G, Martel AY. Effectiveness and tolerability of oral administration of low-dose salmon oil to HIV patients with HAART associated dyslipidemia. HIV Clin Trials 2007;8:400–11.

[37] Woods MN, Wanke CA, Ling PR, Hendricks KM, Tang AM, Knox TA, et al. Effect of a dietary intervention and *n*-3 fatty acid supplementation on measures of serum lipid and insulin sensitivity in persons with HIV. Am J Clin Nutr 2009;90:1566–78.

[38] Oliveira JM, Rondo PH. Omega-3 fatty acids and hypertriglyceridemia in HIV-infected subjects on antiretroviral therapy: systematic review and meta-analysis. HIV Clin Trials 2011;12:268–74.
[39] Peters BS, Wierzbicki AS, Moyle G, Nair D, Brockmeyer N. The effect of a 12-week course of omega-3 polyunsaturated fatty acids on lipid parameters in hypertriglyceridemic adult HIV-infected patients undergoing HAART: a randomized, placebo-controlled pilot trial. Clin Ther 2012;34:67–76.
[40] Miller TL, Somarriba G, Orav EJ, Mendez AJ, Neri D, Schaefer N, et al. Biomarkers of vascular dysfunction in children infected with human immunodeficiency virus-1. J Acquir Immune Defic Syndr 2010;55:182–8.
[41] Miller TI, Borkowsky W, Di Meglio LA, Dooley L, Geffner ME, Hazra R, et al. Metabolic abnormalities and viral replication are associated with biomarkers of vascular dysfunction in HIV-infected children. HIV Med 2012;13:264–75.
[42] Bonfanti P, De Socio GV, Ricci E, Antinori A, Martinelli C, Vichi F, et al. The feature of metabolic syndrome in HIV naive patients is not the same of those treated: results from a prospective study. Biomed Pharmacother 2012;66:348–53.
[43] Stanley TL, Grinspoon SK. Body composition and metabolic changes in HIV-infected patients. J Infect Dis 2012;205:383–90.
[44] Brown TT. Approach to the human immunodeficiency virus-infected patient with lipodystrophy. J Clin Endocrinol Metab 2008;93:2937–45.
[45] Milinkovic A, Martinez E. Current perspectives on HIV-associated lipodystrophy syndrome. J Antimicrob Chemother 2005;56:6–9.
[46] Moyle G, Moutschen M, Martinez E, Domingo P, Guaraldi G, Raffi F, et al. Epidemiology, assessment, and management of excess abdominal fat in persons with HIV infection. AIDS Rev 2010;12:3–14.
[47] Mallewa JE, Wilkins E, Vilar J, Mallewa M, Doran D, Back D, et al. HIV-associated lipodystrophy: a review of underlying mechanisms and therapeutic options. J Antimicrob Chemother 2008;62:648–60.
[48] Sattler FR. Pathogenesis and treatment of lipodystrophy: what clinicians need to know. Top HIV Med 2008;16:127–33.
[49] Villaroya F, Domingo P, Giralt M. Drug-induces lipotoxicity: lipodystrophy associated with HIV-1 infection and antiretroviral treatment. Biochim Biophys Acta 2010;1801(3):392–9. http://dx.doi.org/10.1016/j.bbalip.2009;09.018.
[50] Agarwal AK, Garg A. Genetic basis of lipodystrophies and management of metabolic complications. Annu Rev Med 2006;57:297–311.
[51] Hegele RA. Monogenic forms of insulin resistance: apertures that expose the common metabolic syndrome. Trends Endocrinol Metab 2003;14:371–7.
[52] Slavin JL. Dietary fiber and body weight. Nutrition 2005;21:411–8.
[53] Bandera EV, Kushi LH, Moore DF, Gifkins DM, Mc Cullough ML. Association between dietary fiber and endometrial cancer: a dose–response metaanalysis. Am J Clin Nutr 2007;86:1730–7.
[54] Schatzkin A, Mouw T, Park Y, Subar AF, Kipnis V, Hollenbeck A, et al. Dietary fiber and whole-grain consumption in relation to colorectal cancer in the NIH-AARP diet and health study. Am J Clin Nutr 2007;85:1353–60.
[55] Schatzkin A, Park Y, Leitzmann MF, Hollenbeck AR, Cross AJ. Prospective study of dietary fiber, whole grain foods, and small intestinal cancer. Gastroenterology 2008;135:1163–7.
[56] Sztam KA, Ndirangu M, Sheriff M, Arpadi SM, Hawken M, Rashid J, et al. Rationale and design of a study using a standardized locally procured macronutrient supplement as adjunctive therapy to HIV treatment in Kenya. AIDS Care 2013;16:1138–44.
[57] Chlebowski RT, Beal G, Grosvenor M, Lillington L, Weintraub N, Ambler C, et al. Long-term effects of early nutritional support with new enterotropic peptide-based formula

vs. standard enteral formula in HIV-infected patients: randomized prospective trial. Nutrition 1993;9(6):507–12.

[58] Sztam KA, Fawzi WW, Duggan C. Macronutrient supplementation and food prices in HIV treatment. J Nutr 2010;140(1):2135–235.

[59] Conference of Retroviruses and Opportunistic Infection. Supplemental multivitamins or vitamin B complex significantly delay progression to AIDS and death in South African patients infected with HIV. Abstract 217. Chicago, IL; 1998.

[60] Woods MN, Gorbach SL. Dietary considerations in HIV and AIDS. Nutr Clin Care 1999;2:95–102.

[61] Fawzi W, Msamanga GI, Spiegelman D, Wei R, Kapiga S, Villamor E, et al. A randomized trial of multivitamin supplements and HIV disease progression and mortality. N Engl J Med 2004;351:23–32.

[62] Deepika A, Seema P. Anthropometric and nutritional profile of people living with HIV and AIDS in India: an assessment. Indian J Community Med 2014;39(3):161–8.

[63] Dalton SD, Rahimi AR. Emerging role of riboflavin in the treatment of nucleoside analogue-induced type B lactic acidosis. AIDS Patient Care STDS 2001;15(12):611–4.

[64] Gay R, Meydani SN. The effects of vitamin E, vitamin B6 and vitamin B12 on immune function. Nutr Clin Care 2001;4:188–98.

[65] Liang B, Chung S, Araghiniknam M, Lane LC, Watson RR. Vitamins and immunomodulation in AIDS. Nutrition 1996;12:1–7.

[66] Burkes RL, Cohen H, Krailo M, Sinow RM, Carmel R. Low serum cobalamin levels occur frequently in the acquired immune deficiency syndrome and related disorders. Eur J Haematol 1987;38:141–7.

[67] Harriman GR, Smith PD, Horne MK, Fox CH, Koenig S, Lack EE, et al. Vitamin B12 malabsorption in patients with acquired immunodeficiency syndrome. Arch Intern Med 1989;149:2039–41.

[68] Baum MK, Shor-Posner G, Bonvehi P, Cassetti I, Lu Y, Manteroatienza E, et al. Influence of HIV infection on vitamin status and requirements. Ann N Y Acad Sci 1990;587:165.

[69] Tang AM, Graham NM, Saeh AJ. Low serum vitamin B12 concentrations are associated with faster human immunodeficiency virus type 1 disease progression. J Nutr 1997;127:345–51.

[70] Jarosz M. Nutrition standards for the polish population—amendment. Warsaw, Poland: Food and Nutrition Institute; 2012.

[71] Murray MF, Langan M, Mac Gregor RR. Increased plasma tryptophan in HIV-infected patients treated with pharmacologic doses of nicotinamide. Nutrition 2001;17:654–6.

[72] Abrams B, Duncan D, Hertz-Picciotto I. A prospective study of dietary intake and acquired immune deficiency syndrome in HIVseropositive homosexual men. J Acquir Immune Defic Syndr 1993;6:949–58.

[73] Tang AM, Graham NM, Saah AJ. Effects of micronutrient intake on survival in human immunodeficiency virus type 1 infection. Am J Epidemiol 1996;143:1244–56.

[74] Aghdassi E, Arendt BM, Salit IE, Mohammed SS, Jalali P, Bondar H, et al. In patients with HIV-infection, chromium supplementation improves insulin resistance and other metabolic abnormalities: a randomized, double-blind, placebo controlled trial. Curr HIV Res 2009;7:1–8.

[75] Davis CM, Vincent JB. Chromium oligopeptide activates insulin receptor tyrosine kinase activity. Biochem J 1997;36:113–20.

[76] Schwenk A, Stenck H, Kremer G. Oral supplements as adjunctive treatment to nutritional counseling in malnourished HIV infected patients; randomized controlled trial. Clin Nutr 1999;18:371–4.

[77] Fox J, Peters B, Praksh M, Arribas J, Hill A, Moecklinghoff C. Improvement in vitamin D deficiency following antiretroviral regime change: results from the MONET trial. AIDS Res Hum Retroviruses 2011;27:29–34.

[78] Viard J-P, Souberbielle JC, Kirk O, Reekie J, Knysz B, Losso M, et al. EuroSIDA study group. Vitamin D and clinical disease progression in HIV infection: results from the EuroSIDA study. AIDS 25. 2011. http://dx.doi.org/10.1097/QAD.0b013e328347f6f7.
[79] Swaminathan S, Padmaprlyadarsini C, Yoojin L, Sukumar B, Iliayas S, Karthipriya J, et al. Nutritional supplementation in HIV-infected individuals in South India: a prospective interventional study. Clin Infect Dis 2010;51(1):51–7.
[80] Olczak A. The importance of metabolic disorders during antiretroviral therapy HAART. Overview Epidemiol 2007;61:639–46.
[81] Marchewka Z, Szymańska B, Płonka J. Potential nephrotoxic effects of antiretroviral drugs. Prog Hig Med Exp 2012;66:603–8.
[82] Winek K, Sikora A, Mikuła T. Advances in the treatment of HIV infection. Prog Sci Med 2010;10:800–4.
[83] Botros D, Somarriba G, Neri D, Miller TL. Interventions to address chronic disease and HIV: strategies to promote exercise and nutrition among HIV-infected individuals. Curr HIV/AIDS Rep 2012;9:351–63.

CHAPTER

10

Zinc Supplementation for Infants and Children with HIV Infection

Lingli Zhang[1,2,3], *Linan Zeng*[1,2,3], *Ge Gui*[1,2,5], *Yanjun Duan*[4,5] *and Zhiqiang Hu*[1,2,5]

[1]Department of Pharmacy, West China Second University Hospital, Sichuan University, Chengdu, China, [2]Evidence-Based Pharmacy Center, West China Second University Hospital, Sichuan University, Chengdu, China, [3]Key Laboratory of Birth Defects and Related Diseases of Women and Children (Sichuan University), Ministry of Education, Chengdu, China, [4]College of Pharmacy, University of Nebraska Medical Centre, [5]West China School of Pharmacy, Sichuan University, Chengdu, China

10.1 INTRODUCTION

According to estimates by World Health Organization (WHO) and the United Nations Joint Programme on HIV/AIDS (UNAIDS), 33.4 million people were living with HIV worldwide at the end of 2008, of whom, 2.1 million were children and 15.7 million were women [1]. Sub-Saharan Africa is hardest hit; nearly 30 million adults and children there had HIV/AIDS in 2004 [2]. It is estimated by the end of 1999, in sub-Saharan Africa, the number of women between 15 and 49 infected with HIV is more than 12 million, many of whom are pregnant women. In developing countries, about 1/3 or 1/4 babies born to HIV-infected mothers are born with HIV themselves, most of whom got infected during pregnancy or at child birth. Thus the risk of mother-to-child HIV transmission seems to be great. (WHO) While antiretroviral drugs are important for those with advanced HIV infection, nutrition is of fundamental importance for all people with HIV infection [3,4].

Health of HIV Infected People, Volume 2.
DOI: http://dx.doi.org/10.1016/B978-0-12-800767-9.00010-8

Adequate zinc status is critical for immune function [5,6]. Zinc is essential for division, maturation and differentiation of T cells [7]. It can bind to thymulin (which enhances T cell maturation, interleukin-2 production and cytotoxicity) and produce conformational changes essential for specific immunity [8]. Besides, zinc affects Th1/Th2 balance, which functions importantly against immune dysregulation related with HIV infection. B lymphocytes, to certain degree, are also regulated by zinc. Zinc also acts as an antioxidant and may protect cells from oxygen radicals produced during the non specific immune response [8].

Reduced zinc level has been reported in HIV-infected adults, associated with HIV progression. While studies focused on the relation between zinc deficiency and HIV infection among children are still few in number [9]. According to the studies available, advanced HIV stages are associated with low zinc level in children [9]. The HIV-related factor CRP slightly affect zinc concentration, while another factor CD4+ is shown to be irrelevant. HIV disease is always accompanied with many complications, like fever, diarrhea, and underweight, which can also contribute to the declining level of zinc status among HIV-infected children [9]. Zinc deficiency during HIV disease progression, in turn, can accelerate the loss of CD4+ T cells through its effect on hormone thymulin, thus further worsening immunologic dysfunction condition [9–12].

Thus, zinc supplementation as a supporting therapeutic intervention seems reasonable for patients with HIV/AIDS [13,14]. However, in other instances, zinc supplementation had no effect on immune response, vaccination, CD4/CD8 ratio or viral load [15]. Two nutritional studies showed that increased intake of zinc in HIV-1-infected patients led to an augmented risk of progression to AIDS [16] and lower survival [17]. The San Francisco Men's Health Study [18] found no association between increased dietary intakes of zinc (from food and supplements) and time to progression to AIDS. It seems that current studies cannot come to a consensus on the benefit of zinc supplementation. The safety and efficacy of zinc supplementation to HIV-infected children still need to be discussed.

10.2 EFFECTS OF HIV INFECTION ON MICRONUTRIENT (ZINC) STATUS

There are 4 WHO clinical stages of HIV according to the disease progression. Advanced HIV disease (WHO stage 3 and 4) is associated with low serum zinc in both children and adults [9,19], for advanced HIV disease is more likely to be correlated with recurrent acute infections and an elevated acute phase response interpreted as low zinc [9]. However, elevated CRP, observed commonly in HIV-infected patients, displays no independent correlation with low zinc level [9,19], though associated [9].

Besides, CD4+ T cell count, surprisingly has no association with zinc status in HIV-infected children [9,20], while in non-HIV-infected children, a correlation is existed [20].

Accompanied with HIV, there are always complications like fever, diarrhea, and underweight. Among them, fever, viewed as an indicator of infection and illustrated being closely related with acute phase proteins (CRP), is a significant independent predictor of low zinc level [9]. Diarrhea was reported to be associated with low zinc status [21] in HIV-infected children, and evidence was given that diarrhea itself significantly decreases serum zinc concentration in children [22]. Underweight, which is a common problem in HIV-infected children compared with their uninfected counterparts [23], is shown to be weakly associated with zinc status [9]. Some also reported underweight as a significant predictor of low zinc level in adults [19].

In short, advanced HIV progression itself is associated with low zinc. Among the two HIV-related factors, CRP and CD4+, CRP is non-independently correlated with zinc level, while CD4+ expresses no association. Fever, diarrhea, and underweight are the common complications of HIV infection, which also exhibit their influence to zinc status in HIV-infected children.

10.3 EFFECTS OF ZINC ON HIV INFECTION

10.3.1 Mechanism

10.3.1.1 Effect of Zinc on the Immune System

Adequate zinc is essential for T-cell division, maturation, and differentiation [7]. Zinc itself is a cofactor for thymulin, a best known zinc-dependent thymic hormone crucial for T-cell formation and maturation [7] which exists in two forms, a zinc-bound active one, and a zinc-free inactive form [24]. What's more, zinc may also prevent the programmed death (apoptosis) of precursor T-cell populations and mature CD4+ T cells through various enzymatic mechanisms and through chronic production of glucocorticoids [10]. That could explain some effects of zinc deficiency on T-cell function. Both in animal and human models, a reduction of the level of biologically active thymulin out of zinc deprivation in the circulation and a restoration after supplementation of serum with zinc have been reported [25,26]. Zinc deficiency is also related to the atrophy of thymus as well as other lymphoid tissues in animals and humans [27]. In fact, acrodermatitis enteropathica, a rare autosomal recessive inheritable disease that causes thymic atrophy, was observed in human models with zinc deficiency in as early as 1975 [28]. As a result, lymphopenia in both the central and peripheral lymphoid tissues is a characteristic feature of zinc deficiency, as T lymphocytes are progressively depleted from the spleen, lymphnodes, and peripheral blood.

Furthermore, the Th1/Th2 balance is affected by zinc [24,29]. CD4+ T cells can differentiate into subsets of effector cells that are distinguished most clearly on the basis of the cytokines they produce. Th1 cells, related to cellular immunity [27], secrete interleutkin-2 (IL-2) and interferon-γ (IFN-γ), which activate macrophages and are involved in delayed-type hypersensitivity responses [10]. Th2 cells, involved in humoral immunity [27], secrete IL-4, IL-5, IL-10, and IL-13, which are responsible for antibody responses and inhibition of several macrophage functions [10], and the pattern of the cytokines secreted by each subset acts by down regulating the functions of the opposite subset [27]. During zinc deficiency, the production of Th1 cytokines in particular IFN-γ, IL-2, and tumor necrosis factor (TNF)-α is reduced, whereas the levels of the Th2 cytokines IL-4, IL-6, and IL-10 were not affected in cell culture models and in vivo [24]. This Th1/Th2 imbalance characterized by low levels of IL-2 may have the effects of decreasing the activity of naturally killing cells and the differentiation and activation of CD8+ T cells, and may contribute to the immune dysregulation associated with HIV infection [10].

B-lymphocytes are less dependent on zinc for its proliferation [27] though, its development in the bone marrow is still blocked during zinc deficiency by reducing pre-B- and immature B-lymphocytes [27]. What's more, B-lymphocyte-mediated antibody responses are also depressed during zinc deficiency [30], both in the primary antibody response process, but also in the secondary antibody response process due to the lack of T helper cells' participation [31].

Besides, it was suggested that a biological decrease in memory cell functions also exists in the appearance of zinc deficiency since the suboptimal zinc groups produced only 43% as many plaque-forming cells (PFCs) per spleen as zinc adequate groups [32]. Moreover, zinc has also been proved to be essential for lymphocyte response to mitogens, and programmed cell death of lymphoid and myeloid origins [7].

Influence of zinc during embryonic immune development: even a marginal zinc deficiency may alter its development [27]. In animal offspring models, reductions in lymphoid organ size, γ-globulin concentrations, mitogenesis of peripheral blood lymphocytes, neutrophil function, and lower responses to T-dependent antigens were reported [27]. These results indicate that marginal levels of zinc during gestation profoundly affected the development of B cells and natural antibodies [27]. Zinc deficiency also affects the placentral transport of maternal antibodies from mother to the fetus, all of which normally provide protection until total maturation of the immune system [6].

Zinc supplementation in preschool children provoked a decrease in the percentage of delayed hypersensitivity anergic and hypoergic children, it raised the geometric means of CD3+, CD4+, and CD4+: CD8+ ratio, which represents an improvement of cellular immune status [33].

Summarizing from studies [34–38] on children recovering from severe malnutrition, the stimulation of immune capacity by zinc was confirmed [27].

Immunologic dysfunction during HIV infection is associated with the loss of critically important CD4+ T cells, which may be accelerated by zinc deficiency via its effect on hormone thymulin. Moreover, zinc-related Th1/Th2 ratio imbalance also accounts for the immune dysregulation associated with HIV-infection [10].

10.3.1.2 Effect of Zinc in Treatment

10.3.1.2.1 Effect of Zinc in the Treatment on HIV Virus

Zinc in vitro may have strong anti-HIV activity through inhibition of HIV-1 RNA transcription [39]. At high concentrations, zinc inhibits the activity of HIV-protease, thus reducing the virus's creation of new infectious particles [40]. Zinc regulates the expression of metallothionein, metallothionein-like proteins with documented antioxidant properties and protects several enzyme sulfhydryls from oxidation by oxidative oxygen species that may induce HIV-replication [10]. Besides, zinc's structural role in Cu–Zn COD contributes to a reduction of HIV-1 replication in TNF-α-activated cell lines [41]. However, negative facts are also needed to be considered. HIV is a zinc-dependent retrovirus and heightened availability of zinc may facilitate HIV replication [10]. Zinc stimulates the activity of the viral enzyme integrase, which integrates viral DNA into host DNA [42]. As for vertical transmission of HIV from mother to child, zinc deficiency may have detrimental effects [10]. Zinc deficiency may influence the maintenance of fetal integrity, which could lower a women's risk of transmitting the virus to the fetus [43], and shorten the duration of fetal exposure to infected cervicovaginal secretions [44].

10.3.1.2.2 Effect of Zinc in the Treatment on HIV Complications

Diarrhea, as a common complication of HIV, could be suppressed through zinc supplementation. The possible physiological principles underlying the effectiveness of zinc might include, inhibition of second messenger (cAMP, Cgmp, Ca^{2+})-induced Cl secretion, by blocking serosal K channel(s); stimulation of Na absorption via NHE3; besides, improved regeneration of intestinal epithelium and possibly enhanced immune response allowing for better clearance of pathogens [45]. Zinc is considered to be a key factor for the preservation of structural integrity of the intestinal. Several key enzymes located in the intestinal epithelial layer including those regulate the secretion of mucosal protective bicarbonate ions are metalloenzymes require zinc for their action. What's more, zinc also expressed to be beneficial for the oxidant-antioxidant balance within the intestinal mucosa as well as in the evolution of IBD thanks to Cu/Zn-SOD, which plays a relevant anti-inflammatory role by triggering the clearance of neutrophils accumulated in the intestinal mucosa [46].

According to the study in Uganda among HIV-infected children, two thirds of the children (170/247, 68.8%) were anaemic with low haemoglobin, which shows the anaemic situation another common complication of HIV [9]. Physiological doses of zinc, however, have the capability to significantly increase erythrocyte, hemoglobin, hematocrit, and leukocyte [47]. It is possible that zinc, which is related to many enzymatic systems, is also related to the formation and maturation of erythrocytes [47].

10.3.2 Effects of Intervention (Zinc): Infant, Children, Fatal Period (Pregnant Women)

10.3.2.1 Effects of Intervention (Zinc) on Zinc Level

Intervention trails, most preferably in the form of randomized-controlled trials, are best suited to examine the causal relationship between zinc status and HIV-related outcomes [10]. Studies conducted in children or pregnant women did not report the change in zinc level during trials, the consistent result also has been acquired in a 2014 study where a higher-than-base value and a comparatively higher-than-placebo median zinc level were observed, though not statistically significant [48]. Considering the scarce research results focused on children, information could also be indirectly gained through investigations on adults. Four trials conducted in HIV-infected adults analyzed the change in zinc concentration [14,49–51]. The zinc status at baseline was almost the same among trials (Table 10.1). Only 2 studies that reported the mean and SD could be combined [14,49]. However

TABLE 10.1 Zinc Status at Baseline

Study ID		Zinc status baseline		
Baum et al. (2010)	Serum zinc level: mean (SD)	All patients: 0.6 (0.1)mg/l Zinc: 0.6 (0.1) Placebo: 0.7 (0.2)		
Carcamo et al. (2006)	N (%)		Zinc	Placebo
		Normal:	6/8 (75)	5/9 (55.6)
		Marginal deficiency:	5/8 (62.5)	3/5 (60)
		Overt deficiency:	19/34 (55.9)	23/40 (57.5)
Green et al. (2005)	Serum zinc: mean (SD)	Zinc: 14.1 (2.8) umol/l Placebo: 13.3 (2.3)		
Mocchegiani et al. (1995)	Serum zinc: mean (SD) (ug/dl)		Fourth	Third
		Zinc	78.0 (4.3)	76.8 (2.7)
		Placebo	80.0 (3.1)	79.8 (3.5)
Bobat et al (2005)		U		
Fawzi et al. (2005) and Villamor et al. (2006)		U		

U: Unclear.

heterogeneity between 2 trials was too great to perform a metaanalysis ($X^2 = 10.22$, $I^2 = 80\%$). Participants in these two trials received moderate-dose, short-duration zinc supplementation. In Green et al. [49], the zinc level rose in both zinc and placebo arm without statistical difference ($P = 0.67$); Mocchegiani et al. [14]. only observed this in the intervention arm (Table 10.2). Participants received low-dose, long-duration zinc supplementation that had significantly higher zinc levels than those in the placebo group ($b = 0.04$; $P = 0.047$) [51]. In addition, participants who received high-dose, short-duration zinc supplementation had a better outcome [50] (Tables 10.1 and 10.2).

TABLE 10.2 Outcomes, Zinc versus Placebo (Continuous Data)

Study of subgroup	Zinc			Placebo			Mean difference IV, random, 95% CI
	Mean	SD	Total	Mean	SD	Total	
CHANGE OF ZINC LEVEL, ZINC VERSUS PLACEBO							
ADULTS							
Green et al. (2005)	0.0043	0.0096	32	0.0038	0.0053	34	0.00 [−0.00, 0.00]
Moccheginai et al. (1995) (stage 3)	0.0008	0.0004	18	−0.0012	0.0006	19	0.00 [0.00, 0.00]
Moccheginai et al. (1995) (stage 4)	0.0006	0.0006	10	−0.0023	0.0006	11	0.00 [0.00, 0.00]
CHANGE OF CD4 COUNTS, ZINC VERSUS PLACEBO							
ADULTS							
Moccheginai et al. (1995) (stage 3)	49	20	17	−111	21	18	160.00 [146.42, 173.58]
Moccheginai et al. (1995) (stage 4)	40	10	12	−30	10	10	70.00 [61.61, 78.39]
CHILDREN							
Bobat et al. (2005) (3 months)	0	9.8	44	−1	8.3	41	1.00 [−2.85, 4.85]
Bobat et al. (2005) (6 months)	1	9.8	44	−1	8.7	41	2.00 [−1.93. 5.93[
Bobat et al. (2005) (9 months)	1	10.1	44	0	9.1	41	1.00 [−3.08, 5.08]
PREGNANT WOMEN							
Fawzi et al (2005)	95	126	200	101	137	200	−6.00 [− 31.80, 19.80]

(Continued)

TABLE 10.2 (Continued)

Study of subgroup	Zinc			Placebo			Mean difference IV, random, 95% CI
	Mean	SD	Total	Mean	SD	Total	
CHANGE OF VIRAL LOADS							
ADULTS							
Green et al. (2005)	2.912	41.832	31	−1.735	43.453	32	4647.00 [−16412.72, 25706.7]
CHILDREN							
Bobat et al. (2005) (3 months)	0.1	0.66	44	0	0.73	41	0.10 [−0.20, 0.40]
Bobat et al. (2005) (6 months)	0.2	0.67	44	0	0.7	41	0.20 [−0.09, 0.49]
Bobat et al. (2005) (9 months)	0.2	0.64	44	0.1	0.79	41	0.10 [−0.21, 0.41]
PREGNANT WOMEN							
Villamor et al. (2006)	−0.18	0.65	50	0.01	0.56	50	−0.19 [−0.43, 0.05]

10.3.2.2 *Effects of Intervention (Zinc) on CD4+ Counts*

There are limited data from trails describing the effect of zinc intervention and treatment outcomes in HIV-infected children. Bobat et al. reported no effect of zinc supplementation on CD4+ counts among 96 HIV-infected children in South Africa [52]. The same result was indicated in Irlam's group. They calculated no difference in the mean percentage of CD4+ between the zinc and placebo groups (Irlam et al., [53]). In a recent randomized and double-blind, placebo-controlled trial, HIV-infected children were randomized to receive 20mg of elemental zinc as sulfate or a similar appearing and tasting preparation of placebo, daily for 24 weeks. Although the median CD4% value of the zinc group rose from 10% to 23% at 12 weeks and to 24.5% at 24 weeks, higher than the placebo group which changed from 11% to 20% at 12 weeks and to 22% at 24 weeks, the trend toward a higher increase in the zinc group is not statistically significant [48]. While other study on adults showed an increase of CD4+ counts in the zinc group, but fell in the placebo or no treatment group [14]. Zinc supplementation was proved effective in preventing immunological failure in adults, which was defined as a drop in CD4+ counts to <200cells/mm^3 [51]. However, CD4+ counts increased in HIV-infected mothers at 6 weeks post-partum in both zinc and placebo groups, without a statistically significant difference ($P = 0.97$) [54] (Table 10.2).

10.3.2.3 *Effects of Intervention (Zinc) on Viral Load*

There was no significant change in HIV viral load in either zinc or placebo group in adult participants during a 28-day intervention [49]. The median viral loads at 12 and 24 weeks in the zinc group and placebo group were comparable [48]. Likewise, log10 viral loads were similar between the zinc supplementation and placebo groups during a 6-month treatment in children [52]. The Villamor et al. [55] selected 100 women for viral load analysis. The baseline sample was collected at gestation week 22 on average and the follow-up measurement at 6 weeks post-partum. Log10 viral loads decreased from baseline to the follow-up measurement in the zinc but not in the placebo group. The risk of having a high viral load (>100 000 copies/ml) at the post-partum visit was not significantly lower in women who received zinc (RR = 0.77; 95% CI: 0.42–1.40; $P = 0.38$) (Table 10.2). All these and other studies lead to a conclusion that zinc, does not affect HIV viral loads [56].

10.3.2.4 *Effects of Intervention (Zinc) on Opportunistic Infections*

In children, the proportion of scheduled and illness visits at which children were diagnosed with watery diarrhea ($P = 0.001$) or pneumonia ($P = 0.07$) was smaller for the zinc group than for the placebo group; the number of illness visits per month was slightly lower in the zinc arm (0.11 illness visits/month) than in the placebo arm (0.16 illness visits/month, $P = 0.05$) [51]. Three studies reported opportunistic infections in HIV-infected adults, of which only two could be combined in a meta-analysis [14,49]. Zinc supplementation seemed to help reduce the risk of infection in HIV-infected adults. An intent-to-treat analysis in Baum et al. [51] showed that zinc supplementation significantly reduced the rate of diarrhea over time by more than half in adult patients (OR = 0.4; 95% CI: 0.183–0.981; $P = 0.019$). Diarrhea was significantly associated with lower mean plasma levels of zinc (0.59 ± 0.11 vs. 0.68 ± 0.21 mg/l).

Mortality of adults and children in the zinc group was slightly lower than that of placebo group, but without statistical significance (RR = 0.79, 95% CI: 0.25–2.44, $P = 0.6$; RR = 0.31, 95% CI: 0.07–1.42, $P = 0.13$, respectively). A randomized-controlled trial in Uganda focused on zinc adjunct therapy in cases of severe pneumonia among children, out of whom 55 were HIV positive (28 in the zinc group and 27 in the placebo group). Once-daily dose of placebo or zinc were given in addition to standard antibiotics for 7 days. This small sampled study showed different mortality rates between two groups, with 7 out of 27 (25.9%) in placebo group versus 0 out of 28 (0%) in zinc group [54]. However, three mothers in a zinc group died after delivery while none died in the placebo group for reasons that remain unclear [54].

10.3.2.5 Effects of Intervention (Zinc) on MTCT

Zinc supplementation had no significant effect on MTCT of HIV at birth (0–21 days) (RR = 1.37; 95% CI: 0.49–3.85; $P = 0.55$) or at 6 weeks post-partum (RR = 1.40; 95% CI: 0.67–2.95; $P = 0.37$). This was determined by testing whole blood samples from babies using the amplicor HIV-1 detection kit version 1.5 [50]. This also agrees with Fawzi's study, which shows no statistically significant difference in the relative risk of mother-to-child transmission between the zinc and placebo groups at birth (RR = 1.37; 95% Cl: 0.49, 3.85; $P = 0.55$) or at six weeks (RR = 1.40; 95% CI: 0.67, 2.95; $P = 0.37$) [54].

Compared with placebo, zinc had no significant effect on risk of death during the foetal (RR = 1.38; 95% CI: 0.70–2.75; $P = 0.35$) and early post-partum periods (RR = 1.48; 95% CI: 0.57–3.79; $P = 0.42$) (Table 10.3). No adverse events attributable to zinc supplementation were observed. However, indicators of zinc toxicity, such as copper status, were not monitored except in one trial, in which zinc supplementation did not induce copper deficiency [50]. Another potential adverse effect of zinc supplementation might lie on concentration of hemoglobin and other hematologic indicators [54]. It is possible this negative effect on hemoglobin is due to zinc's interaction with iron thus making adverse effects on iron absorption [57]. What's more, zinc intervention was even reported related to a threefold increase in the risk of wasting [55].

10.4 IMPLICATION FOR FUTURE RESEARCH

Most current studies mainly focused on the effect and safety of micronutrient supplementation or dietary supplementation in patients with HIV infection [58–60]. Micronutrients, however, often interact with each other [61], and thus, the efficacy of a particular trace element should be evaluated in single-interventional trials. Studies evaluating zinc supplementation as single interventions may have been underpowered to assess efficacy outcomes. There is a tremendous need for clinical research on this (Table 10.3) issue by intervention trials and the influence of treatment dose and duration on the efficacy. More trials are needed in resource-limited countries where the burden of disease is greatest, as the initial nutritional status and other characteristics of participants may influence the efficacy of zinc supplementation [62]; studies should consider investigating its role in patients at particular HIV stages.

TABLE 10.3 Outcomes, Zinc Versus Placebo (Dichotomous Data)

Study or subgroup	Zinc		Placebo		Weight (%)	Risk ratio M-H, random, 95% CI
	Events	Total	Events	Total		
OPPORTUNISTIC INFECTION						
ADULTS						
Green et al. (2005)	4	32	3	34	18.4	1.42 [0.34,5.84]
Mocchegiani et al. (1995)	9	29	13	28	81.6	0.67 [0.34, 1.31]
Subtotal (95% CI)	13	61	16	62	100.0	0.77 [0.42, 1.41]
Heterogeneity: $s^2 = 0.00$; $v^2 = 0.90$, df = 1 ($P = 0.34$); I2 = 0%						
Test for overall effect: $Z = 0.85$ ($P = 0.39$)						
MORTALITY						
ADULTS						
Baum et al. (2010)	11	115	8	116	35	1.39 [0.58, 3.32]
Carcamo et al. (2006)	0	81	0	78		Not estimable
Green et al. (2005)	0	32	0	34		Not estimable
Mocchegiani et al. (1995)	5	29	11	28	33.9	0.44 [0.17, 1.10]
Subtotal (95% CI)	16	257	19	256	69.0	0.79 [0.25, 2.44]
Heterogeneity: s2 = 0.45; v2 = 3.17, df = 1 ($P = 0.08$); I2 = 68%						
Test for overall effect: $Z = 0.41$ ($P = 0.68$)						
CHILDREN						
Bobat et al. (2005)	2	46	7	50	22.2	0.31 [0.07, 1.42]
Test for overall effect: $Z = 1.51$ ($P = 0.13$)						
PREGNANT WOMEN						
Fawzi et al. (2005)	3	200	0	200	8.8	7.00 [0.36, 134.64]
Test for overall effect: $Z = 1.29$ ($P = 0.20$)						
total (95% CI)	21	503	26	506	100.0	0.78 [0.29, 2.05]
MOTHER-TO-CHILD TRANSMISSION OF HIV						
AT BIRTH (0–21 DAYS)						
Villamor et al. (2006)	8	141	6	145	100.0	1.37 [0.49, 3.85]
Test for overall effect: $Z = 0.60$ ($P = 0.55$)						

(Continued)

TABLE 10.3 (Continued)

Study or subgroup	Zinc		Placebo		Weight (%)	Risk ratio M-H, random, 95% CI
	Events	Total	Events	Total		
BY 6 WEEKS						
Villamor et al. (2006)	15	141	11	145	100.0	1.40 [0.67, 2.95]
Test for overall effect: $Z = 0.89$, ($P = 0.37$)						
FOETAL OUTCOMES						
MISARRIAGE						
Villamor et al. (2006)	5	198	3	199	100.0	1.68 [0.41, 6.91]
Test for overall effect: $Z = 0.71$ ($P = 0.48$)						
STILL BIRTH						
Villamor et al. (2006)	13	198	10	199	100.0	1.31 [0.59, 2.91]
Test for overall effect: $Z = 0.65$ ($P = 0.51$)						
FOETAL DEATH						
Villamor et al. (2006)	18	198	13	198	100.0	1.31[0.70, 2.75]
Test for overall effect: $Z = 0.93$ ($P = 0.35$)						
NEONATAL DEATH						
Villamor et al. (2006)	10	180	7	186	100.0	1.48 [0.57, 3.79]
Test for overall effect: $Z = 0.81$ ($P = 0.42$)						

References

[1] UNAIDS and World Health Organization: AIDS Epidemic Update. Geneva, Switzerland, 2009.

[2] UNAIDS and World Health Organization: AIDS Epidemic Update. Geneva, Switzerland, 2006.

[3] Semba R, Tang A. Micronutrients and the pathogenesis of human immunodeficiency virus infection. Br J Nutr 1999;81:181–9.

[4] Baeten JM, McClelland RS, Richardson BA, et al. Vitamin A deficiency and the acute phase response among HIV-1-infected and -uninfected women in Kenya. J Acquir Immune Defic Syndr 2002;31:243–9.

[5] Wellinghausen N, Kirchner H, Rink L. The immunobiology of zinc. Immunol Today 1997;18:519–21.

[6] Shankar AH, Prasad AS. Zinc and immune function: the biological basis of altered resistance to infection. Am J Epidemiol 1998;68:447S–63S.

[7] Baum MK, Shor-Posner G, Campa A. Zinc status in human immunodeficiency virus infection[J]. J Nutr 2000;130(5):1421S–23S.

[8] Coovadia HM, Bobat R. Zinc deficiency and supplementation in HIV/AIDS. Nutr Res 2002;22:179–91.
[9] Ndeezi G, Tumwine JK, Bolann BJ, et al. Zinc status in HIV infected Ugandan children aged 1–5 years: a cross sectional baseline survey[J]. BMC Pediatr 2010;10(1):68.
[10] Kupka R, Fawzi PH. Zinc nutrition and HIV infection[J]. Nutr Rev 2002;60(3):69–79.
[11] Baum MK, Campa A, Lai S, et al. Zinc status in human immunodeficiency virus type 1 infection and illicit drug use. Clin Infect Dis 2003;37:S117–23.
[12] Fufa H, Umeta M, Taffess S, et al. Nutritional and immunological status and their associations among HIV-infected adults in Addis Ababa, Ethiopia. Food Nutr Bull 2009; 30:227–32.
[13] Zazzo JF, Rouveix B, Rajagopalon P. Effect of zinc on the immune status of zinc-depleted AIDS related complex patients. Clin Nutr 1989;8:259–61.
[14] Mocchegiani E, Veccia S, Ancarani F, et al. Benefit of oral zinc supplementation as an adjunct to zindovudine (AZT) therapy against opportunistic infections in AIDS. Int J Immunopharmacol 1995;17:719–27.
[15] Deloria-Knoll M, Steinhoff M, Semba RD, et al. Effect of zinc and vitamin A supplementation on antibody responses to a pneumococcal conjugate vaccine in HIV-positive injection drug users: a randomized trial. Vaccine 2006;24:1670–9.
[16] Tang AM, Graham NM, Kirby AJ, et al. Dietary micronutrient intake and risk of progression to acquired immunodeficiency syndrome (AIDS) in human immuno- deficiency virus type 1 (HIV-1)-infected homosexual men. Am J Epidemiol 1993;138:937–51.
[17] Tang AM, Graham NM, Saah AJ. Effects of micronutrient intake on survival in human immunodeficiency virus type 1 infection. Am J Epidemiol 1996;143:1244–56.
[18] Abrams B, Duncan D, Hertz-Picciotto I. A prospective study of dietary intake and acquired immune deficiency syndrome in HIV-seropositive homosexual men. J Acquir Immune Defic Syndr 1993;6:949–58.
[19] Visser ME, et al. Plasma vitamin A and zinc levels in HIV-infected adults in Cape Town, South Africa. Br J Nutr 2003;89(4):475–82.
[20] Ndagije F, Baribwira C, Coulter JBS. Micronutrients and T-cell subsets: a comparison between HIV-infected and uninfected, severely malnourished Rwandan children[J]. Ann Trop Paediatr 2007;27(4):269–75.
[21] Bhandari N, Bahl R, Hambidge KM, et al. Increased diarrhoeal and respiratory morbidity in association with zinc deficiency—a preliminary report[J]. Acta Paediatr 1996; 85(2):148–50.
[22] Arora R, Kulshreshtha S, Mohan G, et al. Estimation of serum zinc and copper in children with acute diarrhea[J]. Biol Trace Elem Res 2006;114(1–3):121–6.
[23] Eley BS, Sive AA, Abelse L, et al. Growth and micronutrient disturbances in stable, HIV-infected children in Cape Town[J]. Ann Trop Paediatr 2002;22(1):19–23.
[24] Haase H, Rink L. The immune system and the impact of zinc during aging[J]. Immun Ageing 2009;6(9):1–17.
[25] Dardenne M, et al. In vivo and in vitro studies of thymulin in marginally zinc-deficient mice. Eur J Immunol 1984;14(5):454–8.
[26] Prasad AS, et al. Serum thymulin in human zinc deficiency. J Clin Invest 1988;82(4):1202.
[27] Salgueiro MJ, Zubillaga M, Lysionek A, et al. Zinc status and immune system relationship[J]. Biol Trace Elem Res 2000;76(3):193–205.
[28] Nelder KH, Hambidge KM, Walravens PA. Zinc therapy of acrodermatitis enteropathica. J Invest Dermatol 1975;64(4), Malden, MA: Blackwell Science Inc.
[29] Prasad AS. Effects of zinc deficiency on immune functions. J Trace Elem Exp Med 2000;13(1):1–20.
[30] Shankar AH, Genton B, Semba RD, et al. Effect of vitamin A supplementation on morbidity due to Plasmodium falciparum in young children in Papua New Guinea: a randomised trial[J]. Lancet 1999;354(9174):203–9.

[31] Ripa S, Ripa R. Zinc and immune function[J]. Minerva Med 1994;86(7–8):315–8.
[32] Fraker PJ, Gershwin ME, Good RA, et al. Interrelationships between zinc and immune function[C]. Fed Proc 1986;45(5):1474–9.
[33] Sazawal S, Black RE, Bhan MK, et al. Efficacy of zinc supplementation in reducing the incidence and prevalence of acute diarrhea—a community-based, double-blind, controlled trial[J]. Am J Clin Nutr 1997;66(2):413–8.
[34] Gibson RS, Huddle JM. Suboptimal zinc status in pregnant Malawian women: its association with low intakes of poorly available zinc, frequent reproductive cycling, and malaria. Am J Clin Nutr 1998;67(4):702–9.
[35] Black RE. Therapeutic and preventive effects of zinc on serious childhood infectious diseases in developing countries. Am J Clin Nutr 1998;68(2):476S–9S.
[36] Ruz M, et al. A 14-mo zinc-supplementation trial in apparently healthy Chilean preschool children. Am J Clin Nutr 1997;66(6):1406–13.
[37] Sempertegui F, et al. Effects of short-term zinc supplementation on cellular immunity, respiratory symptoms, and growth of malnourished Equadorian children. Eur J Clin Nutr 1996;50(1):42–6.
[38] Grazioso CF, et al. The effect of zinc supplementation on parasitic reinfestation of Guatemalan schoolchildren. Am J Clin Nutr 1993;57(5):673–8.
[39] Haraguchi Y, Sakurai H, Hussain S, et al. Inhibition of HIV-1 infection by zinc group metal compounds[J]. Antiviral Res 1999;43(2):123–33.
[40] Sprietsma JE. Cysteine, glutathione (GSH) and zinc and copper ions together are effective, natural, intracellular inhibitors of (AIDS) viruses. Med Hypotheses 1999; 52(6):529–38.
[41] Edeas MA, Peltier E, Claise C, et al. Immunocytochemical study of uptake of exogenous carrier- free copper-zinc superoxide dismutase by peripheral blood lymphocytes. Cell Mol Biol (Noisy-le-grand) 1996;42:1137–43.
[42] Frankel AD, Bredt DS, Pabo CO. Tat protein from human immunodeficiency virus forms a metallinkeddimer. Science 1988;240:70–3.
[43] O' Dell BL. Role of zinc in plasma membrane function. J Nutr 2000;130:1432S–36S.
[44] Sikorski R, Juszkiewicz T, Paszkowski T. Zinc status in women with premature rupture of membranes at term. Obstet Gynecol 1990;76:675–7.
[45] Hoque KM, Sarker R, Guggino SE, et al. A new insight into pathophysiological mechanisms of zinc in diarrhea[J]. Ann N Y Acad Sci 2009;1165(1):279–84.
[46] Faa G, Nurchi VM, Ravarino A, et al. Zinc in gastrointestinal and liver disease[J]. Coord Chem Rev 2008;252(10):1257–69.
[47] Kilic M, Baltaci AK, Gunay M. Effect of zinc supplementation on hematological parameters in athletes. Biol Trace Elem Res 2004;100(1):31–8.
[48] Lodha R, Shah N, Mohari N, Mukherjee A, Vajpayee M, Singh R, et al. Immunologic effect of zinc supplementation in HIV-infected children receiving highly active antiretroviral therapy: a randomized, double-blind, placebo-controlled trial. J Acquir Immune Defic Syndr 2014;66(4):386–92.
[49] Green JA, Lewin SR, Wightman F, et al. A randomized controlled trial of oral zinc on the immune response to tuberculosis in HIV-infected patients. Int J Tuberc Lung Dis 2005; 9:1378–84.
[50] Carcamo C, Hooton T, Weiss NS, et al. Randomized controlled trial of zinc supplementation for persistent diarrhea in adults with HIV-1 infection. J Acquir Immune Defic Syndr 2006;43:197–201.
[51] Baum MK, Lai S, Sales S, et al. Randomized, controlled clinical trial of zinc supplementation to prevent immunological failure in HIV-infected adults. Clin Infect Dis 2010;50:1653–60.
[52] Bobat R, Coovadia H, Stephen C, et al. Safety and efficacy of zinc supplementation for children with HIV-1 infection in South Africa: a randomised double-blind placebo-controlled trial. Lancet 2005;366:1862–7.

[53] Irlam JH, Siegfried N, Visser ME, Rollins NC. Micronutrient supplementation for children with HIV infection. Cochrane Database Syst Rev 2013(10) Art. No.: CD010666. http://dx.doi.org/10.1002/14651858.CD010666
[54] Fawzi WW, Villamor E, Msamanga GI, et al. Trial of zinc supplements in relation to pregnancy outcomes, hematologic indicators, and T cell counts among HIV-1–infected women in Tanzania[J]. Am J Clin Nutr 2005;81(1):161–7.
[55] Villamor E, Aboud S, Koulinska IN, et al. Zinc supplementation to HIV-1-infected pregnant women: effects on maternal anthropometry, viral load, and early mother-to-child transmission[J]. Eur J Clin Nutr 2006;60(7):862–9.
[56] McHenry MS, Dixit A, Vreeman RC. A systematic review of nutritional supplementation in HIV-infected children in resource-limited settings. J Int Assoc Provid AIDS Care 2014. http://dx.doi.org/10.1177/2325957414539044
[57] Solomons NW, Ruz M. Zinc and iron interaction: concepts and perspectives in the developing world. Nutr Res 1997;17(1):177–85.
[58] Kelly P, Musonda R, Kafwembe E, et al. Micronutrient supplementation in the AIDS diarrhoea-wasting syndrome in Zambia: a randomized controlled trial. AIDS 1999; 13:495–500.
[59] Jiamton S, Pepin J, Suttent R, et al. A randomized trial of the impact of multiple micronutrient supplementation on mortality among HIV-infected individuals living in Bangkok. AIDS 2003;17:2461–9.
[60] Irlam JJH, Visser MME, Rollins NN, Siegfried N. Micronutrient supplementation in children and adults with HIV infection. Cochrane Database Syst Rev 2005(4) Art. No.: CD003650. http://dx.doi.org/10.1002/14651858.
[61] Wieringa FT, Dijkhuizen MA, West CE. Redistribution of vitamin A after iron supplementation in Indonesian infants. Am J Epidemiol 2003;77:651–7.
[62] Dardenne M, Savino W, Gagnerault MC, et al. Neuroendocrine control of thymic hormonal production. I. Prolactin stimulates in vivo and in vitro the production of thymulin by human and murine thymic epithelial cells[J]. Endocrinology 1989;125(1):3–12.

CHAPTER

11

HIV AIDS in India: A Nutritional Panorama

Deepika Anand and Seema Puri

Department of Food and Nutrition, Institute of Home Economics, University of Delhi, New Delhi, India

One out of every six people in the world is an Indian, and this mammoth population of India makes tackling health issues a huge challenge. Human immunodeficiency virus/acquired immunodeficiency syndrome (HIV/AIDS) poses a major public health threat in India and has the potential to undermine the significant progress that has been made in poverty alleviation and agriculture and rural development over the past 50 years [1].

11.1 HIV/AIDS IN INDIA: STABILIZATION OF THE EPIDEMIC

The first HIV-positive case was reported in 1986 in Chennai, Tamil Nadu. Since then, the infection has spread rapidly from urban to rural areas and from high-risk groups (HRGs) to the general population. With numerous efforts the spread of infection has stabilized over the years but even today, in a country of more than 1.2 billion people, an estimated 2.1 million people were living with HIV/AIDS in 2011 (PLHIV) [2]. The adult (age 15–49 years) HIV prevalence at the national level has declined from 0.41% in 2001 to 0.36% in 2006 to 0.27% in 2011 (0.32% in males and 0.22% in females). According to the UNAIDS [3] report, India is estimated to have the third highest number of PLHIV (6%), after South Africa (18%) and Nigeria (9%).

Of 2.1 million PLHIV in India in 2011, children (younger than age 15 years) account for 7% of all infections and 86% are between ages 15 and 49 years. Of all HIV infections, 39% occur in women. It is estimated that approximately 1.48 lakh (1.12 lakhs to 1.78 lakhs) people died of

Health of HIV Infected People, Volume 2.
DOI: http://dx.doi.org/10.1016/B978-0-12-800767-9.00011-X

AIDS-related causes in 2011, and deaths among HIV-infected children account for 7% of all AIDS-related deaths. The estimated number of new HIV infections has also declined steadily over the past decade by approximately 57% from 2000 to 2011.

India's initial response to the HIV/AIDS challenge was in the form of setting up of an AIDS Task Force by the Indian Council of Medical Research (ICMR) and a National AIDS Committee (NAC) in 1990. A Medium Term Plan (MTP 1990–1992) was launched in four states, namely, Tamil Nadu, Maharashtra, West Bengal, and Manipur, and four metropolitan cities, namely, Chennai, Kolkata, Mumbai, and Delhi. In 1992, the government launched the first National AIDS Control Programme (NACP-I, 1992–1999) with the objective of slowing the spread of HIV infections to reduce morbidity, mortality, and impact of AIDS in the country. An autonomous National AIDS Control Organization (NACO) was set up to implement the project in 1993, which holds the responsibility of national coordination of the AIDS control programs. Each state has a State AIDS Control Society that works with nongovernmental organizations and private-sector organizations that implement targeted interventions. In 1999, the second National AIDS Control Programme (NACP-II) was launched, with the focus shifted from raising awareness to changing behavior, decentralization of program implementation at the state level, and greater involvement of the NGOs. NACP-III (2007–2012) had the overall goal of halting and reversing the epidemic in India by integrating programs for prevention, care, support, and treatment. Currently, NACP-IV is operational, with the objectives of 80% reduction in new infections in high-prevalence states and 60% in low-prevalence states. It is estimated that the scale-up of free ART since 2004 has saved more than 1.5 lakh lives in the country (until 2011) by averting deaths due to AIDS-related causes. With the current scale-up of ART services, it is estimated it will avert approximately 50,000–60,000 deaths annually in the next 5 years.

With the stabilization of the epidemic and with better availability and use of ART medications, the country is faced with newer challenges. The country is already facing the dual burden of nutrition. There is a huge undernourished population and there are increasing incidences of noncommunicable diseases (NCDs). With a large percentage of the population facing the problem of undernutrition, especially children and women, improvement in the nutritional status of PLHIV holds utmost priority for improving their quality of life (QoL) and also breaking the vicious cycle of malnutrition.

This chapter intends to provide the readers with a panoramic view of the infection in the country. It touches on the priorities in adults and in pediatric HIV patients. It primarily focuses on the nutritional status and knowledge, attitude, and practices (KAP) of infected individuals, and it also provides a glimpse of the QoL. Although a number of studies have examined KAP regarding HIV/AIDS, there is scant information on nutrition-specific KAP of HIV-positive individuals in India. The chapter also touches on the progress and the challenges the country has made with reference to pediatric HIV infection.

11.2 QoL OF PLHIV

WHO [4] defines QoL as individuals' perceptions of their position in life in the context of the culture and value systems in which they live and in relation to their goals, expectations, standards, and concerns. It is a multidimensional concept, and Figure 11.1 depicts the four major domains of QoL that are often affected in HIV/AIDS patients [5]. HIV infection and psychiatric disorders present a complex relationship and have received special attention in the past decade because of their impact in the personal, sexual, social, and occupational lives of PLHIV [6]. Among the various psychiatric disorders frequently identified in PLHIV, depression is the most prevalent.

HIV/AIDS patients struggle with numerous psychosocial problems such as stigma, poverty, depression, substance abuse, and culture beliefs,

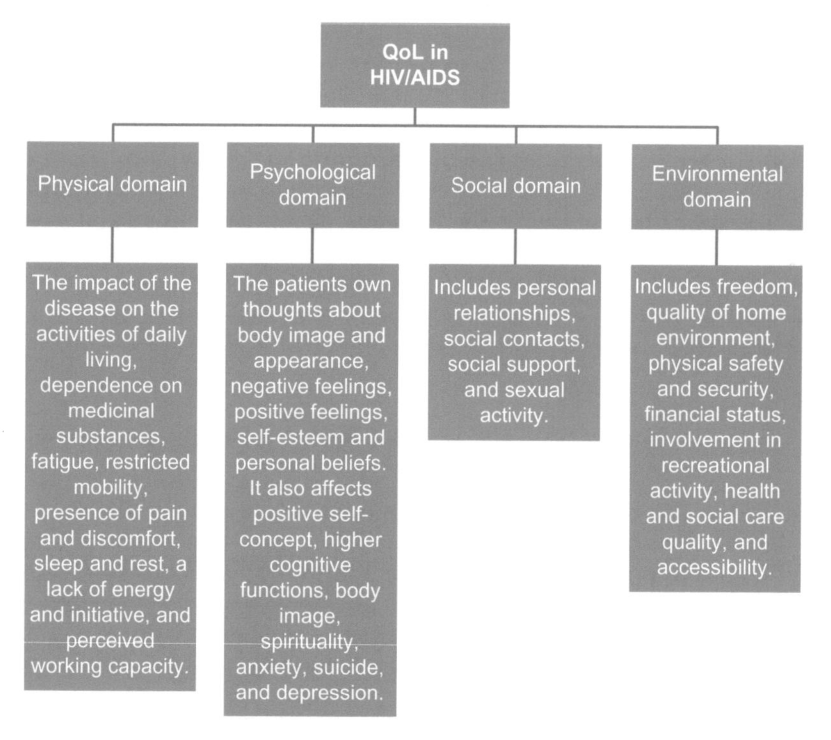

FIGURE 11.1 QoL domains. *Source: Adapted from Basavaraj et al. (2010) [5].*

which can affect their QoL not only from a physical health aspect but also from mental health and social health points of view and cause numerous problems in the activities and interests of the patients [7]. A study by Anand and Puri [8] among HIV-positive adults in India using the WHO QoL-HIV BREF scale found that the sample scored the maximum in the domain of spirituality, religion, and personal beliefs (14.5 ± 2.9) and the minimum in the level of independence (11.9 ± 3.3). They believed that they were suffering because they were chosen to suffer by the supreme power and it was their destiny. However, this did not affect their faith in the supreme power. Spirituality among HIV-positive individuals is perceived as a bridge between hopelessness and meaningfulness in life.

Wig et al. [9] studied the impact of HIV/AIDS on the QoL of such patients in Northern India. They concluded that QoL is associated with education, income, occupation, family support, and clinical categories of the patients. Another study from India reported that the QoL of PLHIV was in the moderate category [10–15], scoring the maximum in SRPB and the minimum in social relationships [8].

The social relationship domain measures personal relationships, social support, sexual activity, and social inclusion. Low score on the social front could be attributed to the fact that the PLHIV restrained themselves from social interactions (i.e., making friends, participating in social gatherings, accepting help from their relatives or friends, etc.) because of their positive status and the social stigma attached. Their study also tried to find an association between the QoL of PLHIV and their nutritional status. It was found that as the subjects changed their nutritional stage from "normal" to "malnourished," the QoL scores in all domains decreased significantly. This indicates that decline in the physical health and nutritional status deteriorates the QoL of PLHIV.

Psychological disturbances, such as mental illness, depression, and personal beliefs, and other sociological factors, such as poverty, family, and food insecurity, amplify and complicate malnutrition and effects of HIV.

11.3 NUTRITIONAL STATUS OF ADULT PLHIV

Nutrition plays a crucial role throughout the course of HIV disease. The links between nutrition and HIV/AIDS amplify the negative effects of HIV infection on human development at individual, household, community, and national levels [16]. BMI is considered an important predictor of survival of PLHIV [17,18]. A study by Anand and Puri [8] among 400 PLHIV from New Delhi, India, indicated 39% of the sample to be underweight, with BMI less than 18.5 kg/m^2. The mean BMI of 19.7 ± 3.6 kg/m^2 was comparable with the data obtained in Thailand by Ludy et al. [19]. HIV infection has been associated with a syndrome of lipoatrophy, which is characterized by the loss of subcutaneous adipose tissue; the legs and lower trunk are most affected in men and women, and the upper trunk is less affected [10,11]. Scherzer et al. [12] suggest that despite the presence of HIV-associated lipoatrophy, the use of waist circumference (WC) and hip circumference (HC) is a highly effective screening method for identifying health and metabolic risk. The mean WC of the sample of 400 PLHIV from India was 73.6 ± 9.8 cm (52–110 cm), which was lower than the recommendations by WHO and IOTF (2000) of less than 90 cm for males and less than 80 cm for females. The study further reported that the subjects with BMI less than 18.5 kg/m^2 had the lowest CD4 count as compared with subjects in higher BMI stages; as the BMI stage improved, the CD4 count also increased significantly ($P < 0.05$). BMI and body circumferences were also found to correlate positively with the CD4 count ($P < 0.01$) [8].

Presence of malnutrition increases the susceptibility to infection, which can impair strength and functional ability and adversely affect the outcome in PLHIV [13–15]. PLHIV requires early identification of risk for malnutrition by including routine nutritional assessments in the management of HIV to determine the level of deficit and appropriate nutrition intervention [20]. This helps to prevent and treat unintentional weight loss and muscle wasting prevalent in HIV patients [21]. In the same sample of 400 PLHIV from India, using the Mini Nutritional Assessment Scale, Anand and Puri [8] found that nearly 50% of the sample were at risk for malnutrition; 34% were malnourished and only approximately 15% were in the normal category. This reiterates the importance of conducting nutritional assessments of PLHIV for early detection of decline in clinical health.

Nutritional intake is often an overlooked factor in the progression of HIV disease, although the relation between nutrition and immune function is well-established. In India, there are limited studies that report the actual intake of nutrients and their quality of diet. Anand and Puri [22] reported that poor dietary energy intakes are prevalent among Indian PLHIV, indicating a direction toward declining nutritional health. For the day's total energy intake, the mean contribution of carbohydrate was 60%, of protein was 15%, and of fat was 25%. However, the contributions were within the prescribed limits but, as cited in literature, the diets of PLHIV should be low in fat and high in protein for overall better diet quality. Therefore, the diets of Indian PLHIV may require alterations in terms of reducing the quantity of fat and increasing the level of protein. Further, they also reported poor micronutrient intakes by Indian PLHIV as follows: 40% for calcium; 73% for riboflavin; 55% for niacin; 95% for folic acid; 73% for vitamin B12; 59% for copper; and 84% for zinc. An interview session with the subjects revealed that the consumption of fresh fruits was low and the majority of diets comprised staples (wheat/rice and pulses). Pulses were the major source of protein for vegetarians; among nonvegetarians, chicken was the major source of protein.

A study by Subbaraman et al. [23] reported the prevalence of anemia among PLHIV to be 41% in the Southern part of India. Anemia is independently associated with decreased QoL, accelerated disease progression, and increased mortality in HIV-infected individuals [24,25]. Low BMI is associated with many nutrient deficiencies, including iron, folate, and B12, that contribute directly to anemia. Three of the strongest factors associated with anemia—TB, immunosuppression, and malnutrition—exacerbate each other in a synergistic manner [23].

11.4 NUTRITIONAL KAP OF HIV-POSITIVE INDIVIDUALS

KAP studies focus specifically on the KAP (behavior) for a certain topic [26]. In India, there are several programs for improving KAP regarding HIV-positive patients. The "Universities Talk AIDS" program (UTA) is run by the Indian government as a strategy to prevent HIV/AIDS by informing students and encouraging discussion about healthy human sexuality. UTA works through the National Service Scheme (NSS) and began on an experimental basis in 1991 in 59 universities [27]. The Family Planning Association of India's Sex Education, Counseling, Research Training/Therapy (SECRT) project spearheads the incorporation of sex education into its family planning activities [28]. The project's focus is on educated urban youth aged 15–29 years—a sector that will become India's future parents and leaders but that has been neglected by the government and voluntary organizations.

A number of KAP studies have been performed among PLHIV in India, but none addresses the issue of nutrition [29–32]. Anand and Puri [33] reported that basic HIV-related knowledge was lacking among PLHIV from New Delhi, India. However, their knowledge of nutritional aspects was moderate. The PLHIV in the present sample had a positive attitude toward the disease and recognized the importance of nutrition in HIV. The study also identified a few areas where PLHIV did not have a positive attitude, and effective messages may be crafted and delivered to remove the negativity and to strengthen the belief that good and nutritious food is important for healthy living. Food safety and healthy food choices are two of these identified areas. Benjamin et al. [34] also reported that there exists a gap in knowledge about AIDS and spread of HIV among PLHIV from Ludhiana, Punjab. Lal et al. [35] identified the need for strengthening national AIDS education and awareness campaigns, especially for girls and those in rural areas to increase the knowledge about HIV/AIDS in the country. Anand and Puri [33] also found that the practices and overall KAP score of those using ART were significantly higher than those not using ART. The reason could be that those using ART are more sensitive toward the issue of HIV/AIDS and, hence, are more attentive toward the HIV-related messages and information and take better care of themselves in terms of better nutrition-related practices.

11.5 HIV-AFFECTED INFANTS AND CHILDREN

The HIV epidemic remains a serious challenge and continues to take its toll, particularly on vulnerable populations such as children. A total of 1.42 lakh children (age 0–14 years) are estimated to be living with HIV in India, with approximately 14,000 new HIV infections annually. Mother-to-child transmission (MTCT) of HIV is the primary route of transmission for HIV among children. It is estimated that without any intervention, the risk of transmission of HIV from an infected mother to her child is between 20% and 45%. With effective use of antiretroviral (ARV) drugs, this risk decreases significantly. The government of India, in turn, has committed itself to work toward achieving the global target of elimination of new HIV infections among children by 2015.

11.6 MOTHER-TO-CHILD TRANSMISSION

MTCT is by far the most significant route of transmission of HIV infection in children younger than age 15 years. HIV can be transmitted during pregnancy, during childbirth, or during breastfeeding with equal frequency. Without intervention, the risk of transmission from an infected mother to her child is much lower in developed countries, ranging from 15% to 25%. This difference is largely attributed to differences in breast-feeding practices. Exposure to HIV transmission continues for as long as a child is breastfed. Prolonged breastfeeding (up to 18–24 months) accounts for increased risk of HIV transmissions to infants compared with shorter periods of breastfeeding (up to 6 months). Mixed feeding, the norm for the majority of women in India (>90%), has been shown to nearly double the risk of postnatal HIV transmission.

The past decade has seen accumulation of a significant amount of research evidence and programmatic experience regarding ARV prophylaxis to prevent PMTCT of HIV infection and treatment eligibility for ARV therapy (ART) initiation in HIV-infected pregnant women. There is enough evidence now that ARV interventions for either the HIV-infected mother or her infant can significantly reduce the risk of postnatal transmission of HIV through breastfeeding. This has major implications on how HIV-infected women might choose to feed their infants because exclusive replacement feedings (ERF) have not been feasible in resource-limited settings, including India. Breastfeeding is a key strategy for infant survival in these settings but has the inherent risk of transmission of HIV infection. Thus, balancing the risk of infants acquiring HIV through breast milk with the risk of death from causes other than HIV, particularly malnutrition and diarrhea, has been a big dilemma. In this context, the availability of evidence that ARV prophylaxis makes breastfeeding safer by reducing the risk of HIV transmission through breast milk is a major breakthrough toward improving HIV-free survival in exposed infants.

Therefore, the NACP launched prevention of parent-to-child (HIV) transmission (PPTCT) of HIV services in 2002. This provided access to HIV testing services for all pregnant women enrolled in antenatal care (ANC), along with provision of ARV prophylaxis with a single dose of nevirapine (SD-NVP) at the time of delivery to mother and baby. These services were rapidly scaled-up across India during the NACP-III (2007–2012). Although implemented effectively in the high HIV prevalence states, the reach of PPTCT services to all pregnant women in the country remains limited [2].

Global evidence suggests that although ARV prophylaxis using SD-NVP is highly effective in reducing risk of transmission from approximately 45% to less than 10%, the 10% uncovered risk is unacceptably high because pediatric HIV can be eliminated if currently available drugs are used effectively. The World Health Organization therefore recommends use of more efficacious ARV regimens using multiple drugs for PPTCT. These regimens can reduce transmission to less than 5% if started early in pregnancy and continued throughout the periods of delivery and breastfeeding. Therefore, lifelong ART is to be provided to all pregnant and breastfeeding women living with HIV: all pregnant women living with HIV receive a triple-drug ART regimen (TDF + 3TC + EFV) regardless of CD4 count or clinical stage for their own health and to prevent vertical HIV transmission, and for additional HIV prevention benefits. These PPTCT services are planned to be scaled-up rapidly across the country in a phased manner to replace currently available SD-NVP prophylaxis.

For early infant diagnosis (EID), it is important for all HIV-exposed infants to have a minimum of 6 weeks of daily infant NVP irrespective of whether the infant is sustained by replacement feeding or breastfeeding. At 6 weeks, during the first immunization visit at ICTC, the DNA PCR (dried blood spot) is collected and cotrimoxazole is provided for all HIV-exposed infants. If the EID results are positive for HIV, then the infant will require initiation of ARV treatment as per national guidelines. For these infants, exclusive breastfeeding is to be performed until 6 months. Breastfeeding, however, can be continued up to 24 months. For HIV-negative infants, it is imperative to advise parents/caregivers that continued monitoring and follow-up of the infant are necessary. Confirmation of HIV status can be performed only at 18 months of age using three rapid tests, even if the first test is negative. Exclusive breastfeeding is to be performed until 6 months of age and complimentary feeding should be started at 6 months of age. Breastfeeding should continue until 12 months only. Stopping of breastfeeding should be done gradually over 1 month according to the comfort of the mother and child. HIV testing needs to be performed again after cessation of breastfeeding according to the EID protocols.

Alvarez-Uria [36] assessed the PMTCT that provided universal ART to all pregnant women regardless of the CD4 lymphocyte count and formula feeding for children at high risk for HIV transmission through breastfeeding in a district of India. The overall rate of HIV transmission was 3.7%. Although breastfeeding added a 3.1% additional risk of HIV acquisition, formula-fed infants had a significantly higher risk of death compared with breastfed infants. The cumulative 12-month mortality was 9.6% for formula-fed infants versus 0.68% for breastfed infants. Anthropometric markers (weight, length/height, weight for length/height, body mass index, head circumference, mid–upper arm circumference, triceps skinfold, and subscapular skinfold) showed that formula-fed infants experienced severe malnutrition during the first 2 months of life. They did not observe any death after rapid weaning at 5–6 months in breastfed infants. The higher rate of HIV-free survival in breastfed infants and the low rate of HIV transmission found in this study support the implementation of PMTCT programs with universal ART to all HIV-infected pregnant women and breastfeeding women to reduce HIV transmission without increasing infant mortality in developing countries.

11.7 HIV AND IYCF

Infant feeding is one of the most critical interfaces between HIV and child survival. The optimal infant feeding choice for women living with HIV continues to be a major concern for health care providers, HIV-infected women, and the families of these women.

Infant feeding in the context of HIV is complex because of the major influence that feeding practices exert on child survival. The dilemma is to balance the risk of infants acquiring HIV through breast milk with the higher risk of death from causes other than HIV.

WHO advice [37] emphasizes that protection of the infant from the risk of death from other causes such as diarrhea and malnutrition is as important as avoiding HIV transmission through breastfeeding. At the same time, the health of mothers should not be undermined in any way because the relationship between maternal health and survival of the infant is well-known. Hence, maternal, newborn, and child health services should promote and support breastfeeding and ARV interventions because the strategy that will most likely give infants born to mothers known to be HIV-infected the greatest chance of HIV-free survival.

11.8 MALNUTRITION AND HIV-AFFECTED CHILDREN

India has high rates of malnutrition among children, and the prevalence of malnutrition is likely to be higher among women and children with HIV than in the general population. Impaired nutritional status is an independent predictor of adverse outcomes among HIV-infected children and adults, including those using ART. Thus, early identification and management of undernutrition, especially among HIV-exposed and HIV-infected children, are critical to achieve optimal impact of other HIV-related care and treatment interventions, including ART. NACP-III focuses on ensuring that HIV-infected children receive medical treatment and aftercare, access to schooling, adequate nutrition, and a safe environment.

Shet et al. [38] analyzed retrospective data from 248 HIV-infected children aged 1–12 years attending three outpatient clinics in South India (2004–2006) to assess the prevalence of malnutrition. The overall prevalence of anemia (defined as hemoglobin <11 g/dL) was 66%, and 8% had severe anemia (Hb <7 g/dL). The proportion of underweight and of stunted children in the population was 55% and 46%, respectively. Independent risk factors of anemia by multivariate analysis included age younger than 6 years (OR, 2.87; 95% CI, 1.45–5.70; $P < 0.01$), rural residence (OR, 12.04; 95% CI, 5.64–26.00; $P<0.01$), advanced HIV disease stage (OR, 6.95; 95% CI, 3.06–15.79; $P < 0.01$), and presence of stunting (height-for-age Z score <−2) (OR, 3.24; 95% CI, 1.65–6.35; $P < 0.01$). Use of iron/multivitamin supplementation was protective against risk of anemia (OR, 0.44; 95% CI, 0.22–0.90; $P = 0.03$). Pulmonary tuberculosis was an independent risk factor in multivariate analysis (OR, 3.36; 95% CI, 1.43–7.89; $P < 0.01$) when correlated variables, such as HIV disease stage and severe immunodeficiency, and nutritional supplement use were not included. Use of ART was associated with a reduced risk of anemia (OR, 0.29; 95% CI, 0.16–0.53; $P < 0.01$). Seth et al. [39] also reported that infants born to HIV-positive mothers had high rates of malnutrition and that there is a need for standardizing feeding counseling.

11.9 INTEGRATING HIV INTERVENTIONS INTO MATERNAL AND CHILD HEALTH SERVICES

In many countries including India, HIV-specific interventions have been implemented as vertical, stand-alone programs rather than integrated services. However, the starting point for all interventions to protect the infant from HIV infection is to identify which pregnant women are HIV-infected and then to offer them the necessary care and support to optimize their health. According to WHO [37], national authorities should aim to integrate HIV testing, care, and treatment interventions for all women into maternal and child health services. Such interventions should include access to CD4 count testing and appropriate ART or prophylaxis for the woman's health and to prevent MTCT of HIV [37]. However, issues of confidentiality and stigma need to be dealt with before integrating the care of HIV-infected pregnant women, infants, and young children with other national maternal and child health programs like the ICDS.

The ability of mothers to successfully achieve a desired feeding practice is significantly influenced by the support provided through formal health services and other community-based groups. This is true for all mothers and their infants and is not specific to settings with high HIV prevalence. Therefore, skilled counseling and support in appropriate infant feeding practices and ARV interventions to promote HIV-free survival of infants should be available to all pregnant women and mothers. Women and mothers known to be HIV-infected should be informed of the infant feeding strategy, along with the suitable alternatives recommended by the national authorities to improve HIV-free survival of HIV-exposed infants and the health of HIV-infected mothers.

11.10 CONCLUSION

Although the prevalence of HIV/AIDS in India has been declining, with a national prevalence of 0.27%, the virus affects the lives of millions, leaving its mark on the financial, social, and health fronts. The country has shown its commitment not only by making remarkable progress reducing new infections but also by making treatment available and affordable to those already infected. Still, there is much that needs to be prioritized, especially the management of disease. There is limited information regarding nutritional practices of these individuals and how they affects their QoL. Few studies have pointed to the fact that, regarding regular psychological and nutritional counseling, the knowledge about basic nutrition is there for adult PLHIVs but the transfer of this knowledge to healthy practices does not take place. Stringent and regular BCC efforts to bring about healthy dietary practices among PLHIV are necessary. With respect to pediatric HIV issues, breastfeeding and especially early breastfeeding are critical for improving child survival. Breastfeeding also confers many benefits other than reducing the risk of child mortality. HIV has created great confusion among health workers regarding the relative merits of breastfeeding for the mother who is known to be HIV-infected. Tragically, this has also resulted in mothers who are known to be HIV-uninfected or whose HIV status is unknown adopting feeding practices that are not necessary for their circumstances, with detrimental effect for their infants. With the clear recommendation of providing ARV prophylaxis and promoting exclusive breastfeeding for the first 6 months for HIV-affected infants by WHO [37], there must be no confusion during counseling regarding infant feeding options.

References

[1] National Aids Control Organization and World Food Programme (NACO/WFP). Nutrition in the fight against HIV and AIDS. Selected papers from the National Consultation on Nutritional Security and the Prevention, Treatment and Mitigation of HIV and AIDS and TB. New Delhi, India; 2004.

[2] NACO. National strategic plan. Multi-drug ARV for prevention of parent-to-child-transmission of HIV (PPTCT) under National AIDS Control Programme in India. Department of AIDS Control, Basic Services Division, MOHFW, Government of India; 2013.

[3] UNAIDS. The GAP Report; 2013.

[4] World Health Organization WHOQOL-HIV instrument, users manual, scoring and coding for the WHOQOL-HIV instruments Mental health: evidence and research department of mental health and substance dependence. Geneva, Switzerland: World Health Organization; 2002.

[5] Basavaraj KH, Navya MA, Rashmi R. Quality of life in HIV/AIDS. Indian J Sex Transm Dis 2010;31(2):75–80.

[6] Chandra PS, Desai G, Ranjan R. HIV and psychiatric disorders. Indian J Med Res 2005;121:451–67.

[7] Aranda-Naranjo B. Quality of life in HIV-positive patients. J Assoc Nurses AIDS Care 2004;15:20–7.

[8] Anand D, Puri S. Effectiveness of nutrition intervention on health and nutrition profile of people living with HIV and AIDS. PhD Dissertation, University of Delhi; 2012 [unpublished].

[9] Wig N, Lekshmi R, Pal H, Ahuja V, Mittal CM, Agarwal SK. The impact of HIV/AIDS on the quality of life: a cross sectional study in north India. Indian J Med Sci 2006;60(1):3–12.

[10] Bacchetti P, Cofrancesco J, Heymsfield S, et al. Fat distribution in women with HIV infection. J Acquir Immune Defic Syndr 2006;42:562–71.

[11] Bacchetti P, Gripshover B, Grunfeld C, Heymsfield S, McCreath H, Osmond D, et al. Fat distribution in men with HIV infection. J Acquir Immune Defic Syndr 2005;40:121–31.

[12] Scherzer R, Shen W, Bacchetti P, Kotler D, Lewis CE, Shlipak MG, et al. Simple anthropometric measures correlate with metabolic risk indicators as strongly as magnetic resonance imaging—measured adipose tissue depots in both HIV-infected and control subjects. Am J Clin Nutr 2008;87:1809–17.

[13] Suttman U, Ockenga J, Selberg O, Hoogestraat L, Helmuth D, Muller MJ. Incidence and prognostic value of malnutrition and wasting in human immunodeficiency virus-infected outpatients. J Acquir Immune Defic Syndr Hum Retrovirol 1995;8:239–46.

[14] Ott M, Lambke B, Fischer H, et al. Early changes of body composition in human immunodeficiency virus infected patients: tetrapolar body impedance analysis indicates significant malnutrition. Am J Clin Nutr 1993;57:15–19.

[15] Kotler DP, Tierney AR, Wang J, Pierson Jr. RN. Magnitude of bodycell-mass depletion and the timing of death from wasting in AIDS. Am J Clin Nutr 1989;50:444–7.

[16] Colecraft E. HIV/AIDS: nutritional implications and impact on human development. Proc Nutr Soc 2008;67:109–13.
[17] Ndekha M, van Oosterhout JJ, Saloojee H, Pettifor J, Manary M. Nutritional status of Malawian adults on antiretroviral therapy 1 year after supplementary feeding in the first 3 months of therapy. Trop Med Int Health 2009;14(9):1059–63.
[18] van der Sande MAB, van der Loeff MFS, Aveika AA, et al. BMI at time of HIV diagnosis: a strong and independent predictor of survival. J Acquir Immune Defic Syndr 2004;37:1288–94.
[19] Ludy MJ, Hendricks K, Houser R, Chetchotisakd P, Mootsikapun P, Anunnatsiri S, et al. Body composition in adults infection with human immunodeficiency virus in Khoan Kaen, Thailand. Am J Trop Med Hyg 2005;73(4):815–9.
[20] Nitenberg G, Raynard B. Nutritional support of the cancer patient: issues and dilemmas. Crit Rev Oncol Hematol 2000;34:137–68.
[21] Crenn PR. Hyperphagia contributes to the normal body composition and protein–energy balance in HIV-infected asymptomatic men. J Nutr 2004;134:2301–6.
[22] Anand D, Puri S. Anthropometric and nutritional profile of people living with HIV and AIDS in India: an assessment. Indian J Community Med 2014;39:161–8.
[23] Subbaraman R, Devaleenal B, Selvamuthu P, Yepthomi T, Solomon SS, Mayer KH, et al. Factors associated with anaemia in HIV infected individuals in southern India. Int J STD AIDS 2009;20(7):489–92.
[24] Semba RD, Martin BK, Kempen JH, et al. The impact of anemia on energy and physical functioning in individuals with AIDS. Arch Intern Med 2005;165:2229–36.
[25] O'Brien ME, Kupka R, Msamanga GI, et al. Anemia is an independent predictor of mortality and immunologic progression of disease among women with HIV in Tanzania. J Acquir Immune Defic Syndr 2005;40:219–25.
[26] Eckman K, Walker R. Knowledge, attitudes and practice (KAP) survey—summary report for the Duluth lakeside storm water reduction project (LSRP). Saint Paul, MN: Water Resources Center, University of Minnesota; 2008.
[27] Bhatt SD, Dhoundiyal NC. Country watch: India. AIDS STD Health Promot Exch 1997;3:11–12.
[28] Watsa M. Sexuallity counselling in India. Plan Parent Chall 1993;2:25–7.
[29] Sanjay S, et al. Evaluation of impact of health education regarding HIV/AIDS on knowledge and attitude among persons living with HIV/AIDS. Indian J Community Med 2003;28(1):30–3.
[30] Gaash B, et al. Knowledge, attitude and belief on HIV/AIDS among female senior secondary students in Srinagar district of Kashmir. Health Popul Perspect Issues 2003;2(3):101–9.
[31] Ahmed M, Gaash B. Awareness of HIV/AIDS in a remotely located conservative district of J&K (Kargil). Indian J Community Med 2002;27(1):12–18.
[32] Paul D, Gopalakrishnan N. Knowledge regarding modes of transmission and prevention of sexually transmitted diseases including HIV/AIDS among child development project officers. Indian J Community Med 2001;26(3):141–4.
[33] Anand D, Puri S. Nutritional knowledge, attitude and practices of HIV-positive individuals in India. J Health Popul Nutr 2013;31(2):195–201.
[34] Benjamin AI, Singh S, Sengupta P, Dhanoa J. HIV seroprevalence and knowledge, behavior and practices regarding HIV/AIDS in specific population groups in Ludhiana, Punjab. Indian J Public Health 2007;51(1):33–8.
[35] Lal SS, Vasan RS, Sarma PS, Thankappan KR. Knowledge and attitude of college students in Kerala towards HIV/AIDS, sexually transmitted diseases and sexuality. Natl Med J India 2000;13(5):231–6.
[36] Alvarez-Uria G, Midde M, Pakam R, Bachu L, Naik PK. Effect of formula feeding and breastfeeding on child growth, infant mortality, and HIV transmission in children

born to HIV-infected pregnant women who received triple antiretroviral therapy in a resource-limited setting: Data from an HIV Cohort Study in India. ISRN Pediatr. 2012; 2012:763591.

[37] WHO. Rapid advice: revised WHO principles and recommendations on infant feeding in the context of HIV; 2009.

[38] Shet A, Mehta S, Rajagopalan N, Dinakar C, Ramesh E, Samuel NM, et al. Anemia and growth failure among HIV-infected children in India: a retrospective analysis. BMC Pediatr 2009;9:37. http://dx.doi.org/10.1186/1471-2431-9-37.

[39] Seth A, Chandra J, Gupta R, Kumar P, Aggarwal V, Dutta A. Outcome of HIV exposed infants: experience of a regional pediatric center for HIV in North India. Indian J Pediatr 2012;79(2):188–93.

CHAPTER

12

Undernutrition, Food Insecurity, and Antiretroviral Outcomes: An Overview of Evidence from sub-Saharan Africa

Patou Masika Musumari[1], Teeranee Techasrivichien[1], S. Pilar Suguimoto[1], Adolphe Ndarabu[2], Aimé Mboyo[3], Baron Ngasia[4], Christina El-Saaidi[1], Bhekumusa Wellington Lukhele[1], Masako Ono-Kihara[1] and Masahiro Kihara[1]

[1]Department of Global Health and Socio-epidemiology, Kyoto University School of Public Health, Yoshida-Konoe-cho, Sakyo-ku, Kyoto, Japan, [2]Centre Hospitalier Monkole, Masangambila, Mont-Ngafula, Kinshasa 817 Kinshasa XI, Democratic Republic of Congo, [3]Multisectoral program of the fight against HIV/AIDS (PNMLS), Ex-Fonames bld, Kasa-Vubu, Kinshasa, Democratic Republic of Congo, [4]Centre Hospitalier Lumbulumbu-Clinique MAPON, Kindu, Maniema, Democratic Republic of Congo

12.1 OVERVIEW OF HIV, NUTRITION, AND FOOD SECURITY IN SUB-SAHARAN AFRICA

Food insecurity, undernutrition, and human immunodeficiency virus/ acquired immunodeficiency syndrome (HIV/AIDS) overlap in sub-Saharan Africa and exercise a negative influence on one another, with an enormous toll in the sub-Saharan African population in terms of morbidity and mortality. Current estimations indicate that sub-Saharan Africa hosts

Health of HIV Infected People, Volume 2.
DOI: http://dx.doi.org/10.1016/B978-0-12-800767-9.00012-1

two-thirds of all people living with HIV/AIDS [1] and is home to 222.7 million (24.8%) people classified as undernourished [2].

Undernutrition is regarded as a state of malnutrition characterized by a deficit in macronutrient and/or micronutrient that leads to changes in body composition and diminished function [3,4]. Food insecurity is variably defined and operationalized, but we note that it is often understood as the limited or uncertain availability of nutritionally adequate safe foods or the inability to acquire personally acceptable foods in socially acceptable ways [5]. Food insecurity is a key contributing factor to undernutrition; however, undernutrition rarely results from food insecurity alone, and it has many other underlying causes, including, but not limited to, inadequate care practices, unclean water, poor hygiene and sanitation, and poor access to health care [6].

The link between HIV/AIDS and undernutrition was obvious from the early era of HIV/AIDS epidemic, where HIV/AIDS was characterized by a profound decline in nutritional status, referred to as "wasting syndrome," defined as the involuntary body weight loss of more than 10% in association with chronic diarrhea and/or fever and/or asthenia for 30 days or longer and in the absence of concurrent illness or condition other than HIV that could explain the wasting [7–10]. Undernutrition during HIV infection is multifactorial, and previous research has consistently related it to decreased caloric intake, malabsorption of nutrients, increased energy need, and expenditure after bacterial and/or systemic opportunistic infections [8–10]. Various indicators exist to assess undernutrition, including anthropometric measures, such as the body mass index (BMI), mid–upper arm circumference (MUAC), skinfolds, or bioelectrical impedance analysis (body cell mass, fat mass, body water), and biochemical nutritional parameters (hemoglobin, albumin, C-reactive protein, etc.) [9,11].

Unlike undernutrition, the relationship between food insecurity and HIV/AIDS has just recently emerged from the literature from both developed and developing settings [12–20]. Food insecurity and HIV/AIDS are viciously linked, and this is well-captured in a conceptual framework advanced by Weiser et al. depicting the pathways involved in the bidirectional links between food insecurity and HIV/AIDS [21]. Diverse scales and indices are used to assess food insecurity at individual or household levels [22] and include, for example, the food consumption score, the dietary diversity score, the Cornell/Radimer hunger scale, and the household food insecurity access scale [22–24].

Although the rapidly expanding free antiretroviral therapy (ART) program in the past decade has resulted in substantially decreased HIV/AIDS-related morbidity and mortality in sub-Saharan Africa, evidence indicates that patients initiating ART in resource-constrained settings are at higher risk for death during the early months of treatment [25,26], and undernutrition is cited as a key contributor of early mortality among

ART-treated patients [26–35]. Undernutrition and food insecurity constitute an important threat to the success of HIV/AIDS programs in sub-Saharan Africa, and that failure to address them accordingly may jeopardize the benefits garnered so far in the fight against HIV/AIDS.

The extent to which food is a central concern among HIV-infected individuals in sub-Saharan Africa is well-illustrated in the following statement from Dr. Peter Piot, the former executive director of the Joint United Nations Programme on HIV/AIDS (UNAIDS) on returning from a trip to southern Africa: *I was in Malawi and met with a group of women living with HIV. As I always do, I asked them what their highest priority was. Their answer was clear and unanimous: food. Not care, not drugs for treatment, not relief from stigma, but food* [36].

As a response to this growing concern, international organizations such as the World Health Organization (WHO), the UNAIDS, the United Nations World Food Program (WFP), and the World Bank have recognized as a matter of priority the need to break the perpetuating cycle between food insecurity/undernutrition and HIV/AIDS, and have initiated programs to offset the negative impact of undernutrition and food insecurity on the health of HIV-infected individuals [37–43]. However, evidence of how effective nutritional programs or interventions are in achieving their intended goals is still not clearly established, particularly among individuals using ART.

This chapter reviews existing evidence of the impact of undernutrition and food insecurity on HIV treatment outcomes, and it examines intervention studies that have addressed food insecurity and undernutrition with respect to their effect on ART outcomes among HIV-infected adults in sub-Saharan Africa. For the purpose of this chapter, we focus on BMI as the parameter to assess nutritional status; for food insecurity, we include any relevant qualitative or quantitative study that explicitly reports food insecurity regardless of the method of assessment that was used. HIV treatment outcomes are behavioral (adherence to ART), nutritional (BMI), clinical (survival/mortality), immunological (CD4 count), and virological (HIV viral load).

12.2 UNDERNUTRITION AND HIV TREATMENT OUTCOMES

12.2.1 The Impact of Undernutrition on Adherence to ART

Adherence to ART is one of the key factors of success of HIV treatment, and studies have consistently linked poor adherence with increased risk of treatment failure and emergence of drug resistance [44,45]. Very few studies have examined the effect of undernutrition on adherence to ART in sub-Saharan Africa. In a recent study from Ethiopia, undernutrition, defined as BMI less than 18.5 kg/m^2, was associated with a 10-fold increased risk of nonadherence to ART [46]. However, a preceding study in the same country found contrasting results in that individuals with good nutritional status were more likely to miss ART doses when compared with those who had poor nutritional status [47]. Although the authors suggested study design differentials to explain the discrepancy in the results of both studies [46], we note that the opposing results underscore the complexity of the relationship between patient nutritional status and adherence to ART, and the need of considering other factors that can potentially act as mediators. For example, poor nutritional status may affect adherence to ART by depriving the patient of the energy required to report to the health facility for ART refill or by potentiating drug toxicity [48,49]. Conversely, patients with poor nutritional status may benefit from closer attention and care from family members ensuring that medication is appropriately collected and used. Social support, stigma/discrimination, and the degree of undernutrition are examples of factors that may serve as mediators. However, good nutritional status may also result in either increased or decreased adherence to ART. Feeling healthy after initiation of ART was reported to be associated with poor adherence to ART. Patients felt they were well and that there was no need to use the medication [50]. Therapeutic education of patients should insist on the lifetime nature of ART to avoid patients thinking that their improvement in health is a permanent cure. It is also possible that patients with improved health are more likely to engage in daily subsistence activities that may result in forgetfulness to use medication. For example, in a study from Uganda, forgetfulness regarding using ART doses resulted from the fact that patients were busy working all day for food [18]. There is definitely a need for more studies to clarify the link between nutritional factors and adherence to ART in sub-Saharan Africa.

12.2.2 The Impact of Undernutrition on Clinical, Immunological, and Virological Response to ART

Rich documentation exists showing the link between poor nutritional status and adverse health outcomes among ART-treated individuals in sub-Saharan Africa [25–35]. For example, studies from Ethiopia [27], Malawi [28], Zambia [29], and Tanzania [30,33] have consistently linked low BMI to an increased risk of mortality, particularly early mortality, which is defined as death occurring within the first 3 months after initiation of ART. In many instances, BMI was related to early death in a dose–response fashion [26,28,30,33]. For example, in Malawi [28], BMI of less than 16, 16–16.9, and 17.0–18.4 kg/m^2 were, respectively, associated with 6.0, 2.4, and 2.1 increased odds of early mortality when compared with individuals who had BMI $\geq$18.5 kg/m^2. Similarly, in Tanzania [33], BMI of less than 16, 16–16.9, and 17.0–18.4 kg/m^2 were, respectively, significantly associated with 2.3, 2.1, and 1.5 increased relative risk of early mortality. However, in another study performed in Tanzania [30], only individuals with BMI less than 16 kg/m^2 had a significant increased risk of death, indicating that severe undernutrition (BMI <16 kg/m^2) is a stronger independent predictor of mortality among HIV-positive individuals initiating ART. In support of the evidence relating undernutrition to early mortality, studies from Kenya [31] and Zambia [32] have shown that weight gain after ART initiation was associated with improved survival and decreased risk of clinical failure. Although theoretical and experimental evidence have indicated poor immune reconstitution as a potential mediator to explain the negative effect of undernutrition on survival among HIV-positive individuals on ART, consensus on the impact of undernutrition on the immune response of ART-treated individuals is yet to be reached, because poor nutritional status at the initiation of ART is also shown to be a predictor of mortality independent of immune status [26–35]. A recently published protocol of a systematic review [11] attempts to clarify the association between undernutrition and immunological response to ART, with the ultimate goal of determining whether ART is suboptimal in undernourished HIV-infected individuals in low- and middle-income countries. We hope this systematic review will provide conclusive facts to shed light on the impact of undernutrition on immune response to ART.

There is a scarcity of studies assessing the relationship between nutritional status and virological response to ART among individuals using antiretroviral medication. Unlike in resource-rich settings, the use of viral load as a routine tool for monitoring the response to ART in resource-constrained settings is not widely expanded, mainly because of the associated cost. This can possibly explain the limited literature on the impact of undernutrition on virological response to ART among HIV-positive individuals.

12.3 FOOD INSECURITY AND HIV TREATMENT OUTCOMES

12.3.1 The Impact of Food Insecurity on Adherence to ART

Initial evidence on the possible negative effects of food insecurity on patient adherence to ART in sub-Saharan Africa mainly emerged from qualitative studies [17–19,51–56], contrasting with studies from resource-rich countries, which were mainly quantitative in nature [12–16,57]. Early qualitative studies in sub-Saharan Africa set the scene by laying out the adverse role of food insecurity on antiretroviral medication adherence, and they were very useful in unveiling possible mechanisms through which food insecurity affects adherence. For example, qualitative studies from the Democratic Republic of Congo (DRC) [17], Uganda [18,52], South Africa [51], Rwanda [53], Kenya [54], Mozambique [55], and Zambia [56] have reported lack of food as an important barrier to ART adherence and documented mechanisms through which limited access to food resulted in poor medication adherence, including the belief that ART is not effective or harmful when taken without food, fear or experience of exacerbated side effects when ART is taken without food, fear of or experience of exacerbated hunger when ART is taken without food, and competing needs between food and demands regarding ART. However, the limited sample size characteristic to qualitative studies restricts the generalizability of these mechanisms to the broader population of food-insecure HIV-infected individuals using ART in sub-Saharan Africa.

We have documented a total of eight quantitative studies examining the link between food insecurity and patient adherence to ART [20,46,58–63]. Three studies were prospective cohorts [20,59,62], cross-sectional [58,60,61,63], or had a case–control design [46]. However, only two of the eight studies used a complete validated scale to measure food insecurity [20,58]. Six of the eight studies reported adjusted estimates [20,46,58–60,62], of which four studies found statistically significant increased odds of nonadherence to ART among food-insecure individuals [20,46,58,60]. For example, the longitudinal study from Uganda has shown a 56% increase in the odds of nonadherence among food-insecure individuals when compared with their counterparts who were food-secure [20]. In the cross-sectional study from DRC, food-insecure individuals were two-times more likely to be nonadherent compared with food-secure individuals [58]. This latter study [58] tested two mechanisms documented in a preceding qualitative research [17], including the beliefs that ART is not effective or harmful when taken without food. Beliefs regarding the effectiveness or harmfulness of ART were not associated with adherence to ART. Nonetheless, a significant proportion (31.3%) of patients held the belief that ART is harmful when used in the absence of food, highlighting the need for adherence counseling to address such beliefs given the potential detrimental effect they may have on medication adherence.

In one study performed in Zambia, food insecurity was not significantly associated with ART adherence [59]; another study in the same country [62], in contrast, found that food-insecure individuals had statically increased odds of being adherent to ART. It was hypothesized that this could reflect the increased social support extended to severely socioeconomically deprived individuals. Overall, studies from sub-Saharan Africa corroborate with results from resource-rich countries [12–16,57], indicating the negative effect of food insecurity on antiretroviral medication adherence. Future research will benefit more from longitudinal quantitative studies, using validated scales for both food insecurity and adherence to

ART, and examining the different postulated mechanisms through which food insecurity affects patient adherence to ART.

12.3.2 The Impact of Food Insecurity on Clinical, Immunological, and Virological Response to ART

In contrast to undernutrition, there is a dearth of studies examining the impact of food insecurity on HIV clinical, immunological, and virological outcomes among HIV-infected individuals using ART in sub-Saharan Africa. Our literature review identified one study from sub-Saharan Africa [20]; most research linking food insecurity to HIV treatment outcomes was conducted in resource-rich settings [13,57,64–66]. The documented study from sub-Saharan Africa consists of a longitudinal study conducted in Uganda [20] that demonstrated the link between food insecurity and incomplete viral suppression and low CD4 cell counts in a cohort of HIV-infected individuals receiving ART in rural Uganda. The relationship between food insecurity and viral suppression was mediated by adherence to ART. After adjusting for adherence status, the association between food insecurity and viral suppression was no longer statistically significant. However, there was no mediating effect of ART adherence in the relationship between food insecurity and low CD4 cell counts. As stated by authors, immunological response to ART may be influenced by other factors such as the nutritional status and the pretreatment CD4 cell counts, which in turn may be affected in food-insecure individuals presenting late to care.

Studies from developed settings have reported similar results showing associations of food insecurity with incomplete virological suppression [13,57,64,65] and low CD4 cell counts [13,57,65] when ART adherence was a weak mediator [57] or showed no mediating effects [13,64,65] between food insecurity and virological/immunological outcomes. A previously published conceptual framework has mapped out pathways explaining the link between food insecurity and HIV treatment outcomes, including nutritional, mental (depression/anxiety), and behavioral (ART adherence) pathways [21]. There is a need for studies to explore these possible pathways and ultimately provide a comprehensive understanding of underlying mechanisms through which food insecurity affects HIV treatment outcomes among HIV-infected individuals on ART.

A remarkable gap in the literature is the lack of studies examining the effect of food insecurity on mortality of individuals receiving ART in sub-Saharan Africa. The only such documented study was conducted in British Columbia and showed that food insecurity at baseline was associated with increased risk of mortality among individuals initiated on ART [66]. The effect of food insecurity on mortality was stronger among individuals who were underweight, defined as BMI less than 18.5 km^2 compared with those who were not underweight. Interestingly, individuals who were food-insecure and were not underweight had increased mortality risk, whereas those who were food-secure and underweight were not more likely to die when compared with individuals who were food-secure and not underweight. The authors made a strong case that mechanisms other than poor nutritional status may, in part, explain the detrimental effect of food insecurity on mortality among ART-treated individuals, and that previously observed associations between nutritional status and mortality among individuals using ART could be, to a certain degree, mediated by food insecurity. Future studies will advance research by examining the interplay of food insecurity and nutritional status on adherence, clinical, virological, and immunological outcomes in ART-treated individuals.

12.4 IMPACT OF NUTRITIONAL SUPPORT ON HIV TREATMENT OUTCOMES

Nutritional support, in the form of macronutrient and/or micronutrient supplementation, is and has been offered by food programs in many parts of the developing world to achieve diverse goals [67]. The need to provide nutritional support to HIV-positive individuals to offset the negative feedback loop between food insecurity/undernutrition and HIV was long recognized and placed in the agenda of global institutions such as the WHO, the UNAIDS, the WFP, and the World Bank [37–43].

We focus on macronutrient supplementation, which includes any intervention given to provide protein and/or energy by replacing or supplementing the normal diet [67,68]. Even though it is well-established from observational studies that food insecurity and undernutrition negatively affect HIV treatment outcomes, studies assessing the impact of nutritional support on ART outcomes among HIV-infected people remain very limited, rendering it difficult to make the claim that food nutritional interventions improve ART outcomes.

We identified 10 food intervention studies conducted in Zambia [69,70], Niger [71], Uganda [72], Mozambique [73], Malawi [74,75], South Africa [76], Kenya [77], and Ethiopia [78]. The studies differ with respect to design, choice of outcomes, type of controls, and nature and duration of the intervention.

In terms of the study designs, five studies were randomized controlled trials, including two from Malawi [74,75], one from South Africa [76], one unpublished randomized trial from Kenya [77], and one from Ethiopia [78]. The other studies were either intervention cohort [69,71] or retrospective intervention cohort [70,72,73] in design. Nonrandomized interventions [69–73] examined clinic-based food assistance programs compared with clinics or regions that did not or were to receive food assistance at a later period. Nutritional support was intended to meet the nutritional needs of the primary beneficiaries or of the entire household and varied in nature. For example, in Niger, the monthly food ration comprised 500 g of cereal, 100 g of legumes (dry peas and not containing vegetables), and 30 g of vegetable oil strengthened with vitamin A [71]. In Mozambique, beneficiaries had individual food rations that included 10 kg of soya, 5 kg of cowpeas, and 25 kg of maize; in Zambia, food assistance consisted of vegetable oil, maize, peas or beans, and corn and soy blended flour [69,70]. Randomized controlled trials either compared two types of nutritional support [74,75] or examined the effects of a specified nutritional support compared with controls who did not receive nutritional assistance [76–78].

Broadly, the intervention period ranged from 3 to 12 months and examined a range of outcomes, including adherence to ART [69–71,73], nutritional outcomes (BMI/weight, fat-free body mass, lean body mass) [69–72,74–78], clinical outcomes (mortality/survival, hospitalization rate, WHO stage) [71,72,74,75], immunological outcomes (CD4, CD3, and CD8 counts) [69–71,74–78], virological outcomes [74,75]), and quality of life [74,75,77].

In this section, we provide an overview of the evidence of the impacts of food supplementation on adherence to ART and nutritional, clinical, immunological, and virological outcomes. The documented randomized trials are addressed separately at the end of the section.

12.4.1 Impact of Nutritional Support on ART Adherence

A total of six studies, including two randomized controlled trials, examined the effect of nutritional support on ART adherence [69–71, 73–75]. However, both randomized trials [74,75] were not considered because they compared two types of food supplementation, which did not allow us to single-out the individual effect of nutritional support on medication adherence.

Three out of the four food supplementations have reached the similar conclusion that food assistance improves ART adherence among HIV-infected individuals in resource-limited settings [69–71,73]. For example, in the pilot study in Zambia, Cantrell et al. [69] found that recipients of food assistance had a 50% higher relative risk of achieving better adherence to ART compared with those who were not nutritionally assisted. Another study in Zambia similarly found that food assistance recipients achieved higher adherence compared with nonrecipients [70]. In Niger, Serrano et al. [71], examining the effect of a family food distribution on ART adherence, reached similar results. In contrast, ART adherence was not significantly different between recipients and nonrecipients of food assistance in a recent study from Mozambique [73].

Important insights regarding the results of these studies merit consideration. Three of the four studies, including the studies from Zambia [69,70] and Mozambique [73], used pharmacy-based methods to assess adherence to ART [79]. The study from Niger [71] used both a pharmacy-based method (pill count) and interviews, but it did not formulate details regarding how both measures were combined to assess adherence. The pharmacy-based methods consisted of the pill pick-up [73] and a measure referred to as the medication possession ratio (MPR) [69], which measures the proportion of days a patient has possession of his/her medication. Pharmacy-based methods are known to be reliable and objective measures of adherence [79,80]. Although it is beyond the scope of this chapter to describe in detail the methods of assessment of adherence, it is important to note that a common feature to most pharmacy-based methods is that the level of adherence is predicated on how regularly and timely patients refill their ART, and that they underestimate adherence in case there is more than one source of ART provision [79]. In this context, the increased adherence observed among recipients of food assistance could simply reflect the incentivizing effect of nutritional support encouraging patients to collect their food ration and medication in time. Food remains a valuable commodity in many resource-limited settings and is enough to motivate regular clinic attendance. We may also extrapolate that any other locally valued incentive could similarly result in increased ART adherence as long as it urges enough motivation to encourage regular and timely visits for medication refill. Considering the negative impact of food insecurity on ART adherence, one would assume that food assistance would result in increased adherence by adjusting the underlying mechanisms to supposedly link food insecurity to poor medication adherence. The fact that the increased adherence among recipients of food assistance might be related to the incentivizing nature of the latter does not *per se* oppose results from previous qualitative studies specifying mechanisms through which food insecurity negatively impacted on ART adherence [17–19,51–56]. As previously mentioned, the beliefs that ART is not effective or harmful when taken without food, fear of or experience of exacerbated side effects when ART is taken without food, fear of or experience of exacerbated hunger when ART is taken without food, and competing needs between food and demands regarding ART were documented as pathways linking food insecurity to suboptimal level of adherence [17–19,51–56]. It is possible that food collected by ART-treated patients ultimately served to alleviate the challenges involved in taking ART on an empty stomach. Future intervention studies assessing the impact of nutritional support on adherence to ART should validate this hypothesis.

A word should be mentioned about the study in Mozambique that failed to demonstrate the effect of nutritional support in improving ART adherence among recipients of food rations [73]. The authors noted that caution is necessary in the interpretation of the results and hypothesized a number of factors likely to explain the failure of the program to improve ART adherence. It was evoked that factors inherent to the program itself, such as some aspects related to the implementation like recipients' satisfaction with the program, could explain the observed results. For example, it turned out that patients were not satisfied with the enrollment period of the program. Transportation difficulties were also cited as a possible explanation because food distributions were not necessarily done in the health facilities; this could incur additional time and money to collect food at a distribution site housed in a different location. Furthermore, reasons other than food insecurity were equally suggested as possible explanations. The type of adherence measure used in the study was also postulated to explain why the program did not work. Adherence in this study was assessed using a pharmacy-based method (pill pick-up) that is reliable when patients have only one source of ART provision; otherwise, they may underestimate the level of adherence [79]. However, authors could not validate this assumption.

12.4.2 Impact of Nutritional Support on Nutritional, Clinical, Immunological, and Virological Outcomes

Four of the five nonrandomized intervention studies examined nutritional, clinical, and immunological outcomes between recipients and nonrecipients of food assistance among HIV-infected adults using ART [69–72]. Both similarities and divergences are noted in their results with respect to the effect of nutritional support on HIV treatment outcomes.

All the studies consistently found no significant effect of food assistance on patients' BMI/weight. There is a range of factors that could potentially explain the lack of significance of the effect of food assistance on the nutritional status. Commonly reported was the issue of food sharing within households. Previous studies have shown that food sharing is very common and often results in failure for the primary beneficiary of food assistance to garner the necessary amount of protein and energy that would induce a gain in weight [67,69,70]. In the pilot study from Zambia [69], there was substantial sharing of food between the recipients of food assistance with the other household members, which led to a programmatic change to indistinctly provide household food rations rather than individual rations. Authors also questioned the nutritional value and the content of the food basket provided to HIV-infected individuals. The use of more nutrient-dense supplements such as the ready-to-use therapeutic foods (RUTFs) in addition to other foods in the basket might have produced different results. The combination of fortified blended foods and RUTFs has shown significant effects on morbidity and nutritional outcomes among refugees in different settings [81]. Another possible reason that could explain the failure of the intervention to improve BMI/weight counts included the inclusion criteria that were used to enroll participants in the food assistance program that were based on the household food insecurity status rather than on the nutritional status of the HIV-infected individuals. Recipients of food assistance were food-insecure, but most of them were not severely undernourished at baseline [69,70,72]. Although one of the eligibility criteria in the Nigerian study included the nutritional status of patients (BMI <18 kg/m^2), patients with BMI ≥18 kg/m^2 could still be recruited based on the other criteria (CD4 counts <200/mm^3, WHO stage 3 or 4). As a result, few patients were undernourished and the median BMI was 19 at baseline [71]. The short duration of interventions, which ranged from 6 to 12 months, could also be a potential reason to explain the failure of the interventions in improving the nutritional status of patients [69–72]. Recovery from undernutrition among HIV-infected individuals generally takes longer than among other individuals [67].

Even though none of the nonrandomized food assistance studies in sub-Saharan Africa have shown a significant effect on patients' nutritional status, a recent study from Haiti found that food supplementation was associated with improved BMI after 12 months of follow-up [82]. It is noteworthy to mention significant points that might have influenced the reported results. In sub-Saharan African studies [69–72], recipients of food assistance and their controls had comparable vulnerability regarding their socioeconomic and food security status, and they were all eligible for the food supplementation program. In the Haiti study, controls were individuals who did not meet the eligibility criteria, and thus they were inherently less vulnerable and more advantageous in terms of socioeconomic, clinical, and nutritional status. Actually, in the Haiti study, food recipients had lower weight and higher food insecurity at baseline compared with controls. Additionally, not all individuals were using ART. The proportion using ART was unbalanced between the two groups, with 82.3% using ART in the food assistance group and 57.8% using ART in the control group. These shortcomings naturally restrict any conclusive evidence regarding benefit of food assistance in improving outcomes among HIV-infected individuals using ART.

Three [69–71] out of the five studies on food assistance examined the effect on immunological response to ART, and only one has shown improved CD4 counts among recipients of nutritional support compared with controls [3]. Only one study assessed survival as one of the outcomes and found better survival among recipients of food assistance [71]. Of the two studies that have assessed the impact of food assistance on disease progression [71,72], none has found significant differences between recipients and nonrecipients of food assistance.

Assessments of nonrandomized intervention studies in sub-Saharan Africa overall support the evidence that emerged from qualitative and observational studies linking food insecurity to poor adherence to ART. However, the effects of food assistance on nutritional, immunological, and clinical outcomes among ART-treated HIV-positive individuals remain to be clarified.

A common weakness to all these studies lies in the nature of their designs, which were not randomized. Therefore, confounding factors might have influenced the reported results in ways that are difficult to predict. Even though some food assistance studies have used propensity score matching with differences in estimation [70,72,73] or have matched intervention clinics to control clinics [70] to approximate the control group to the ideal "counterfactual," these techniques are still not free of bias because matching can only be based on measured variables, and unmeasured variables can account for many differences observed between the intervention and control groups.

A significant gap in the literature of nutritional support among HIV-infected individuals using ART in developing countries, and in sub-Saran Africa in particular, is the remarkable lack of randomized controlled trials. We have documented five randomized controlled trials from sub-Saharan Africa [74–78], including one randomized pilot trial [76] and one unpublished trial from Kenya [77].

Two randomized trials compared two types of food supplementation: ready-to-use fortified spread (RUFS) and corn–soy blend supplementation [74,75]. RUFS is an energy-dense, lipid-based product that resists bacterial infection and requires no cooking [83]. Corn–soy blend is a standard supplementary food provided in many food programs; it needs to be cooked before being eaten. Both randomized trials were conducted in Malawi, and both compared BMI, CD4 counts, adherence to ART, fat-free body mass, mortality, and quality of life in wasted HIV-positive individuals using ART allocated to receive either RUFS or corn–soy blend. Additional outcomes included HIV viral load [74] and hospitalization rate [75]. In one of the trials [74], recipients of RUFS experienced a greater increase in BMI and fat-free body mass after 14 weeks of follow-up, whereas other outcomes were not significantly different between the two groups. The other trial [75] examined, after 9 months, the effects of 3 months of supplementary feeding and found that although BMI was significantly higher in the RUFS arm during the supplementation period, both arms were similar in terms of BMI and other outcomes after 9 months of follow-up, suggesting that the nutritional benefits of RUFS are not maintained once the food supplementation stops. This also raises the question of how long the duration of food supplementation should last to maximize its nutritional benefits. A similar and recently published randomized trial from Haiti, however, reported contrasting results [84]. In this study, BMI and CD4 counts were similar in both groups receiving either RUFS or corn–soy blend plus fortified oil and sugar after 12 months of follow-up. This trial particularly differs from those in sub-Saharan Africa [74,75] in that food insecurity status was used as the criterion for eligibility rather than the wasting syndrome. The baseline BMI between the two groups was within normal range.

A major limitation of these trials is that they assessed the effectiveness of nutritional support between two different forms of food supplementation rather than using a control group that is not nutritionally assisted. As a consequence, there was no possibility to measure the true benefits that food supplementation of any kind could confer. Ethical considerations restricted the use of such a control group in Malawi given that the Malawian national policy demands that wasted HIV-positive patients be offered food supplementation. Ethical considerations require that patients enrolled as controls in clinical trials should be offered the standard of care, which at one extreme is understood as the standard prevailing locally and at the other extreme is understood as the best current proven intervention [85]. In the absence of national policy compelling food supplementation to HIV-positive individuals, one of the strategies to circumvent ethical restrictions could be the use of a wait-list control. This strategy has been used in a recently published randomized controlled trial from Ethiopia [78]. The Ethiopian trial was designed to compare the lean body mass, physical activity, weight, viral load, and CD4 counts among ART-treated patients allocated to receive lipid-based nutritional supplements with either soy protein or whey and a control group of ART-treated patients without nutritional support followed-up for a period of 3 months. Overall, nutritional support was associated with improved weight, lean body mass, and grip strength. Additionally, patients who received the whey-based supplement experienced an improvement in their immune status. However, there were no differences in suppression of viral load between the groups. This is one of the rare published trials demonstrating the effect of nutritional support on weight gain and CD4 counts in sub-Saharan Africa. Unfortunately, the study was not powered sufficiently to assess the effect of nutritional support on survival, and other important outcomes such as adherence to ART were not examined. A preceding randomized pilot trial from South Africa found similar results when patients commencing ART who were randomized to receive nutritional support had improved weight, immune response, and physical activity after 6 months of follow-up compared with the control group of ART-treated individuals [76]. However, this pilot study was limited by its very small sample size. Data from an unpublished randomized trial from Kenya reported in a recent Cochrane review indicated significant gain in weight among patients allocated to receive nutritional support in the form of fortified blended food compared with patients with no nutritional support [77].

The current landscape of research of nutritional support among HIV-positive individuals in sub-Saharan Africa portrays that there is bourgeoning evidence from randomized controlled trials demonstrating the positive effect of nutritional support on a number of HIV treatment outcomes [76–78]; however, it is too early to draw any conclusion because of the limited number of trials. There is a salient need for more evidence from well-crafted randomized trials to ascertain the effect of food intervention on an exhaustive range of ART outcomes.

A recently published Cochrane systematic review reported that based on the current evidence, no firm conclusion can be drawn about the effects of macronutrient supplementation on morbidity and mortality of people living with HIV [68]. However, most of the trials included in the review were conducted in Europe or in the United States, and those that were conducted in sub-Saharan Africa; only one unpublished trial included ART-treated individuals as the target population [77]; the rest targeted children [86,87] or ART-naïve patients [88].

One of the limitations of the current trials from sub-Saharan Africa is the short duration; consequently, study endpoints such as mortality, BMI/weight, CD4 count, and viral load may not appropriately capture the effect of the interventions. This is true for randomized trials and for nonrandomized studies documented in this chapter. Longer and larger trials are needed to shed light on the effect of food supplementation on HIV treatment outcomes; however, it should be balanced with cost and other factors related to the nature of the intervention. For example, high-energy lipid-based nutrients such as RUFS are associated with increase in fat-free body mass and MUAC [74]. Therefore, long-term use of high-energy lipid-based nutrients should carefully be considered in settings where stavudine-based ART regimens are still in use to avoid possible metabolic complications. Stavudine is known to be associated with increased metabolic side effects such as dyslipidemias, lipodystrophy, and insulin resistance [89].

Several other factors might have limited the ability of some intervention studies to show an effect. For example, coinfection with other endemic pathogens is known to affect immunological and virological responses to ART [25]. ART itself is known to improve nutritional status of people living with HIV, even in the absence of any nutritional support [31]. This may dampen the effect size of the intervention if for any reason adherence to ART in the control group is better than in the intervention group, leading to failure to demonstrate the effectiveness of an intervention, especially when the study is not sufficiently powered. Another important threat to the effectiveness of food intervention studies is the issue of food sharing. Food intervention studies target individuals who come from socioeconomically deprived households. This means that individuals who receive food rations may share them with other household members, therefore reducing or annihilating the benefits that food assistance could confer. To circumvent this issue, some programs have suggested provision of household food rations in addition to the individual rations [67,69], as well as counseling and education about the importance of the food ration to the targeted individuals [67].

Food intervention studies to improve ART outcomes can benefit from lessons learned from other intervention studies in sub-Saharan Africa. For example, evidence from studies to improve adherence to ART in sub-Saharan Africa indicates that interventions targeting most at-risk individuals were more likely to show positive results than those that did not [44]. Even though the degree to which this may extend to food interventions is not certain, it underscores the need to define appropriate criteria for eligibility of nutritional support programs. Different eligibility and targeting strategies will incur different implications in terms of the resourced required, types of food products needed, and dissemination strategies [90] and criteria, and may influence to a certain extent the effect on the measured outcomes.

It is important to note that nutritional support programs are hardly sustainable over the long-term and generally are intended to serve as short-term formal sources of support to HIV-positive individuals; therefore, parallel efforts should be channeled to find sustainable food and livelihood approaches that fit contextual factors and address upstream drivers of food insecurity and undernutrition among HIV-infected individuals in sub-Saharan Africa. It also appears that none of the nutritional intervention studies had integrated a cost-effectiveness component in its design. A recent study has used the Zambian national ART program data to model the cost-effectiveness of nutrition supplementation by estimating the improvements in 6-month survival and program retention among undernourished HIV-infected adults starting ART and found that even though nutritional interventions were cost-effective across all the categories of undernutrition compared with standard treatment (ART alone), interventions were more likely to be cost-effective when targeted to severely undernourished individuals [91]. Future research would be strengthened by incorporating cost-effectiveness analyses to allow a more insightful interpretation of the results in light of both cost and the ability of the intervention to achieve the desired outcome.

Although it was not within the scope of this chapter to assess the current literature of nutritional support for ART outcomes in children, there is a strong indication that this area of research is poorly documented in sub-Saharan Africa [68], and research is urgently needed to fill the gap.

12.5 SUMMARY

The negative impact of food insecurity and undernutrition on HIV treatment outcomes in sub-Saharan Africa is widely recognized and documented in both qualitative and quantitative studies. There is emerging evidence from randomized trials that nutritional support improves ART outcomes; however, there is salient need for more evidence from well-crafted randomized trials comparing a full range of outcomes between recipients and nonrecipients of nutritional support to ascertain the benefits of food provision among ART-treated HIV-infected individuals in sub-Saharan Africa. Trials assessing different types of food interventions of varying duration, incorporating cost-effectiveness analyses, and targeting HIV-positive individuals with varying duration of ART may benefit future policy decisions on how to eliminate food insecurity and undernutrition among people living with HIV in sub-Saharan Africa.

References

[1] Joint United Nations Programme on HIV/AIDS. Global report: UNAIDS report on the global AIDS epidemic 2012. Available from: http://www.unaids.org/en/media/unaids/contentassets/documents/epidemiology/2012gr2012/20121120_UNAIDS_Global_Report_2012_with_annexes_en.pdf.

[2] Food and Agriculture Organization of the United Nations. The state of food insecurity in the world: economic growth is necessary but not sufficient to accelerate reduction of hunger and malnutrition. Available from: http://www.fao.org/docrep/016/i3027e/i3027e.pdf; 2012 [accessed 25.01.13].

[3] Seres DS. Surrogate nutrition markers, malnutrition, and adequacy of nutrition support. Nutr Clin Pract 2005;20:308–13.

[4] Soeters PB, Reijven PL, van Bokhorst-de van der Schueren MA, et al. A rational approach to nutritional assessment. Clin Nutr 2008;27:706–16.

[5] Radimer KL, Olson CM, Greene JC, et al. Understanding hunger and developing indicators to assess it in women and children. J Nutr Educ 1992;24(Suppl. 1):36S–45S.

[6] Black RE, Allen LH, Bhutta ZA, et al. Maternal and child undernutrition: global and regional exposures and health consequences. Lancet 2008;371(9608):243–60. 19.

[7] Centers for Disease Control Revision of the CDC surveillance case definition for acquired immunodeficiency syndrome. J Am Med Assoc 1987;258(Suppl. IS):1143–53.

[8] Grunfeld C, Kotler DP. Pathophysiology of the AIDS wasting syndrome. AIDS Clin Rev 1992:191–224.

[9] Keithley JK, Swanson B. HIV-associated wasting. J Assoc Nurses AIDS Care 2013;24:S103–11.

[10] Salomon J, De Truchis P, Melchoir J-C. Nutrition and HIV infection. Br J Nutr 2002;87(Suppl. 1):S111–9.

[11] Sicotte M, Langlois EV, Aho J, et al. Association between nutritional status and the immune response in HIV + patients under HAART: protocol for a systematic review. Syst Rev 2014;3:9.

[12] Weiser SD, Fernandes KA, Anema A, et al. Food insecurity as a barrier to antiretroviral adherence among HIV-infected individuals in British Columbia. Presented at 5th International AIDS Society (IAS) Conference on HIV Pathogenesis, Treatment and Prevention. Cape Town, South Africa; 2009. Available from: http://caps.ucsf.edu/uploads/pubs/presentations/pdf/Weiser1_IAS09.pdf [accessed 20.06.14].

[13] Weiser S, Frongillo E, Ragland K, et al. Food insecurity is associated with incomplete HIV RNA suppression among homeless and marginally housed HIV-infected individuals in San Francisco. J Gen Intern Med 2009;24:14–20.

[14] Kalichman S, Cherry C, Amaral C, et al. Health and treatment implications of food insufficiency among people living with HIV/AIDS, Atlanta, Georgia. J Urban Health 2010;87:631–41.

[15] Kalichman S, Pellowski J, Kalichman M, et al. Food insufficiency and medication adherence among people living with HIV/AIDS in urban and peri-urban settings. Prev Sci 2011;12:324–32.

[16] Peretti-Watel P, Spire B, Schiltz MA, et al. Vulnerability, unsafe sex and non-adherence to HAART: evidence from a large sample of French HIV/AIDS outpatients. Soc Sci Med 2011;62:2420–33.

[17] Musumari PM, Feldman MD, Techasrivichien T, et al. If I have nothing to eat, I get angry and push the pills bottle away from me: a qualitative study of patient determinants of adherence to antiretroviral therapy in the Democratic Republic of Congo. AIDS Care 2013;25(10):1271–7.

[18] Weiser SD, Tuller DM, Frongillo EA, et al. Food insecurity as a barrier to sustained antiretroviral therapy adherence in Uganda. PLoS One 2010;5(4):e10340. http://dx.doi.org/10.1371/journal.pone.0010340.

[19] Hardon AP, Akurut D, Comoro C, et al. Hunger, waiting time and transport costs: time to confront challenges to ART adherence in Africa. AIDS Care 2007;19:658–65.
[20] Weiser SD, Palar K, Frongillo EA, et al. Longitudinal assessment of associations between food insecurity, antiretroviral adherence and HIV treatment outcomes in rural Uganda. AIDS 2013;28(1):115–20.
[21] Weiser SD, Young SL, Cohen CR, Kushel MB, Tsai AC, Tien PC, et al. Conceptual framework for understanding the bidirectional links between food insecurity and HIV/AIDS. Am J Clin Nutr 2011;94(Suppl.):1729S–39S.
[22] World Food Program (WFP). Emergency food security assessment handbook. 2nd ed.; 2009. Available from: http://documents.wfp.org/stellent/groups/public/documents/manual_guide_proced/wfp203244.pdf.
[23] Radimer KL, Olson CM, Frongillo EA. Validation of the radimer/cornellmeasures of hunger and food insecurity. J Nutr 1995;125:2793–801.
[24] Coates J, Swindale A, Bilinsky P. Household food insecurity access scale (HFIAS) for measurement of food access: indicator guide. Washington, DC: Food and Nutrition Technical Assistance Project, Academy for Educational Development; 2007.
[25] Braitstein P, Brinkhof MW, Dabis F, et al. Mortality of HIV-1-infected patients in the first year of antiretroviral therapy: comparison between low-income and high-income countries. Lancet 2006;367(9513):817–24.
[26] Marazzi MC, Liotta G, Germano P, et al. Excessive early mortality in the first year of treatment in HIV type 1-infected patients initiating antiretroviral therapy in resource-limited settings. AIDS Res Hum Retroviruses 2008;24:555–60.
[27] Jerene D, Endale A, Hailu Y, et al. Predictors of early death in a cohort of Ethiopian patients treated with HAART. BMC Infect Dis 2006;6:136.
[28] Zachariah R, Fitzgerald M, Massaquoi M, et al. Risk factors for high early mortality in patients on antiretroviral treatment in a rural district of Malawi. AIDS 2006;20:2355–60.
[29] Stringer JS, Zulu I, Levy J, et al. Rapid scale-up of antiretroviral therapy at primary care sites in Zambia: feasibility and early outcomes. JAMA 2006;296:782–93.
[30] Johannessen A, Naman E, Ngowi BJ, et al. Predictors of mortality in HIV-infected patients starting antiretroviral therapy in a rural hospital in Tanzania. BMC Infect Dis 2008;8:52.
[31] Madec Y, Szumilin E, Genevier C, et al. Weight gain at 3 months of antiretroviral therapy is strongly associated with survival: evidence from two developing countries. AIDS 2009;23(7):853–61.
[32] Koethe JR, Lukusa A, Giganti MJ, et al. Association between weight gain and clinical outcomes among malnourished adults initiating antiretroviral therapy in Lusaka, Zambia. J Acquir Immune Defic Syndr 2010;53(4):507–13.
[33] Liu E, Spiegelman D, Semu H, et al. Nutritional status and mortality among HIV-infected patients receiving antiretroviral therapy in Tanzania. J Infect Dis 2011;204(2):282–90.
[34] Palombi L, Marazzi MC, Guidotti G, et al. Incidence and predictors of death, retention, and switch to second-line regimens in antiretroviral- treated patients in Sub-Saharan African sites with comprehensive monitoring availability. Clin Infect Dis 2009;48(1):115–22.
[35] Gupta A, Nadkarni G, Yang WT, et al. Early mortality in adults initiating antiretroviral therapy (ART) in low- and middle-income countries (LMIC): a systematic review and meta-analysis. PLoS One 2011;6(12):e28691.
[36] World Food Program (WFP). Statement to the 32nd Session of UN Food and Agriculture Organization's Governing Conference, Rome, Italy; 2006. Available from: http://wfp.org/content/statement-32nd-session-un-food-and-agriculture-organizations-governing-conference-rome-italy.
[37] UNAIDS. Political declaration on HIV/AIDS. In Joint United Nations Programme on HIV/AIDS; 2006. Available from: http://data.unaids.org/pub/report/2006/20060615_hlm_politicaldeclaration_ares60262_en.pdf.

[38] UNAIDS. Report on the global AIDS epidemic. Geneva, Switzerland: Joint United Nations Programme on HIV/AIDS; 2008. Available from: http://unaids.org/en/media/unaids/contentassets/dataimport/pub/globalreport/2008/jc1510_2008globalreport_en.pdf.
[39] World Food Program (WFP). HIV, AIDS, TB and Nutrition. In World Food Program; 2012. Available from: http://documents.wfp.org/stellent/groups/public/documents/communications/wfp248909.pdf.
[40] Programming in the Era of AIDS. WPF's response to HIV/AIDS. Rome, Italy: World Food Program; 2003. Available from: http://wfp.org/content/programming-era-aids-wfps-responses-hivaids.
[41] Nutrition and HIV/AIDS. Statement by the Administrative Committee on Coordination, Sub-committee on Nutrition at its 28th Session. Nairobi, Kenya: United Nations Administrative Committee on Coordination, Sub-Committee on Nutrition; 2001.
[42] The World Bank. HIV/AIDS, nutrition, and food security: what we can do. A synthesis of international guidance. Washington, DC: The World Bank; 2007. Available from: http://siteresources.worldbank.org/NUTRITION/Ressources/281846-1100008431337/HIVAIDSNutritionFoodSecuritylowerres.pdf.
[43] United Nations World Food Program. HIV, food security, and nutrition. Policy Brief; 2008. Available from: http://one.wfp.org/food_aid/doc/JC1515-Policy_Brief_Expanded.pdf.
[44] Bärnighausen T, Chaiyachati K, Chimbindi N, et al. Interventions to increase antiretroviral adherence in Sub-Saharan Africa: a systematic review of evaluation studies. Lancet Infect Dis 2011;11(12):942–51.
[45] Chaiyachati KH, Ogbuoji O, Price M, et al. Interventions to improve adherence to antiretroviral therapy: a rapid systematic review. AIDS 2014;28(Suppl. 2):S187–204.
[46] Berhe N, Tegabu D, Alemayehu M. Effect of nutritional factors on adherence to antiretroviral therapy among HIV-infected adults: a case control study in Northern Ethiopia. BMC Infect Dis 2013;13:233.
[47] Abiy S. Impact of food and nutrition security on adherence to anti-retroviral therapy (ART) and treatment outcomes among adult plwha in dire dawa provisional administration. : Addis Ababa University [Internet]; 2007. Available from: http://hdl.handle.net/123456789/861.
[48] Marston B, De Cock KM. Multivitamins, nutrition, and antiretroviral therapy for HIV disease in Africa. N Engl J Med 2004;351:78–80.
[49] Casey KM. Malnutrition associated with HIV/AIDS. Part one: definition and scope, epidemiology, and pathophysiology. J Assoc Nurses AIDS Care 1997;8:24–32.
[50] Olowookere SA, Fatiregun AA, Akinyemi JO, et al. Prevalence and determinants of adherence to highly active antiretroviral therapy among people living with HIV/AIDS in Ibadan, Nigeria. J Infect Dev Countries 2008;2(5):369–72.
[51] Goudge J, Ngoma B. Exploring antiretroviral treatment adherence in an urban setting in South Africa. J Public Health Policy 2011;32(Suppl. 1):S52–64.
[52] Senkomago V, Guwatudde D, Breda M, et al. Barriers to antiretroviral adherence in HIV-positive patients receiving free medication in Kayunga, Uganda. AIDS Care 2011;23(10):1246–53.
[53] Au JT, Kayitenkore K, Shutes E, et al. Access to adequate nutrition is a major potential obstacle to antiretroviral adherence among HIV-infected individuals in Rwanda. AIDS 2006;20(16):2116–8.
[54] Nagata JM, Magerenge RO, Young SL, et al. Social determinants, lived experiences, and consequences of household food insecurity among persons living with HIV/AIDS on the shore of Lake Victoria, Kenya. AIDS Care 2012;24(6):728–36.
[55] Groh K, Audet CM, Baptista A, et al. Barriers to antiretroviral therapy adherence in rural Mozambique. BMC Public Health 2011;11:650.
[56] Sanjobo N, Frich JC, Fretheim A. Barriers and facilitators to patients' adherence to antiretroviral treatment in Zambia: a qualitative study. Sahara J 2008;5:136–43.

[57] Weiser SD, Yuan C, Guzman D, et al. Food insecurity and HIV clinical outcomes in a longitudinal study of urban homeless and marginally housed HIV-infected individuals. AIDS 2013;27(18):2953–8.
[58] Musumari PM, Wouters E, Kayembe PK, et al. Food insecurity is associated with increased risk of non-adherence to antiretroviral therapy among HIV-infected adults in the Democratic Republic of Congo: a cross-sectional study. PLoS One 2014;9(1):e85327.
[59] Birbeck GL, Kvalsund MP, Byers PA, et al. Neuropsychiatric and socioeconomic status impact antiretroviral adherence and mortality in rural Zambia. Am J Trop Med Hyg 2011;85(4):782–9.
[60] Boyer S, Clerc I, Bonono CR, et al. Non-adherence to antiretroviral treatment and unplanned treatment interruption among people living with HIV/AIDS in Cameroon: individual and healthcare supply-related factors. Soc Sci Med 2011;72(8):1383–92.
[61] Marcellin F, Boyer S, Protopopescu C, et al. Determinants of unplanned antiretroviral treatment interruptions among people living with HIV in Yaoundé, Cameroon (EVAL survey, ANRS 12–116). Trop Med Int Health 2008;13(12):1470–8.
[62] Sasaki Y, Kikimoto K, Dube C, et al. Adherence to antiretroviral therapy (ART) during the early months of treatment in rural Zambia: influence of demographic characteristics and social surroundings of patients. Ann Clin Microbiol Antimicrob 2012;11:34.
[63] Van Dyk AC. Treatment adherence following national antiretroviral rollout in South Africa. Afr J AIDS Res 2010;9(3):235–47.
[64] Weiser SD, Bangsberg DR, Kegeles S, et al. Food insecurity among homeless and marginally housed individuals living with HIV/AIDS in San Francisco. AIDS Behav 2009;13:841–8.
[65] Wang EA, McGinnis KA, Fiellin DA, et al. Food insecurity is associated with poor virologic response among HIV-infected patients receiving antiretroviral medications. J Gen Intern Med 2011;26:1012–8.
[66] Weiser SD, Fernandes KA, Brandson EK, et al. The association between food insecurity and mortality among HIV-infected individuals on HAART. J Acquir Immune Defic Syndr 2009;52:342–9.
[67] Food and Nutrition Technical Assistance (FANTA) Project and World Food Program (WFP). Food assistance programming in the context of HIV. Washington, DC: FANTA Project, Academy for Educational Development; 2007. Available from: http://fantaproject.org/focus-areas/infectious-diseases/food-assistance-programming-hiv.
[68] Grobler L, Siegfried N, Visser ME, et al. Nutritional interventions for reducing morbidity and mortality in people with HIV. Cochrane Database Syst Rev 2013;2:CD004536.
[69] Cantrell RA, Sinkala M, Megazinni K, et al. A pilot study of food supplementation to improve adherence to antiretroviral therapy among food-insecure adults in Lusaka, Zambia. J Acquir Immune Defic Syndr 2008;49(2):190–5.
[70] Tirivayi N, Koethe JR, Groot W. Clinic-based food assistance is associated with increased medication adherence among HIV-infected adults on long-term antiretroviral therapy in Zambia. J AIDS Clin Res 2012;3(7):171.
[71] Serrano C, Laporte R, Ide M, et al. Family nutritional support improves survival, immune restoration and adherence in HIV patients receiving ART in developing country. Asia Pac J Clin Nutr 2010;19(1):68–75.
[72] Rawat R, Kadiyala S, McNamara PE. The impact of food assistance on weight gain and disease progression among HIV-infected individuals accessing AIDS care and treatment services in Uganda. BMC Public Health 2010;10:316.
[73] Posse M, Tirivayi M, Sasha UR, et al. The effect of food assistance on adherence to antiretroviral therapy among HIV/AIDS patients in Sofala Province, in Mozambique: a retrospective study. J AIDS Clin Res 2013;4(3):1000198.

[74] Ndekha MJ, Oosterhout JJ, Zijlstra EE, et al. Supplementary feeding with either ready-to-use fortified spread or corn–soy blend in wasted adults starting anti-retroviral therapy in Malawi: randomised, investigator blinded, controlled trial. BMJ 2009;338:b1867.
[75] Ndekha M, Oosterhout JJ, Saloojee H, et al. Nutritional status of Malawian adults on antiretroviral therapy 1 year after supplementary feeding in the first 3 months of therapy. Trop Med Int Health 2009;14(9):1059–63.
[76] Evans D, McNamara L, Maskew M, et al. Impact of nutritional supplementation on immune response, body mass index and bioelectrical impedance in HIV-positive patients starting antiretroviral therapy. Nutr J 2013;12:111.
[77] Castleman T, Mwadime R, et al. Randomised controlled trial of the impact of supplementary food on malnourished adult ART clients and adult pre-ART clients in Kenya. Final report; June 2011.
[78] Olsen MF, Abdissa A, Kæstel P, et al. Effects of nutritional supplementation for HIV patients starting antiretroviral treatment: randomised controlled trial in Ethiopia. BMJ 2014;348:g3187.
[79] McMahon JH, Jordan MR, Kelley K, et al. Pharmacy adherence measures to assess adherence to antiretroviral therapy: review of the literature and implications for treatment monitoring. Clin Infect Dis 2011;52:493–506.
[80] Chi BH, Cantrell RA, Zulu I, et al. Adherence to first-line antiretroviral therapy affects non-virologic outcomes among patients on treatment for more than 12 months in Lusaka, Zambia. Int J Epidemiol 2009;38:746–56.
[81] Ivers LC, Cullen KA, Freedberg KA, et al. HIV/AIDS, undernutrition, and food insecurity. Clin Infect Dis 2009;49(7):1096–102.
[82] Ivers LC, Chang Y, Jerome JG, et al. Food assistance is associated with improved body mass index, food security and attendance at clinic in an HIV program in central Haiti: a prospective observational cohort study. AIDS Res Ther 2010;7:33.
[83] US Agency for International Development. Ready-to-use therapeutic food commodity fact sheet. Available from: http://www.usaid.gov/what-we-do/agriculture-and-food-security/food-assistance/resources/ready-use-therapeutic-food.
[84] Ivers LC, Teng JE, Jerome JG, et al. A randomized trial of ready-to-use supplementary food versus corn–soy blend plus as food rations for HIV-infected adults on antiretroviral therapy in rural Haiti. Clin Infect Dis 2014;58(8):1176–84.
[85] World Medical Association. Declaration of Helsinki—ethical principles for medical research involving human subjects; 2013. Available from: http://www.wma.net/en/30publications/10policies/b3/index.html.
[86] Rollins NC, van den Broeck J, Kindra G, et al. The effect of nutritional support on weight gain of HIV-infected children with prolonged diarrhoea. Acta Paediatr 2007;96:62–8.
[87] Simpore J, Zongo F, Kabore F, et al. Nutrition rehabilitation of HIV-infected and HIV-negative undernourished children utilizing spirulina. Ann Nutr Metab 2005;49:373–80.
[88] Yamani E, Kaba-Mebri J, Mouala C, et al. Use of spirulina supplement for nutritional management of HIV-infected patients: study in Bangui, Central African Republic. Med Trop 2009;69(1):66–70.
[89] Van Griensven J, De Naeyer L, Mushi T, et al. High prevalence of lipoatrophy among patients on stavudine-containing first-line antiretroviral therapy regimens in Rwanda. Trans R Soc Trop Med Hyg 2007;101:793–8.
[90] Singer AW, Weiser SD, McCoy SI. Does food insecurity undermine adherence to antiretroviral therapy? A systematic review. AIDS Behav 2014 [Epub ahead of print].
[91] Koethe JR, Marseille E, Giganti MJ, et al. Estimating the cost-effectiveness of nutrition supplementation for malnourished, HIV-infected adults starting antiretroviral therapy in a resource-constrained setting. Cost Eff Resour Alloc 2014;12:10.

CHAPTER

13

How the HIV Epidemic Carved an Indelible Imprint on Infant Feeding

Hoosen Coovadia[1] *and Heena Brahmbhatt*[2]

[1]MatCH Health Systems a Division of the University of the Witwatersrand, Emeritus Professor of Paediatrics and Child Health, University of KwaZulu-Natal Commissioner, National Planning Commission at the Presidency, Republic of South Africa, [2]Johns Hopkins Bloomberg School of Public Health, Department of Population, Family and Reproductive Health, Baltimore, MD, USA

13.1 IMPACT OF BREASTFEEDING ON CHILD SURVIVAL

Almost 7 million children younger than age 5 years died in 2012, mostly from preventable diseases [1]. Although, globally, mortality rates for those younger than 5 have declined by almost 50% from 90 deaths in 1990 to 48 deaths per 1,000 live births in 2012, rates in sub-Saharan Africa continue to be unacceptably high at more than 100 deaths per 1,000 live births [2]. One of the millennium development goals (MDGs) is to reduce child mortality by two-thirds by 2015 by reducing the five major causes of child mortality globally: diarrhea, malaria, neonatal infection, pneumonia, and preterm delivery [3]. Malnutrition and lack of safe water contribute to more than half of these child deaths [1].

There is incontrovertible evidence that breastfeeding is the best form of infant feeding for all women everywhere, with very few and only marginal exceptions [4,5]. The long-term beneficial impact of breastfeeding for both the mother and child are well-documented; for women,

Health of HIV Infected People, Volume 2.
DOI: http://dx.doi.org/10.1016/B978-0-12-800767-9.00013-3

breastfeeding has been shown to reduce obesity, breast cancer, ovarian cancer, type 2 diabetes, and myocardial infarction [6], and for infants and children, breastfeeding has been shown to reduce morbidities and child mortality, improve child growth and development, reduce risks of childhood obesity, type 1 diabetes, and type 2 diabetes, improve learning, and improve productivity [7–10]. The practice of exclusive breastfeeding provides more than an ideal food source; exclusively breastfed infants are less likely to die from diarrhea, acute respiratory infections, and other diseases [4,8,11], and exclusive breastfeeding has been found to support infants' immune systems and protect from chronic diseases later in life such as obesity and diabetes [11].

The World Health Organization (WHO) estimates that modifiable nutritional risk factors such as underweight and deficiency of zinc and iron are responsible for more than 6 million childhood deaths per year [8]. An additional almost 2 million child deaths are due to environmental risk factors such as unsafe water and lack of sanitation [2]. It is estimated that approximately 1.4 million child deaths could be prevented in high-mortality countries by increasing breastfeeding among infants [5]. Although the evidence of the benefits of breastfeeding is indubitable, the advent of the HIV epidemic challenged breastfeeding practices because HIV can be vertically transmitted from the infected mother to the infant *in utero*, intrapartum, and postnatally via breastfeeding [12].

13.2 BREASTFEEDING AND MOTHER-TO-CHILD TRANSMISSION OF HIV

HIV prevalence rates among women of reproductive age continue to be high, with rates between 20% and 40% in countries in southern Africa such as Botswana, Lesotho, Swaziland, and South Africa [13]. In developing countries, HIV/AIDS continues to be a leading cause of mortality among women of reproductive age, and without treatment approximately 50% of HIV-positive children die by their second birthday [14]. HIV transmission rates prior to antiretroviral therapy (ART) for the prevention of mother-to-child-transmission (PMTCT) have been estimated at 15–25% in industrialized countries where breastfeeding is not the norm, compared with rates as high as 45% in developing countries where breastfeeding is the usual practice [12,13]. Factors shown to increase the risk of MTCT are maternal HIV viral load, maternal advanced disease, mode of delivery, prolonged rupture of membranes, chorioamnionitis, type of breastfeeding (exclusive, mixed, or replacement feeding), duration of breastfeeding, and use of ARTs for PMTCT [12,13].

Advances in ART regimens for PMTCT reduced *in utero* and intrapartum vertical transmission rates by almost 50% [15] but increased the numbers of infants who would then potentially be infected via breastfeeding, which is estimated to be between 5% and 20%, with an attributable risk of 40% [16,17]. The biological explanations for vertical transmission of HIV through breastfeeding are based on several putative mechanisms; HIV is present in human breast milk as cell-associated or cell-free virus and both have been found to be involved in breast milk HIV transmission [16]. Postnatal HIV transmission is thought to increase with maternal seroconversion during lactation (when maternal viral loads are high), increased maternal RNA and low CD4 levels, clinical and subclinical mastitis, and nipple bleeding and abscesses [12,18–21]. Once the milk is ingested by the infant, transmission is thought to occur through the infant gut mucosal surface [18].

Postnatal HIV transmission via breastfeeding has been shown by many studies [15,18,19]. A landmark randomized trial in Nairobi, Kenya, where women were randomized to breastfeeding or formula feeding, demonstrated that the risk of MTCT was 44% higher among breastfed compared with formula-fed infants and that 75% of all breastfeeding transmission occurred in the first 6 months of the infant's life [22]. However, despite exclusive breastfeeding being recommended in this trial, it was likely not exclusive and no information was collected regarding mode of feeding. A meta-analysis of data from randomized controlled trials that assessed the risk of postnatal HIV transmission found that the overall risk of late postnatal transmission (after 4–6 weeks) was 8.9 transmissions per 100 child-years of breastfeeding and late postnatal transmission could contribute as much as 42% to the overall rate of MTCT [23]. High rates of postnatal HIV transmission are a particular concern in sub-Saharan Africa, where breastfeeding is practiced almost universally. However, prevention of breastfeeding transmission of HIV has to be considered in a broader context, taking into account the known and significant benefits of breast milk to infant health and growth as well as for fertility control for the mother. In addition, the estimates of the mortality risk from breastfeeding may be confounded; a study analyzing DHS data from multiple countries found that rates of child mortality due to breastfeeding are probably overestimates because in cultures where lactation is normative, the decision not to breastfeed or wean early is probably involuntary and due to a preceding illness in the mother or infant [24]. This study found that preceding morbidity in the mother–infant pair was the most common reason for not breastfeeding (64%) and that the cumulative hazard of child mortality at 24 months was more than seven-times higher among infants who were never breastfed due to a preceding illness in the mother compared with those who did not breastfeed by maternal choice, and more than two-times higher among children weaned due to preceding morbidity compared with children who weaned due to nonhealth-related reasons. Therefore, child mortality rates from voluntary weaning should be used as a benchmark for counseling HIV-positive women regarding the risks of nonbreastfeeding or weaning for the prevention of MTCT.

As the breast versus formula feeding debate raged in the late 1990s, another landmark study from Durban, South Africa, by Coutsoudis et al. [25,26] was published, which highlighted the role of mixed feeding (breast milk plus other solids or liquids) in postnatal transmission of HIV. The hypothesis was that the risk of postnatal HIV transmission was increased due to mixed feeding, probably because the solids disrupt the functional integrity of the gut mucosa of the developing infant and facilitate transmission of the virus. This study demonstrated that the cumulative risk of MTCT was similar by 6 months of age between never and exclusively breastfed infants (0.194; 95% CI, 0.136 $\pm$ 0.260; and 0.194; 95% CI, 0.125 $\pm$ 0.274, respectively), but it was significantly higher among mixed-fed infants (0.261; 95% CI, 0.205 $\pm$ 0.319). This observational study highlighted the importance of mode of feeding on MTCT and raised questions about findings from previous studies on postnatal MTCT that did not differentiate between exclusive and mixed feeding. The Durban KwaZulu Natal studies [25–27] now provided HIV positive mothers an option to exclusively breastfeed their children, thereby providing the known benefits of breast milk and, at the same time, minimizing the risk of HIV transmission by avoiding mixed feeding that could increase the risk of transmission.

The risk of vertical transmission estimated by duration and mode of breastfeeding was calculated at approximately 6% for infants exclusively breastfed for 6 months and weaned abruptly, 11% if mixed-fed for 6 months and weaned abruptly, and 15% if breastfed for 2 years [28]. However, despite the recommendation to exclusively breastfeed, it is not commonly practiced for 6 months because women often introduce liquids and solids within the first few months of the infant's life; therefore, other interventions such as prolonged ARTs during the breastfeeding period are necessary to minimize postnatal vertical transmission of HIV [28–30].

In addition to the reduction in risk of MTCT, there were additional benefits for the health of the infant from exclusive breastfeeding. A review on the optimal duration of breastfeeding for infant health found that exclusive breastfeeding for 6 months resulted in lower rates of morbidity and gastrointestinal infection and no deficits in growth compared with breastfeeding for 3–4 months [31]. In addition, mortality rates among nonbreastfed children were seven-fold higher, and the risks for diarrhea and pneumonia were more than five-fold higher [9] compared with infants who were exclusively breastfed during the first 6 months. Infants who are not exclusively breastfed have a more than two-fold higher risk of death from diarrhea and pneumonia [32], mainly due to drinking contaminated water, lack of sanitation, and poor hygiene.

Based on studies demonstrating transmission of HIV via breastfeeding [30], and given the high mortality rates of HIV-infected infants and children [5], WHO recommended that women breastfeed their children exclusively for up to 6 months unless replacement feeding is acceptable, feasible, affordable, sustainable, and safe [30]. However, given the risks of high rates of morbidity and mortality from vertical transmission of HIV, the WHO recommended avoidance of all breastfeeding by HIV-infected mothers if these conditions were not met. The 2013 WHO guidelines were revised to recommend the introduction of complementary foods at 6 months and weaning by 12 months of age [33].

13.2.1 Antiretroviral Therapy for the Prevention of Postnatal HIV Transmission

Given the role of maternal HIV viral load in increasing the risk of MTCT [34], ARTs to reduce maternal viral load levels have been a successful strategy in PMTCT. Use of single-dose nevirapine (sd NVP) for PMTCT in the late 1990s resulted in MTCT rates decreasing to approximately 12% [13]. Subsequently, use of combined ART regimes, delivery of infants via cesarean, and avoidance of breastfeeding in developed countries resulted in marked reduction in MTCT rates [34]. MTCT soon became a preventable disease in many of these settings. As the success of ARTs for the prevention of *in utero* and intrapartum MTCT became evident in the 1990s, the issue of HIV transmission through breastfeeding became more critical and led to several trials assessing the impact of postpartum ART regimes for the prevention of vertical postnatal transmission (Table 13.1).

Several randomized clinical trials assessed the impact of ART initiation during late gestation through the postpartum period on HIV transmission via breastfeeding. The PETRA (prevention of early and late transmission of HIV-1) randomized trial in Tanzania, South Africa, and Uganda [47] was one of the earliest studies assessing the impact of ARTs during late gestation and up to 7 days postpartum. The goal of the study was to assess the impact of four ART regimes on postnatal HIV transmission. At 6 weeks, the lowest HIV transmission and mortality rates were among mothers who had HAART starting during pregnancy (36 weeks of gestation), continued in the intrapartum period, and for 7 days postpartum. After the PETRA study, the MASHI (means milk in the local language) randomized clinical trial in Botswana [46] assessed the impact of ARTs during late gestation and, unlike the PETRA study, extended postnatal ARTs to 6 months to assess the impact of extended ARTs on HIV transmission via breastfeeding. The study found that at 1 month there was no difference in MTCT rates between breastfed and formula-fed babies; hence, breastfeeding was not a risk for MTCT within the first month of life for mothers and infants receiving ART. However, at 7 months formula-fed babies had significantly higher mortality rates compared with breastfed babies, but this difference was no longer statistically significant by

TABLE 13.1 Summary of Trials on ARTs for Prevention of Postnatal HIV Transmission

Study	Trial site	ART regime for mother	ART regime for infant	Breast-fed counseling	HIV transmission rates	Reference
HPTN 046	South Africa, Uganda, Zimbabwe	Local ART regimen for PMTCT within 7 days of delivery	Control: sd NVP[a] for first 6 weeks Intervention: Control + extended NVP till 6 months or till breast-fed cessation, whichever came first	Exclusive breast-fed for up to 6 months and then wean	6 weeks to 6 months: Control: 2.4% Intervention: 1.1% 54% reduction in HIV transmission	[35,36]
BAN study	Malawi [37]	CD4 > 250 cells/μL Triple ART (NVP + 3TC[b]+ZDV[c]) initiated after delivery for 28 weeks or till cessation of breast-fed	*Control*: sd NVP + 2 times-daily ZDV and 3TC for 1 week *Intervention*: Control + daily NVP for 28 weeks	Exclusive breast-fed to 24 weeks, then rapid weaning	28 weeks: 8.2% 48 weeks: Control: 7%, Maternal ART: 4% Infant NVP: 4%	[37]
Kesho-Bora study	Burkina Faso, Kenya, South Africa [38]	Randomized at 28–36 weeks gestation with CD4 200–500 cells/mm^3, with triple ART (ZDV + 3TC + Lopinavir/ritonavir) till cessation of breast-fed/6.5 months PP OR ZDV + SD NVP until 1 week PP	sd NVP + ZDV at birth and up to 1 week after birth	Supported and counseled to exclusively breast-feed and rapidly wean by 6 months	*Triple therapy*: 6 weeks: 3.3% 12 months: 5.4% *sd NVP/ZDV*: 6 weeks: 5.0% 12 months: 9.5% *Cumulative HIV transmission/death at 12 months*: Triple therapy: 10.2% Sd NVP/ZDV: 16.0% *Breast-fed infants*: HIV transmission 12 months: 5.6% in triple therapy vs 10.7% sd NVP/ZDV	[38]

KiBS	Kenya [39]	ZDV, 3TC, and NVP/ nelfinavir 34–36 weeks' gestation to 6 months PP	SD NVP at birth	Exclusively breast-feed for the first 5.5 months and abrupt weaning by 6 months	6 weeks: 4.2% 4 month: 4.6% 6 months: 5% 12 months: 5.7% 18 month: 6.7% Cumulative transmission between 6 weeks and 24 months, attributable to breast-feeding, was 3.2%	[39]
Mma Bana study	Botswana [40]	Women with CD4 > 500 cells/mm^3; (abacavir + ZDV + 3TC) OR lopinavir-ritonavir + ZDV-3TC) from 28 to 34 weeks gestation through 6 months of breast-feeding	sd NVP and 4 weeks of ZDV		6 months: 1.1%	[40]
Mitra Plus study	Tanzania [41]	ZDV, 3TC, and either NVP or NFV during late pregnancy (34 weeks gestation) through 6 months of breast-feeding	ZDV + 3TC for 1 week after birth	Exclusively breast-feed and abrupt weaning between 5 and 6 months	HIV Transmission rate: cumulative at 6 weeks: 4.1% 6 months: 5% 18 months: 6% HIV Transmission/death: 6 months: 8.6% 18 months: 13.6%	[41]
Amata study	Rwanda [42]	D4T[d]+3TC + NVP from 28 weeks gestation and for up to 7 PP	NVP at birth and ZDV for 7 days	Exclusively breast-feed until 6 months and then abrupt weaning	Overall 9 months: 1.3% 9-month cumulative risk of breast-feeding transmission: 0.5% 9-month cumulative mortality: Breast-fed: 3.3%; FF: 5.7%	[42]
PEPI study	Malawi [43]	sd NVP during labor	Control: sd NVP + ZDV for 1 week intervention: A: Control + NVP for 14 weeks B: Control + NVP + ZDV for 14 weeks	Exclusive breast-fed to 6 months, then weaning	9 months: Control: 10.6% Extended NVP: 5.2% Extended dual group: 6.4%	[43]

(*Continued*)

TABLE 13.1 (Continued)

Study	Trial site	ART regime for mother	ART regime for infant	Breast-fed counseling	HIV transmission rates	Reference
SWEN study	Ethiopia, India, Uganda [44]	sd NVP + optional ART per local standard of care at labor	Control: sd NVP Intervention: Control + daily NVP for 6 weeks	Encouraged to wean between 4 and 6 months	6 months: sd NVP: 8.98%, extended dose: 6.91% No difference between single and extended dose	[44]
DREAM study	Mozambique, Tanzania, Malawi [45]	ARTs from 25 weeks gestation. Comparison of observational cohort receiving Formula and water filters for 6 months versus exclusive breast-fed and (ZDV + 3TC + NVP) for 6 PP		Exclusive breast-fed till 6 months and weaning	1 month: FF: 0.8%; breast-fed: 1.2% 6 months: FF:1.8% breast-fed: 0.8%	[45]
MASHI study	Botswana [46]	ZDV from 34 weeks gestation till delivery	Breast-fed + ZDV for 6 months OR FF + ZDV for 1 month	Exclusive breast-fed was recommended and instructed to wean between 5 to 6 months	1 month: FF: 1.1%; breast-fed: 1.2% 7 months: FF:5.6%; breast-fed: 9.0% *Cumulative mortality at 7 months* FF: 9.3%; breast-fed: 4.9% *Cumulative mortality/HIV transmission at 18 months*: FF: 13.9%; breast-fed: 15.1% (not significant by 18 months)	[46]
PETRA study	Tanzania, South Africa, Uganda [47]	A: ZDV + Lamivudin starting at 36 weeks gestation + intrapartum ARTs + 7 days PP B: same as A without prepartum ARV C: intrapartum ZDV + 3TC D: Placebo	A: ARTs till 7 days PP B: same as A, C, and D: no ARTs		6 weeks: A: 5.7%; B: 8.9%; C: 14.2%; Placebo: 15.3% 6-week HIV transmission and mortality rates: A: 7%; B: 11.6%; C: 17.5%; Placebo: 18.1%	[47]

[a] *sd NVP: single dose nevirapine.*
[b] *3TC: lamivudine.*
[c] *ZDV: zidovudine.*
[d] *D4T: stavudine.*

18 months. MTCT rates at 1 month in the MASHI study were significantly lower than 6-week HIV transmission rates in the PETRA study, indicating that extended ARTs during pregnancy continued to lower postnatal HIV transmission rates. In a later randomized trial in Botswana, the Mma Bana (meaning mother of the baby in the local language) study [40] women with CD4 more than 500 cells/mm^3 were initiated on two different ART regimens from 28 to 34 weeks of gestation through 6 months of breastfeeding and infants received sd NVP at birth and 4 weeks of ZDV. The 6-month cumulative HIV transmission rates were low at 1.1%, and similar rates of virologic suppression were achieved at delivery and during breastfeeding among women in both HAART groups. Starting women on HAART at higher CD4 levels in the Mma Bana study [40] resulted in low MTCT rates at 1.1%, compared with the MASHI study [46] in a similar population where HIV transmission rates in breastfeeding women at 7 months were 9.0%.

However, given that a majority of women in resource-poor countries present to health facilities only once labor has initiated, several studies assessed the impact of ART initiation during labor and the breastfeeding period on MTCT. The Kesho Bora (meaning a better future in the local language) study in Burkina Faso, Kenya, and South Africa [38] randomized women at 28–36 weeks of gestation to receiving triple ART until 6 months postpartum and provided infants with sd NVP at birth. The HIV transmission rates were 42% lower in the triple ART group compared with ZDV and sd NVP regimens, and there was no significant difference according to infant feeding pattern. The Breastfeeding, Antiretrovirals, and Nutrition (BAN) study in Malawi [37] was another study assessing the impact of triple ART during breastfeeding on postnatal HIV transmission, although ARTs were only initiated after delivery. The 12-month HIV transmission rates were more than 40% lower in the triple extended ART compared with the control group and slightly lower at 4% compared with the Kesho Bora study [38]. The Six Week Extended Dose NVP (SWEN) randomized trial conducted in Ethiopia, India, and Uganda [44] provided sd NVP during labor to all HIV-positive women without previous exposure to ART and newborns received either sd NVP (control) or control plus extended daily NVP for 6 weeks postpartum. At the end of 6 months, there was no significant difference in HIV transmission rates between the single and extended NVP groups. However, HIV transmission rates were higher in the SWEN compared with the earlier trials [38,46,47] in which ART was initiated earlier in pregnancy. The Post-Exposure Prophylaxis of Infant (PEPI) study [35] was a phase III randomized clinical study conducted in Malawi; all mothers received intrapartum sd NVP and aimed to assess the impact of three infant ART regimens: sd NVP and zidovudine (ZDV) for 1 week (control); control plus NVP from day 8 to 14 weeks; and control plus NVP and ZDV from day 8 to 14 weeks. At 14 weeks, compared with the control group, HIV transmission rates were 67% lower for infants who received the extended NVP plus ZDV regimen. At 9 months, HIV transmission rates were 51% lower among the NVP plus ZDV group and 39% lower among the extended NVP group compared with the control group. Although the majority of the breastfeeding trials compared different regimens during breastfeeding to sd NVP given at birth, none examined the incremental benefit of extending prophylaxis to 6 months compared with shorter courses, which was performed by the HPTN 046 randomized, multisite trial. At 6 months, the HIV transmission rates were significantly lower in the extended NVP compared with placebo arm [36,45].

There were also several observational cohort studies assessing the impact of ART during pregnancy and the breastfeeding period on MTCT. In the Drug Resource Enhancement against AIDS and Malnutrition (DREAM) observational study in Mozambique, Tanzania, and Malawi [43], ART was initiated earlier, at 25 weeks of gestation, and mother–infant pairs who received formula feeds and water filters were compared with breastfeeding mothers who received triple ART therapy for 6 months and were advised to breastfeed exclusively up to 6 months and then wean abruptly. The study found no increased risk of HIV transmission among breastfed infants at 1 or 6 months postpartum and concluded that the earlier exposure to ART during pregnancy did not increase side effects among the mothers. The Amata observational cohort study (means milk in the local language) in Rwanda [42] provided mothers with triple HAART from 28 weeks of gestation to 7 days postpartum and sd NVP at birth and ZDV for 7 days postpartum to the infant. The study found no significant difference in HIV transmission or mortality rates at 9 months between breastfed and formula-fed infants. The Mitra Plus nonrandomized cohort study in Tanzania [41] provided triple therapy to mothers starting at 34 weeks of gestation until 6 months postpartum and provided ZDV and lamivudine to infants until 1 week postpartum. Cumulative HIV transmission rates were 5% at 6 months and 6% at 18 months, which were similar to the other randomized trials on breastfeeding HIV transmission. The Kisumu Breastfeeding study (KiBS) was a single arm clinical intervention study in Kenya [39], and the objective was to assess the feasibility and safety of extended ART use among women in resource-poor settings. Women, irrespective of CD4 levels, initiated triple ART at 34–36 weeks of gestation through 6 months of gestation and infants received sd NVP at birth. HIV transmission rates went from 4.2% at 6 weeks, to 5% at 6 months, to 6.7% at 18 months. There was no difference in HIV transmission by baseline maternal CD4 count. This study demonstrated that a simple regimen that does not rely on CD4 testing can be used for women who present late in pregnancy and does lower HIV transmission rates.

These trials on postnatal ART use started either during pregnancy or during the intrapartum period and extended through the breastfeeding period; all provide evidence of the efficacy of extended ARTs through 6 months of breastfeeding as well as of triple ART therapy and indicate that this is an effective strategy for the prevention of postnatal vertical transmission of HIV while at the same time providing the benefits of breast milk to infants born to HIV-positive mothers. However, postnatal transmission occurred after NVP cessation among breastfed children in several trials, raising the issue of potentially providing postexposure prophylaxis in breastfed children over the entire breastfeeding duration.

13.2.2 Lifelong Antiretroviral Treatment for Pregnant and Breast-Feeding Women: Option B+

In 2010, WHO released new PMTCT Guidelines that recommended lifelong ART with two options for HIV-positive women—Option A and Option B—both requiring CD4 measurements to distinguish women who required ART for their own health from those requiring it for PMTCT [48]. To date, studies find similar efficacy between Options A and B [48,49]. UNAIDS has a Global Plan to eliminate all new HIV infections in children by 2015 and keep their mothers alive [50]. This goal seemed possible given the success shown by the trials demonstrating reductions of MTCT rates to less than 2%, even in breastfeeding populations with provision of ART up to 6 months postnatally. However, given that transmission of HIV continues during breastfeeding once ARTs have been stopped at 6 months, there is considerable debate regarding whether the only way to truly *eliminate* MTCT is to give all HIV positive pregnant and breastfeeding women lifelong ARTs—Option B+—irrespective of clinical status.

Given the costs, logistics, and complications related to ongoing measurement of CD4 levels to assess treatment eligibility, Malawi proposed Option B+, with all pregnant women, irrespective of CD4 cell count, initiated a lifelong, once daily, triple ART regimen [51]. As the debate around Option B+ continues and more countries either have adopted it or are considering adopting it for all HIV-positive pregnant women, a review of evidence of the Option B+ approach was conducted by Ahmed et al. [49] and colleagues to assess the advantages and weaknesses of Option B+. Much of the debate around the impact of Option B+ on maternal health has centered on the initiation of lifelong ART for women who are healthier and have CD4 cell counts of more than 350 cells/mm. Given that Option B+ has been introduced fairly recently, there are no data from randomized trials on the long-term risks or benefits of lifelong ARTs for maternal health or of the impact on the child's health of ART use until the end of the breastfeeding period. Modeling studies, however, find Option B+ to be more cost-effective in the long-term and demonstrate an increase in the mother's life expectancy [52]. The concern about extended ART use for child health is based on several studies finding that compared with monotherapy, exposure to combination therapy increases the risk of poor birth outcomes such as still birth, preterm delivery, and low weight for gestational age [53,54]. However, some studies have demonstrated that longer duration of ART use among HIV-exposed and infected children results in reduction of some neurologic impairment [55]. When considering the most effective strategies for PMTCT, the issue of adherence continues to be debated as studies have shown that adherence decreases from more than 80% to 75% during pregnancy, and even lower to 53% during breastfeeding [56]. However, despite some of the challenges, Option B+ does have other benefits of reduced HIV transmission in serodiscordant couples [57], and this is significant given that HIV incidence has been shown to be higher during pregnancy [58]. It will be critical to get longer-term data on the efficacy of Option B+ as well as some of the intended and unintended consequences of putting all pregnant infected women on lifelong prophylaxis.

13.3 IMPLEMENTATION OF INFANT FEEDING AND ART GUIDELINES FOR PMTCT

There have been considerable advances over the past few decades in PMTCT with increased access and availability of ART for prevention of vertical transmission of HIV *in utero* and during the intrapartum and postnatal periods. However, despite incredible gains in PMTCT, by the end of 2012, more than 35% of pregnant women living with HIV did not receive ART and 260,000 children were newly infected with HIV and in need of lifelong HIV treatment [59]. The Joint UNAIDS Global Plan to eliminate new HIV infections in children by 2015 will require the support and coordination of multiple partners in each country to reach the goal of elimination of all new infections to children by 2015 [50].

This brings us to what we see as a natural progression toward the expanding scope of national and global programs for PMTCT. We visualize a four-level enlargement of the scale and scope of the subject:

1. Prevention of transmission of HIV to infants without substantial support for the pregnant women, the mothers, and their infants.
2. Pregnancy and delivery-related interventions: antenatal, peripartum, and postnatal interventions.
3. Care for the mother (antenatal, postnatal) and for the infants.
4. Social determinants of health.

The descriptions of the decisive trials on prevention of breastfeeding transmission of HIV, together with references to the numerous studies on the prevention of intrauterine and intrapartum transmission, illustrate only a few components (levels 1 and 2) of a much wider dimension of

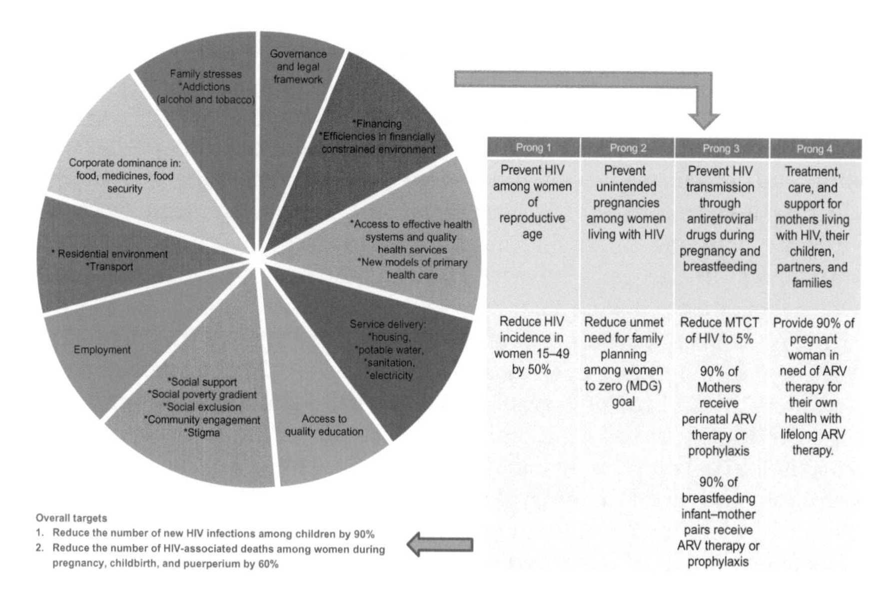

FIGURE 13.1 Social determinants and the WHO 4 Prongs approach for a comprehensive approach.
Source: Adapted from Watts and Mofenson (2012). P39 of the Global Plan toward the elimination of new HIV infections among children by 2015 and keeping their mothers alive.

the transmission of HIV from infected women to their babies. Level 3 has been adequately described by WHO [60]. We now turn to the contextual aspects of the subject, the social determinants (Figure 13.1).

13.4 COMBINATION AND CONVERGENCE OF HEALTH SERVICE PROGRAMS

Programs for the prevention and management of HIV in children cannot be effectively implemented without assessing the impact of their national and global contexts. The immediate health system in which these programs are located is the bedrock on which the quality of these services is constructed. Health systems are constituted by an intersecting system of building blocks such as personnel, facilities, governance, financing, and service delivery, which are embedded within a framework of social determinants such as the burden of disease, education, basic services, poverty, political factors, the economy, and food security [60]. The articulation of these various elements has historically resulted in multiple fragmentations, for example, along the lines of burden of disease, financing, location, and types of facilities; the best known is the gap between Primary Health Care (PHC) and Tertiary or Quaternary Care. Interventions across the continuum of care for mothers and their newborn babies are stratified by vertical divisions through the preconception, antenatal, intrapartum, and postnatal periods, and in community engagement. Attempts at combining some of the cognate fragments of the system into comprehensive health care programs have been widely reported, although convincing evidence of sustainability has been weak [61]. These weaknesses may be overcome with the increasing attention regarding combining different components of the health services and convergence of programs geared toward sustainable development.

There has been a resurgence of interest in overcoming fragmentation on the eve of the global evaluation of the MDGs in 2015, and *The Lancet* advocates "...the idea of a grand convergence—a reduction in preventable infectious, maternal, and child deaths to universally low levels—as a sustainable development goal after 2015" [62]. The journal suggests that except for "Universal Coverage," which is fundamental to PMTCT implementation, there has been no unifying all-encompassing global objective. A global goal, defined for grand convergence, is simplified as "16–8–4": a mortality rate for those younger than 5 of 16/1,000 live births, an annual AIDS mortality rate of 8 per 100,000 population, and an annual death rate from tuberculosis of 4 per 100,000 population. Ann Starrs, writing on "Survival Convergence..." [63] as a post-2015 goal, includes effective interventions for maternal newborn and child health (MNCH), accessible health facilities, and greater country control. She refers to "... a cohesive set of targets on reproductive, maternal, newborn, and child health (which) will be clustered in the agenda so that their linkages across the continuum of care are clear" [63].

Barriers to the fulfillment of these MNCH targets have been addressed recently [64–67]. These articles, and other works in progress, describe the combination of the following elements providing PHC and specialist services throughout the continuum of care for newborns and their mothers, which are potential points of discontinuities in a seamless health service: PMTCT; neonatal care; postnatal care; maternal mental health; home-based care; types of mid-level health personnel employed; and the range of locations for care, from home and family through outpatients toward district and regional hospitals. We have emphasized the ineffectiveness of stand-alone services and the need to expand access to pediatric prevention and treatment by building clinical delivery mechanisms [66].

Combined services specifically for PMTCT were tested and recommended by WHO approximately a decade ago through the very useful "4 Prongs" approach and captured in levels 1–3 in the formulation provided. Table 13.2 [68] provides the efficacy and effectiveness data from the "4 Prongs approach." The research evidence for synergy between multiple discrete interventions for PMTCT is suggestive but needs to be strengthened by studies on sustainability and population level impact

TABLE 13.2 Economic Aspects and Outcomes of a Comprehensive "4 Prongs" Prevention of Mother to Child Transmission of HIV-1 Program—WHO [68]

Programme Costs (average, annual)	$4.8 m
Infant HIV infections averted (average)	1898
Costs; per HIV infection averted	$2517
per Daly averted	$84
Equivalents to total HIV infections averted:	
*Lowering female HIV prevalence	by 1.25%
*Reducing unintended pregnancies in HIV infected women	by 16%

in post-MDG sustainability policies and programs. Although the most efficacious ARV regimens for PMTCT are necessary, they may be insufficient because there are social determinants that influence outcomes. We use a few examples to illustrate this last point There are a number of well-recognized prevention measures to reduce HIV incidence in all women regardless of their pregnancy state, for example, condoms and microbicides, which are beyond the scope of this chapter. A reduction of unintended pregnancies, which are a serious social problem in many African countries, may lead to a similar outcome [69]. Family planning has multiple benefits; the prevention of new infant HIV infections is an added benefit. It has been shown that at the same level of expenditure, a contraceptive strategy averts 28.6% more HIV-positive births than nevirapine alone for PMTCT [69]. Aluisio et al. [70] have shown in Cape Town that male partner testing for HIV and attendance at an antenatal clinic is associated with a more than a two-fold decreased rate of HIV transmission to infants born to HIV-positive mothers, adjusted for maternal viral load and infant feeding modality. Seroconversions during pregnancy may be missed during routine antenatal care [71]. In Botswana, 43% of 1,082 new HIV transmissions were due to HIV infection during this gestational period; introducing an intervention for more frequent testing for HIV may reduce MTCT [72,73]. It appears that PMTCT is enhanced when the service providers improve the quality of antenatal care and delivery services [74] and the program is integrated into MCH services [72]. These operational aspects are discussed in more detail elsewhere [74–76].

13.4.1 Prevention of MTCT of HIV and Childhood HIV in the Context of the MDGs

The MDGs, which are some of the most ambitious of the grand global programs to improve health and social and economic conditions in the world, were finalized by 2000, with targets by 2015, compared with the position for the various indicators of 1990. It is instructive to assess progress in the contextual factors embodied within the MDGs, which are likely to impact on PMTCT and maternal and child health. The case for bringing together many different sources of information and activities for the public good has already been made and the MDGs take the scale of inclusion even higher. There are fundamental philosophical reasons attesting to the superiority of collective rather than individual action, from C. P. Snow's "Two Cultures" (humanities and the sciences) [77], to E. O. Wilson's "Consilience" [78], which derives meaning from a collective understanding and synthesis of knowledge from many diverse fields of human endeavor, including health. The specific MDG Goal 4A, which relates to a two-thirds reduction of mortality for those younger than 5 between 1990 and 2015, provides a suitable context for the factors affecting PMTCT [79]. Progress is as follows:

1. The number of deaths in children younger than 5 years worldwide declined from 12.6 million in 1990 to 6.6 million in 2012.
2. As a consequence, the proportion of deaths during the first month after birth is increasing.
3. An increasing proportion (4 out of 5 child deaths) occurs in sub-Saharan Africa and Southern Asia.
4. Poor children younger than 5 years are almost twice as likely to die as are wealthy children.
5. Children of educated mothers are more likely to survive than children of mothers with no education.

There are excellent recent reviews [80,81] of the global and local progress in reaching the 2015 overall goals of the MDGs, and these should be consulted by those interested.

The most recent evaluation of the advances made in the MDGs overall demonstrates the several different stages of progress [80]. Some "...targets have either already been met or are within close reach."

Faster progress is needed in other areas such as child survival, maternal mortality, access to ARVs, knowledge of HIV, access to primary education for children, sanitation, and financial support from aid agencies. Many inequities, including gender-based inequalities, rural–urban gaps, and the vulnerability of the poorest children, persist.

In an evaluation on the MDGs that impact of MNCH [81], the key message is: achievement of high, sustained, and equitable coverage of life-saving interventions for women and children is insufficient.

Although most countries will not achieve MDGs 4 and 5, progress has accelerated in recent years, suggesting that further gains are possible with continued, intensified actions.

Some of the most important coverage gaps are in family planning, interventions addressing newborn mortality, and case management of childhood diseases. Massive inequalities in intervention coverage and health outcomes, including stunting, must be tackled for progress to continue. Progress has occurred in country adoption of evidence-based policies and strategies to improve women's and children's health. Accountability cannot exist without data. Baseline data must be collected now for the post-2015 era.

13.5 THE AGENCY OF CULTURE AND POLITICAL ORGANIZATION ON HIV

Local governments will play a crucial role in curbing this epidemic and eliminating MTCT globally. There are significant logistical and organizational impediments to modernizing the health care system, especially in some southern African countries where the HIV epidemic has hit the strongest. The impact of cultural and political factors on the HIV epidemic is widely recognized. In many developing countries, including those on the African continent, culture is often the handmaiden to political development, the exercise of power, social institutions, and governance. We illustrate these issues by briefly recounting the unusual, bizarre, and possibly unique experience of HIV denialism by President Thabo Mbeki and his Minister of Health Mantoo Shabalala. These events had a direct impact on prevention of MTCT of HIV and the acquisition of HIV by parents and their children. The details of this devastating episode in the country's history have been published [82].

The South African government's attack on evidence-based proposals to reduce MTCT of HIV was unexpectedly far-reaching. President Mbeki and his Minister Shabalala warned of the presumed toxicity of antiretroviral drugs: "The fact is some of the mice (tested with AZT) have contracted cancer. It attacks the bone marrow. It is very toxic." This resulted in probably thousands of babies being infected with HIV, and HIV in infants at that time was a lethal disease because drugs were unaffordable.

Investment in useless causes such as "Sarafina," a play that was amateurish, superficial, and worthless as an instrument to inform, educate, and encourage safe sex. Predictably, the show failed miserably and vanished into the realm of lost causes.

The Virodene Saga was an example of the use of science for chauvinistic purposes. It was a major blunder associated with the African National Congress' first years in power. Senior government figures trumpeted the local discovery of a wonder drug for AIDS. Three University of Pretoria medical and scientific individuals, with no credible prior research record, suddenly announced a successful treatment for AIDS. The scientific evidence for this claim was nonexistent. The wonder drug turned out to be an industrial solvent (dimethylformamide)!

The Presidential AIDS Advisory Panel (Mbeki Panel, 2001) was a so-called independent panel assembled by Mbeki to pit scientists against pseudo-scientists. This dalliance with a group of "dissidents" was a monumental miscalculation on the part of Mbeki that dented his image irrevocably. The country wasted significant resources and squandered an opportunity for taking early steps to halt the spread of the infection.

At that time we wrote, "What will be remembered is the failure of a newly democratic government...to appreciate the scientific process ... of translating research into practice, in the throes of an unprecedented national crisis" [82]. The process to challenge the existing data on the cause of HIV/AIDS, by Mbeki "was constructed as an extension of the methodologies of politics such as negotiation and compromise, into the realms of scientific debate. It was a false and superficial understanding of the experimental, observational, and theoretical, paths followed by scientists" [79].

13.5.1 Reorganization of Primary Health Services

Key data suggest that the models of PHC devised during "Alma Ata" need to be reformulated; reorganization of primary health care services, extending from those envisaged by Alma-Ata to the integrated management of chronic diseases, requires a major shift [83]. On the basis of our experiences in KwaZulu-Natal, South Africa in dealing, at different locations, with either fragmented or unified services for tuberculosis and PMTCT, such shifts include the need for changes in the current legal framework to allow more tasks to be done by alternative cadres of health workers and careful assessment. This will include other issues in dealing with Health Services and Health Systems appropriate for PMTCT such as the delivery of a newborn package of care. Recently, there have been substantial decreases in global deaths in children younger than 5 years, mostly due to reductions in postneonatal deaths [84]. There has been no similar progress in reduction of mortality in neonates. This lack of progress has prompted investigators to direct interventions not only at staff in health facilities but also at communities.

13.5.2 The Durban Declaration [85]

More than 5,000 scientists from around the world, including 12 Nobel Laureates, as well directors of leading research institutes and presidents of academies and medical societies were moved by these events to sign the "Durban Declaration." The Declaration affirmed "...the evidence that AIDS is caused by HIV-1 or HIV-2 is clear-cut, exhaustive, and unambiguous, meeting the highest standards of science."

References

[1] UNICEF. State of the world's children 2014 in numbers: every child counts. Revealing Disparities, Advancing Children's Rights. Division of Communication, UNICEF. Geneva, Switzerland; 2014.

[2] WHO. Global health observatory: under 5 mortality rates; 2012.

[3] UNICEF. Millennium development goals: reduce child mortality; 2014.

[4] Jenkins JM, Foster EM. The effects of breastfeeding exclusivity on early childhood outcomes. AJPH 2014;104:S128–35.

[5] Jones G, Steketee RW, Black RE, Bhutta ZA, Morris SS. How many child deaths can we prevent this year? Lancet 2003;362:65–71.

[6] Stuebe AM, Schwarz EB. The risks and benefits of infant feeding practices for women and their children. J Perinatol 2010;30:155–62.

[7] Victora CG, Smith PG, Vaughan JP, et al. Evidence for protection by breast-feeding against infant deaths from infectious diseases in Brazil. Lancet 1987;2:319–22.

[8] Effect of breastfeeding on infant and child mortality due to infectious diseases in less developed countries: a pooled analysis. WHO Collaborative Study Team on the Role of Breastfeeding on the Prevention of Infant Mortality. Lancet 2000;355:451–5.

[9] Black RE, Morris SS, Bryce J. Where and why are 10 million children dying every year? Lancet 2003;361:2226–34.

[10] Ip S, Chung M, Raman G, Trikalinos TA, Lau J. A summary of the agency for healthcare research and quality's evidence report on breastfeeding in developed countries. Breastfeed Med 2009;4(Suppl. 1):S17–30.

[11] Lamberti LM, Fischer Walker CL, Noiman A, Victora C, Black RE. Breastfeeding and the risk for diarrhea morbidity and mortality. BMC Public Health 2011;11(Suppl. 3):S15.

[12] Mofenson LM. Mother–child HIV-1 transmission: timing and determinants. Obstet Gynecol Clin North Am 1997;24:759–84.

[13] Taha TE. Mother-to-child transmission of HIV-1 in Sub-Saharan Africa: past, present and future challenges. Life Sci 2011;88:917–21.

[14] Brahmbhatt H, Kigozi G, Wabwire-Mangen F, et al. Mortality in HIV-infected and uninfected children of HIV-infected and uninfected mothers in rural Uganda. J Acquir Immune Defic Syndr 2006;41:504–8.

[15] Coovadia H. Current issues in prevention of mother-to-child transmission of HIV-1. Curr Opin HIV AIDS 2009;4:319–24.

[16] Van de PP. Breast milk transmission of HIV-1. Laboratory and clinical studies. Ann N Y Acad Sci 2000;918:122–7.

[17] Taha TE, Hoover DR, Kumwenda NI, et al. Late postnatal transmission of HIV-1 and associated factors. J Infect Dis 2007;196:10–14.

[18] WHO WHO HIV transmission through breastfeeding: a review of available evidence—2007 update. WHO Press; 2008.

[19] Nduati RW, John GC, Richardson BA, et al. Human immunodeficiency virus type 1-infected cells in breast milk: association with immunosuppression and vitamin A deficiency. J Infect Dis 1995;172:1461–8.

[20] Miotti PG, Taha TE, Kumwenda N, et al. HIV transmission through breastfeeding. J Am Med Assoc 1999;282:744–9.

[21] Semba RD, Kumwenda N, Hoover DR, et al. Human immunodeficiency virus load in breast milk, mastitis, and mother-to-child transmission of human immunodeficiency virus type 1. J Infect Dis 1999;180:93–8.

[22] Nduati RW, John GC, Mbori-Ngacha D, et al. Effect of breastfeeding and formula feeding on transmission of HIV-1. JAMA 2000;283:1167–74.

[23] The Breastfeeding and HIV International Transmission Study Group (BHITS). Late postnatal transmission of HIV in breast-fed children: an individual patient data meta-analysis. J Infect Dis 2004;189:2154–66.

[24] Brahmbhatt H, Gray RH. Child mortality associated with reasons for non-breastfeeding and weaning: is breastfeeding best for HIV-positive mothers? AIDS 2003;17:879–85.
[25] Coutsoudis A, Pillay K, Spooner E, Kuhn L. South African Vitamin A study group. Influence of infant feeding patterns on early mother-to-child transmission of HIV-1 in Durban, South Africa: a prospective cohort study. Lancet 1999;354(9177):471–6.
[26] Coutsoudis A, Pillay K, Kuhn L, Spooner E, Tsai WY, Coovadia HM. Method of feeding and transmission of HIV-1 from mothers to children by 15 months of age: prospective cohort study from Durban, South Africa. AIDS 2001;15:379–87.
[27] Coovadia HM, Rollins N, Bland R, Little K, Coutsoudis A, Bennish ML, et al. Mother-to-child transmission of HIV-1 infection during exclusive breastfeeding in the first 6 months of life: an intervention cohort study. Lancet 2007;369:1107–16.
[28] Kourtis AP, Lee FK, Abrams EJ, Jamieson DJ, Bulterys M. Mother-to-child transmission of HIV-1: timing and implications for prevention. Lancet Infect Dis 2006;6:726–32.
[29] Coutsoudis A, Kuhn L, Pillay K, Coovadia HM. Exclusive breast-feeding and HIV transmission. AIDS 2002;16:498–9.
[30] WHO. HIV and infant feeding: a review of HIV transmission through breastfeeding; 1998.
[31] Kramer MS, Kakuma R. Optimal duration of exclusive breastfeeding. Cochrane Database Syst Rev 2012:8. CD003517.
[32] Arifeen S, Black RE, Antelman G, Baqui A, Caulfield L, Becker S. Exclusive breastfeeding reduces acute respiratory infection and diarrhea deaths among infants in Dhaka slums. Pediatrics 2001;108:E67.
[33] WHO WHO consolidated ARV guidelines. Summary of major recommendations and estimated impact. HIV Department. Geneva, Switzerland: WHO; 2013.
[34] Bulterys M, Lepage P. Mother-to-child transmission of HIV. Curr Opin Pediatr 1998;10:143–50.
[35] Kumwenda NI, Hoover DR, Mofenson LM, et al. Extended antiretroviral prophylaxis to reduce breast-milk HIV-1 transmission. N Engl J Med 2008;359:119–29.
[36] Fowler MG, Coovadia H, Herron CM, et al. Efficacy and safety of an extended nevirapine regimen in infants of breastfeeding mothers with HIV-1 infection for prevention of HIV-1 transmission (HPTN 046): 18-month results of a randomized, double-blind, placebo-controlled trial. J AIDS 2014;65:366–74.
[37] Jamieson DJ, Chasela CS, Hudgens MG, et al. Maternal and infant antiretroviral regimens to prevent postnatal HIV-1 transmission: 48-week follow-up of the BAN randomised controlled trial. Lancet 2012;379:2449–58.
[38] de Vincenzi I, Kesho Bora Study Group Triple antiretroviral compared with zidovudine and single-dose nevirapine prophylaxis during pregnancy and breastfeeding for prevention of mother-to-child transmission of HIV-1 (Kesho Bora study): a randomised controlled trial. Lancet Infect Dis 2011;11:171–80.
[39] Thomas TK, Masaba R, Borkowf CB, et al. Triple-antiretroviral prophylaxis to prevent mother-to-child HIV transmission through breastfeeding—the Kisumu breastfeeding study, Kenya: a clinical trial. PLoS Med 2011;8:e1001015.
[40] Shapiro RL, Hughes MD, Ogwu A, et al. Antiretroviral regimens in pregnancy and breast-feeding in Botswana. N Engl J Med 2010;362:2282–94.
[41] Kilewo C, Karlsson K, Ngarina M, et al. Prevention of mother-to-child transmission of HIV-1 through breastfeeding by treating mothers with triple antiretroviral therapy in Dar es Salaam, Tanzania: the Mitra plus study. J Acquir Immune Defic Syndr 2009;52:406–16.
[42] Peltier CA, Ndayisaba GF, Lepage P, et al. Breastfeeding with maternal antiretroviral therapy or formula feeding to prevent HIV postnatal mother-to-child transmission in Rwanda. AIDS 2009;23:2415–23.

[43] Palombi L, Marazzi MC, Voetberg A, Magid NA. Treatment acceleration program and the experience of the DREAM program in prevention of mother-to-child transmission of HIV. AIDS 2007;21(Suppl. 4):S65–71.
[44] Bedri A, Gudetta B, Isehak A, et al. Extended-dose nevirapine to 6 weeks of age for infants to prevent HIV transmission via breastfeeding in Ethiopia, India, and Uganda: an analysis of three randomised controlled trials. Lancet 2008;372:300–13.
[45] Coovadia HM, Brown ER, Fowler MG, et al. Efficacy and safety of an extended nevirapine regimen in infant children of breastfeeding mothers with HIV-1 infection for prevention of postnatal HIV-1 transmission (HPTN 046): a randomised, double-blind, placebo-controlled trial. Lancet 2012;379:221–8.
[46] Thior I, Lockman S, Smeaton LM, et al. Breastfeeding plus infant zidovudine prophylaxis for 6 months vs formula feeding plus infant zidovudine for 1 month to reduce mother-to-child HIV transmission in Botswana: a randomized trial: the Mashi study. JAMA 2006;296:794–805.
[47] Petra Study Team Efficacy of three short-course regimens of zidovudine and lamivudine in preventing early and late transmission of HIV-1 from mother to child in Tanzania, South Africa, and Uganda (Petra study): a randomised, double-blind, placebo-controlled trial. Lancet 2002;359:1178–86.
[48] WHO. Antiretroviral drugs for treating pregnant women and preventing HIV infections in infants: recommendations for a public health approach. Geneva, Switzerland; 2010.
[49] Ahmed S, Kim MH, Abrams EJ. Risks and benefits of lifelong antiretroviral treatment for pregnant and breastfeeding women: a review of the evidence for the option B+ approach. Curr Opin HIV AIDS 2013;8:474–89.
[50] Countdown to Zero. Global plan towards the elimination of new HIV infections among children by 2015 and keeping their mothers alive (2011–2015). UNAIDS/JC2137E. Geneva, Switzerland; 2011.
[51] Schouten EJ, Jahn A, Midiani D, et al. Prevention of mother-to-child transmission of HIV and the health-related millennium development goals: time for a public health approach. Lancet 2011;378:282–4.
[52] Fasawe O, Avila C, Shaffer N, et al. Cost-effectiveness analysis of option B+ for HIV prevention and treatment of mothers and children in Malawi. PLoS One 2013;8:e57778.
[53] Watts DH, Mofenson LM. Antiretrovirals in pregnancy: a note of caution. J Infect Dis 2012;206:1639–41.
[54] Watts DH, Williams PL, Kacenek D. Combination antiretroviral use and preterm birth. J Infect Dis 2013;207:612–21.
[55] Brahmbhatt H, Boivin M, Ssempiija V, et al. Neurodevelopmental benefits of antiretroviral therapy in Ugandan children 0–6 years of age with HIV. JAIDS 2014;67:316–22.
[56] Nachega JB, Uthman OA, Anderson J, et al. Adherence to antiretroviral therapy during and after pregnancy in low-income, middle-income, and high-income countries: a systematic review and meta-analysis. AIDS 2012;26:2039–52.
[57] Cohen MS, Chen YQ, McCauley M, et al. Prevention of HIV-1 infection with early antiretroviral therapy. N Engl J Med 2011;365:493–505.
[58] Gray RH, Li X, Kigozi G, et al. Increased risk of incident HIV during pregnancy in Rakai, Uganda: a prospective study. Lancet 2005;366:1182–8.
[59] UNAIDS. Global report: UNAIDS report on the global AIDS epidemic 2013. UNAIDS. UNAIDS/JC2502/1/E; 2013.
[60] Murray CJL, Frenk J. A framework for assessing the performance of health systems. Bull World Health Organ 2000;78(6):717–31.
[61] Leveraging HIV Scale-up to Strengthen Health Systems in Africa. International Centre for AIDS care and treatment [ICAP], Bellagio Conference Report; September 2008.

[62] Grand convergence: a future sustainable development goal? The Lancet 01/2014; 383 (9913):187. http://dx.doi.org/10.1016/S0140-6736(14)60051-9 [Published Online: January 15, 2014].
[63] Starrs AM. Survival convergence: bringing maternal and newborn health together for 2015 and beyond. The Lancet, 2014. http://dx.doi.org/10.1016/S0140-6736(14)60838-2 [Early Online Publication].
[64] Chopra M, Daviaud E, Pattinson R, et al. Saving the lives of South Africa's mothers. Babies and children: can the health system deliver? Lancet 2009;374:835–46.
[65] Kerber KJ, de Graft-Johnson JE, Bhutta ZA, et al. Continuum of care for maternal newborn and child health: from slogan to service delivery. Lancet 2007;370:1358–69.
[66] Cluver L, Sherr L, Grimwood A, et al. Assembling an effective paediatric HIV treatment and prevention toolkit. Lancet 2014. http://dx.doi.org/10.1016/S2214-109X(14)70267-0 [Published Online: June 4, 2014].
[67] WHO UNICEF Global monitoring framework and strategy for the global plan towards the elimination of new HIV infections among children by 2015 and keeping their mothers alive (EMTCT). Geneva, Switzerland: World Health Organization; 2012.
[68] Sweat MD, O'Reilly KR, Schmid GP, et al. Cost-effectiveness of nevirapine to prevent mother to child HIV transmission in eight African countries. AIDS 2004;18(12):1661–71.
[69] Reynolds HW, Janowitz B, Homan R, et al. The value of contraception to prevent perinatal HIV transmission. Sex Transm Dis 2006;33(6):350–6. http://dx.doi.org/10.1097/01.olq.0000194602.01058.e1.
[70] Aluisio A, Bosire R, Stewart GJ, et al. Male partner HIV-1 testing and antenatal clinical attendance associated with reduced infant HIV-1 acquisition and mortality. 5th (IAS) International AIDS Society Conference. Cape Town, South Africa; 2009 [Abstract TuAC105. iasociety.org/Default.aspx?pageId=12&abstractId=200721751].
[71] Moodley D, Esterhuizen TM, Pather T, et al. High HIV incidence during pregnancy: compelling reason for repeat HIV testing. AIDS 2009;23(10):1255–9. http://dx.doi.org/10.1097/QAD.0b013e32832a5934.
[72] Lu L, Legwaila K, Motswere C, et al. HIV incidence in pregnancy and the first postpartum year and implications for PMTCT programs, Francistown, Botswana, 2008. [Abstract 91]. Presented at: 16th Conference on Retroviruses and Opportunistic Infections; Montreal, Canada; 2009.
[73] Motswere-Chirwa C, Voetsch A, Lu L, et al. Follow-up of infants diagnosed with HIV—early infant diagnosis program, Francistown, Botswana, 2005–2012. MMWR Morb Mortal Wkly Rep. 2014 ;63(7):158–60.
[74] Delvaux T, Konan JP, Aké-Tano O, et al. Quality of antenatal and delivery care before and after the implementation of a prevention of mother-to-child HIV transmission programme in Côte d'Ivoire. Trop Med Int Health 2008;13(8):970–9. http://dx.doi.org/10.1111/j.1365-3156.2008.02105.x.
[75] El-Sadr WM, Abrams EJ, et al. Scale-up of HIV care and treatment: can it transform healthcare services in resource-limited settings. AIDS 2007;21:S65–70. http://dx.doi.org/10.1097/01.aids.0000298105.79484.62.
[76] Aizir J, Fowler MG, Coovadia H. Operational issues and barriers to implementation of prevention of mother-to-child transmission of HIV (PMTCT) interventions in Sub-Saharan Africa. Curr HIV Res 2013.
[77] Snow CP. The two cultures. London: Cambridge University Press; 2001. 1993, p3. ISBN 0-521-45730-0.
[78] Wilson EO. Consilience: the unity of knowledge 1998. ISBN 9780679450771.
[79] United Nations Millennium Development Goals. Goal 4: Child mortality. Target4A. http://www.un.org/millenniumgoals/childhealth.shtml.
[80] United Nations. The millennium development goals 2013. We Can End Poverty 2015. United Nations, New York, NY; 2013.

[81] Requejo JH, Bryce J, Barros AJD, et al. Countdown to 2015 and beyond: fulfilling the health agenda for women and children. Lancet. http://dx.doi.org/10.1016/S0140-6736(14)60925-9 [Early Online Publication: 30 June 2014.07.14].

[82] Coovadia HM, Coovadia I. Science and society: the HIV epidemic and South African political responses. Contribution for: hot topics in infection and immunity. Pollard Andrew J.Finn Adam, editors. Advances in experimental medicine and biology, 609. New York, NY; Boston, MA; Dordrecht, the Netherlands; London; Moscow, Russia: Kluwer Academic/Plenum Publishers; 2008. pp. 16–28.

[83] Coovadia H, Bland R. From Alma-Ata to Agincourt: primary health care in AIDS. Lancet 2008;372:866–8.

[84] Wang H, Liddell CA, Coates MM. et al. Global, regional, and national levels of neonatal, infant, and under-5 mortality during 1990–2013: a systematic analysis for the Global Burden of Disease Study 2013. Lancet. http://dx.doi.org/10.1016/S0140-6736(14)60497-9 [Published Online: May 2, 2014].

[85] Anonymous Commentary The durban declaration. Nature 2000;406:15–16. http://dx.doi.org/10.1038/35017662.

CHAPTER

14

Nutrition Care of the HIV-Exposed Child

Anju Seth and Rohini Gupta

Pediatric Center of Excellence in HIV Care, Lady Hardinge Medical College, New Delhi, India

14.1 INTRODUCTION

Childhood, especially infancy, is a period of rapid physical growth. This is also the period when maximum brain growth and development occurs. Adequate nutrition is critical to ensure both. Nutritional deficits during this vulnerable phase lead to long-term deficits in growth, which cannot be counteracted by subsequent rehabilitative efforts.

An infant born to a woman with HIV infection (HIV-exposed infant) is vulnerable to suboptimal nutrition irrespective of his/her own HIV status. Various studies have reported a high prevalence of wasting and stunting in these children [1–3]. Many factors contribute toward poor nutritional status in these children. These include:

- Increased likelihood of replacement feeding (RF), which may often be inappropriate and overdiluted, leading to poor intake of calories, macronutrients, and micronutrients.
- Unhygienic feed preparation due to ignorance, poor environmental sanitation, unavailability of clean drinking water, and bottle feeding, causing increased likelihood of gastrointestinal infections. These lead to poor appetite, decreased nutrient absorption, and increased catabolism.
- Delayed introduction and poor quality of complementary feeds.
- Adverse social and economic factors associated with parental HIV infection like poverty, broken families, parental sickness/drug abuse, and stigmatization by society.

Exposed infants who themselves have HIV infection are even more vulnerable to malnutrition because of increased energy needs, nutrient

Health of HIV Infected People, Volume 2.
DOI: http://dx.doi.org/10.1016/B978-0-12-800767-9.00014-5

malabsorption, impaired storage, and an altered metabolism. Presence of an immune-compromised state leads to repeated infections that further impact on the nutritional status. Malnutrition is an important risk factor for mortality in all children, and those born to HIV-infected women are no exception [4,5]. Thus, providing optimal nutritional care to these infants is critical to their survival and achievement of optimum health.

14.2 NUTRITIONAL NEEDS OF HIV-EXPOSED INFANTS

Like all children, HIV-exposed infants need energy, proteins, vitamins, and minerals to ensure normal growth. Nutritional needs of an HIV-exposed infant depend on age, growth pattern, HIV infection status, and presence of other comorbidities. An uninfected exposed infant has same nutritional requirements as an infant unexposed to HIV infection. Presence of HIV infection increases the energy requirement by 10% in case of an asymptomatic infant with adequate growth, by 20% in an infant with growth faltering, and by 50–100% in the presence of severe malnutrition [6]. Whereas the former two groups of infants may be provided these extra calories by appropriate home modification of feeds, the latter would require therapeutic feeding under supervision.

14.3 FEEDING OPTIONS FOR HIV-EXPOSED INFANTS YOUNGER THAN 6 MONTHS OF AGE

The role of breastfeeding in ensuring child survival and prevention of infant/child morbidity, especially in resource-constrained circumstances, is well-established. The pattern of infant feeding is a significant predictor of child morbidity and mortality [7,8]. However, in the setting of maternal HIV infection, it carries with it the inherent risk of transmission of HIV virus to her newborn. Thus, choosing the correct feeding option for HIV-exposed infants has been a contentious issue and extensive research has been performed to assess impact of breast versus RF on HIV-free survival in infants, especially under resource-constrained circumstances. WHO has defined various feeding options for HIV-exposed infants (Box 14.1). These are discussed along with the current evidence and recommendations.

14.3.1 Exclusive Breastfeeding

Breastfeeding is the most important determinant of infant survival in developed as well as resource-constrained nations of the world [9,10]. Breast milk is uniquely suited to meet all nutritional requirements of

BOX 14.1

WHO DEFINITIONS OF TERMS USED FOR INFANT FEEDING

1. *Exclusive breastfeeding*
   Giving the infant no other food or drink, not even water, apart from breast milk (including expressed breast milk), with the exception of drops or syrups consisting of vitamins, mineral supplements, or prescribed medicines.
2. *Mixed feeding*
   Giving a baby some breast milk and also any other fluid or solids; even a teaspoon of water would be called mixed feeding.
3. *Replacement feeding*
   The process of feeding a child who is not receiving breast milk with a diet that provides all the nutrients the child needs until the child is fully fed by family foods.

young infants during the first 6 months of life; it also continues to be an important source of nutrition during the second half of infancy and beyond. It provides several critical micronutrients like vitamins A, C, and B12 and folate and copper. It also provides the young infant with a variety of anti-infective and immunological factors. Studies suggest decreased rate of SIDS during the first year of life [11] and reduction in the incidence of diabetes [12], obesity [13], asthma [14], and hematological malignancies [15] in older children and adults who were breastfed. Thus, breastfeeding is the reference model for young infants against which all alternative feeding methods must be measured with regard to growth, development, health, and other short-term and long-term outcomes. It is particularly important in the resource-poor regions of the world where limited access to clean water increases the risk of diarrhea with RF.

HIV-exposed infants are at higher risk for morbidity [16] and mortality [17] than their nonexposed peers. They are also more likely to be born low birth weight [18], thus increasing their vulnerability to sickness and death. In HIV-exposed infants, not breastfeeding or a shorter duration of breastfeeding has been associated with increased morbidity, especially because of diarrhea [19], increased risk of malnutrition [20], and increased mortality [21].

However, there is clear scientific evidence that HIV virus gets transmitted through breast milk. A higher rate of HIV infection among breastfed as compared with formula-fed children is reported in several studies [22,23]. A systematic review of published studies revealed an estimated risk of HIV transmission through breastfeeding by women who acquired infection postnatally to be 29% (95% CI, 16–42%) [24]. In mothers with chronic HIV infection, a similar analysis of published studies estimated that breastfeeding confers a further risk of transmission of HIV by 14% (95% CI, 7–22%), in addition to risk of acquisition during the *in utero*/intrapartum period [25]. Studies have subsequently confirmed detection of HIV-1 in human milk as both a cell-free virus and a cell-associated virus [26,27].

In resource-constrained settings, where sustained exclusive RF may be neither feasible nor safe, evidence has shown that exclusive breastfeeding for the first 4–6 months reduces the risk of HIV transmission as compared with mixed feeding [28,29] and may have survival benefits at 18–24 months similar to those for exclusive RF [30]. Thus, the decision to breastfeed an HIV-exposed infant and duration of breastfeeding has to be made by balancing the benefits versus the risks of breastfeeding in each individual case, with the aim of ensuring the best possible chance of HIV-free survival for the infant.

Making breastfeeding safer would give the infant all its benefits while reducing the associated risk of HIV transmission. Strategies for making breastfeeding safer include the following.

- Heat treatment of breast milk. HIV virus is heat-labile. Thus, heat treatment of breast milk using a variety of techniques has been used to sterilize it. These include Pretoria pasteurization, in which a jar of breast milk is placed in water that has been brought to a boil immediately after removal from heat source [31], and flash heating, which involves heating a jar of breast milk in a pan of water until the water boils and then removing the jar [32]. These heat treatment techniques have been shown to inactivate HIV virus while retaining its nutritional, immunological, and antimicrobial properties [33,34]. Although heat-treated expressed milk as a sole feeding option for a young infant may be difficult to sustain on a long-term basis and its safety and feasibility beyond its short-term use in research settings has not been established, it can be a useful option for interim use during periods of maternal sickness/breast abscess and for low-birth-weight/sick infants unable to suckle. Its feasibility during the period of transition from exclusive breastfeeding to complementary feeding when the chance of infection transmission to the infant may be high due to mixed feeding has been demonstrated [35,36].
- Breast milk banking. Human milk banks have been used to provide donor milk to sick and vulnerable infants for a long time [37,38]. Because the milk is pasteurized, the chance of transmission of HIV or other infectious agents is prevented. However, availability of human

milk banks is extremely limited at present, especially in low-income countries. Even in resource-replete countries, the cost of banked human milk is far more than infant feeding formula, limiting its long-term use for infant feeding [39].

- Wet nursing. In regions of the world where wet nursing may be culturally acceptable and is being practiced, it may be another viable option of providing an HIV-exposed infant with all the benefits of fresh breast milk without associated risk of HIV transmission. However, wet nursing has challenges of its own, including ensuring that the lactating woman (wet nurse) herself is HIV-negative and follows safe sexual practices throughout the period of lactation to avoid acquiring HIV infection, and her being aware of the very small risk of reverse transmission of HIV infection to her in case the infant is HIV-infected. There is no published evidence of use of wet nursing for HIV-exposed infants.
- Use of antiretroviral (ARV) drugs during breastfeeding. An exciting development in the past decade has been emergence of scientific evidence that extended use of ARV drugs given throughout the period of breastfeeding reduces the risk of HIV transmission while providing the young infant all the benefits of breastfeeding. Although peri-partum prophylaxis with a single dose/short course of ARV agents effectively reduces intrapartum transmission [40], its protective effect does not extend much beyond 4–6 weeks in breastfed infant [41,42]. ARV drugs taken through the pregnancy and lactation with full compliance are shown to reduce the HIV infection rate to up to 2% [43–46]. Before these newer ARV interventions were available, it was considered necessary to rapidly wean the breastfed infants after 4–6 months to minimize exposure to mixed feeding. Thus, the WHO, in their 2000 guidelines, recommended that for infants exclusively breastfed during the first months of life, breastfeeding should be discontinued as soon as feasible, taking into account local circumstances, the individual woman's situation, and risk of RF [47]. ARV prophylaxis covering the period of lactation and continued until 1 week after complete cessation of breastfeeding makes the weaning period safe. Thus, duration of the weaning period can be extended, with breastfeeding continued until 12 months of age, thereby reducing infant morbidity and mortality. The new WHO 2013 treatment guidelines have recommended that in the areas with generalized HIV epidemic, all pregnant women, irrespective of their clinical and immunological stage, should be initiated on lifelong ARV therapy (ART). Combined with nevirapine prophylaxis to the infant during the first 6–12 weeks of life and proper breast health management, this makes breastfeeding an even safer option for HIV-exposed infants [48,49].

14.3.2 Exclusive RF

In the setting of maternal HIV infection, RF appears to be a logical option, given the risk of HIV transmission to the infant through breastfeeding. In regions of the world where clean water is available and RF is affordable and culturally acceptable, it is usually promoted as the only feeding option. A guidance from the Department of Health, United Kingdom, states that "under exceptional circumstances and after seeking expert professional advice on reducing the risk of transmission of HIV through breastfeeding, a highly informed and motivated mother might be assisted to breast-feed" [50]. Likewise, in the United States, the Centers for Disease Control and Prevention (CDC) has recommended that HIV-positive women should not breastfeed [51]. Options for RF include the following.

- Commercial infant feeding formula. Infant feeding formulas that have a standard composition especially formulated to meet the nutritional needs of an infant younger than 6 months are the RF of choice for HIV-exposed infants. In many countries affected by HIV, infant feeding formula has been made available free of cost to mothers with HIV as part of government policy or under research protocols of many ongoing scientific studies [52,53]. However, exclusive formula feeding is expensive, more so as the child grows and the requirement increases. Thus, without free supply of formula or a concurrent financial support for the formula, exclusive RF is difficult to sustain, especially under resource-constrained circumstances. This is likely to lead to overdilution of feed and resultant poor nutritional intake and malnutrition in the infants. Also, unless accompanied by a thorough and ongoing nutritional counseling regarding hygienic feed preparation and administration, formula feeding is fraught with danger.
- Fresh animal milk. Animal milk differs substantially in composition from human milk. Most international organizations do not recommend its use for feeding infants younger than 6 months of age because of inappropriate macronutrient and micronutrient content, concerns about safe storage, and risk of gut bleeding [54]. However, fresh animal milk is easily available, is economical, and is culturally acceptable in many parts of the world. Thus, in India, use of fresh boiled animal milk or prepacked processed animal milk (toned, containing 3% fat, 3.1% protein, and providing 58 kcal/100 mL), both of which are freely available commercially, are approved for use in HIV-exposed infants who are using RF and cannot afford formula feeds. It is also recommended that these infants receive iron and multivitamin supplements [55]. However, there is scant

literature regarding the use of fresh animal milk as a replacement to breastfeeding in young infants, nor is there any literature comparing its safety and utility as compared with infant feeding formula in young HIV-exposed infants.

The strategy of RF, optimum use of ARV medicines and preventive obstetric strategies for HIV-infected women have led to a very low mother-to-child HIV transmission rates in high-income countries [56,57]. However, in low-income and middle-income countries, RF has not yielded the same positive results. With little access to clean water, sanitation, and health services, the risk of disease and death are high in infants who are not breastfeeding. No net benefit in HIV-free survival has been seen in sub-Saharan Africa, even if the formula has been provided free of cost [58]. Mortality among HIV-exposed infants on RF has been high and has negated the decreased risk of HIV transmission in such babies [59,60]. A study from Pune, India, has shown that infants on RF had high rates of hospitalization within the first 6 months of life for gastroenteritis, pneumonia, septicemia, and jaundice [61]. Thus, for HIV-infected women in lower-income and middle-income countries, advice regarding infant feeding may differ from that of high-income countries, reflecting limitations in resources and infrastructure.

14.3.3 Mixed Feeding

Feeding an infant both breast milk and RF combines the disadvantages of both strategies without providing the young infant with the benefits of either. Thus, the risk of HIV transmission remains because of exposure to breast milk, and administering RF confers increased risk of gastrointestinal infections. In fact, many studies have reported a higher HIV transmission with mixed feeding as compared with either exclusive breastfeeding or RF [29,62,63]. The reasons for this may include RF-induced damage to the integrity of gut mucosa- pathogens cause intestinal inflammation, whereas foreign antigens activate intestinal immune reactions. The damaged mucosa becomes more permeable to HIV virus present in breast milk, facilitating its transfer to the infant [64].

14.3.4 Current Feeding Recommendations for HIV-Exposed Infants Younger Than 6 Months of Age

It has increasingly been recognized that given the markedly different personal, social, economic, and cultural backgrounds and circumstances to which HIV-infected women may belong, no single point of advice regarding feeding their infants may be the correct choice for all. In each case, the option that ensures the best possible chance, not only of HIV-free survival but also "thrival," that is, healthy survival with normal growth and development, should be advised. Rapid emergence of scientific evidence has seen an equally rapid change in feeding advice for exposed infants. Thus, in 1998, WHO acknowledged that replacement-fed HIV-exposed infants were at less risk for illness and death as long as they had "uninterrupted access to nutritionally adequate breast milk substitutes that are safely prepared and fed to them" [65]. In 2001, WHO introduced the concept of AFASS (acceptable, feasible, affordable, sustainable, and safe) criteria for RF, recommending that all breastfeeding by HIV-infected mothers should be avoided when RF was considered to be AFASS [66]. In 2003, WHO shifted the focus of advice from RF to breastfeeding, stating that HIV-infected mothers should exclusively breastfeed for the first months of life and then rapidly wean their infants as soon as RF is AFASS [67]. Scientific evidence over subsequent years showed that HIV-exposed infants weaned early sustained higher rates of diarrheal morbidity and mortality over time and were more likely to be underweight than those who were breastfed longer [20,68]. Recognizing this, WHO changed its recommendation yet again in 2007 and advised that HIV-infected women exclusively breastfeed for 6 months and continue breastfeeding thereafter, unless RF without any breastfeeding is AFASS [69]. Because further evidence of efficacy and safety of ARV use during breastfeeding in prevention of HIV transmission emerged, WHO provided new guidelines in 2010. These guidelines list only two feeding options for exposed infants—exclusive breastfeeding with maternal and infant ARV interventions or complete avoidance of all breastfeeding. The recommendations further state that "national authorities should decide whether health services will principally counsel and support mothers known to be HIV-infected to either breast-feed and receive ARV interventions, or avoid all breastfeeding as the strategy that will most likely give infants the greatest chance of HIV free survival" [70]. With these recommendations, the onus of decision-making has shifted from individual mother and counselor to national authorities who can make a decision based on the strategy best-suited and feasible for their country and train their health workers to counsel HIV-infected mothers regarding feeding options by using a more directive approach. The WHO 2013 HIV treatment recommendations endorse these recommendations while advising lifelong ART for all pregnant and breastfeeding women with HIV infection, irrespective of their clinical or immunological state.

Breastfeeding remains the feeding option of choice even when ARV interventions are not available, unless all environmental and social conditions suitable for sustained, exclusive RF are met. These conditions are presented in Box 14.2. Mothers are also advised to follow safe breastfeeding practices (Box 14.3).

BOX 14.2

CONDITIONS NEEDED TO SAFELY FORMULA-FEED HIV-EXPOSED INFANTS [69]

Mothers known to be HIV-infected should only give commercial infant formula milk as a replacement feed to their HIV-uninfected infants or infants who are of unknown HIV status when specific conditions are met:

a. Safe water and sanitation are assured at the household level and in the community.
b. The mother, or other caregiver, can reliably provide sufficient infant formula milk to support normal growth and development of the infant.
c. The mother or caregiver can prepare it cleanly and frequently enough so that it is safe and carries a low risk of diarrhea and malnutrition.
d. The mother or caregiver can, during the first 6 months, exclusively provide infant formula milk.
e. The family is supportive of this practice.
f. The mother or caregiver can access health care that offers comprehensive child health services.

BOX 14.3

SAFE BREASTFEEDING PRACTICES FOR MOTHERS REGARDING EXCLUSIVE BREASTFEEDING DURING THE FIRST 6 MONTHS [71]

1. Mothers should use dual protection (condom) to avoid reinfection with HIV and other STIs during pregnancy and breastfeeding.
2. Practice exclusive breastfeeding for the first 6 months.
3. Avoid mixed feeding.
4. Avoid non-nutritive or comfort suckling.
5. Check for and treat oral thrush and sores in child's mouth immediately.
6. Practice good breast care.
7. Recognize and promptly manage breast conditions like mastitis, sore nipples, and abscesses. Do not breastfeed the infant from the affected breast. Seek medical help if the need arises.

14.4 FEEDING OF HIV-EXPOSED INFANTS OLDER THAN 6 MONTHS OF AGE

Although breast milk alone is sufficient to meet the nutritional requirements of infants up to 6 months of age, for an older infant an additional source of energy and nutrients is needed. The energy needed in addition to breast milk is approximately 200 kcal/day for infants 6–8 months, 300 kcal/day for infants 9–11 months, and 550 kcal/day for children 12–23 months. Thus, introduction of complementary food is advised for all infants at 6 months of age. The guidelines hold true for HIV-exposed infants as well, as reiterated in the WHO 2010 guidelines. Because breast milk has a relatively high fat content compared with most complementary foods, it remains a key source of energy and essential fatty acids in older infants. Its fat promotes utilization of provitamin A carotenoids in predominantly plant-based diets. It continues to provide substantial amounts of micronutrients like vitamin A, calcium, and riboflavin intake during the second year of life. The nutritional impact of breastfeeding is most evident during periods of illness, when the child's appetite for other foods decreases but breast milk intake is maintained. Thus, it is recommended that breastfeeding be continued for as long as possible, even until 2 years of age and beyond, along with other foods.

However, longer duration of breastfeeding by HIV-infected women is associated with an increased risk of HIV transmission to the infant. In a study conducted in Malawi, the cumulative risk of infection for infants breastfed beyond 1 month of age was 3.55% at 5 months, 7% after 11 months, 8.9% at 17 months, and 10.3% at end of 23 months [72]. Therefore, it was thought that because exclusive breastfeeding has a lower risk of HIV transmission than mixed feeding, abruptly stopping breastfeeding with introduction of complementary foods at approximately 6 months of age would offer the infants maximum health benefits while minimizing the risk. However, limiting the duration of breastfeeding to 4–6 months with abrupt cessation thereafter has been shown to increase morbidity and mortality due to diarrhea and growth faltering and is not practically feasible [20,73,74]. Breast milk viral load has also been shown to spike with rapid cessation of breastfeeding [75]. After the age of 12 months, a child's nutritional needs can be met more easily by family foods, including animal milk. Although breast milk may continue to provide significant benefits at this age, its withdrawal has not been seen to lead to growth faltering or increased mortality. Thus, there is no compelling need to continue it, especially in the setting of maternal HIV infection, when the risk of HIV transmission cannot be entirely eliminated despite all interventions to make it safe. The WHO 2010 exposed infant feeding guidelines therefore recommend breastfeeding until 12 months of age for HIV-negative infants under cover of continued maternal ARV drugs. This lowers the risk of HIV transmission associated with mixed feeding while allowing breastfeeding to continue over a longer period of time. Mothers who decide to stop breastfeeding can do so gradually over a period of 1 month once a nutritionally adequate and safe diet without breast milk can be provided. It is recommended that the maternal ARV prophylaxis should continue for at least 1 week after the breastfeeding has fully stopped, unless the mother is on ART.

For breastfeeding infants diagnosed as HIV-positive, ART should be started and breastfeeding should be continued until 2 years of age, along with the usual complementary foods advisable for children of this age. This will ensure optimum growth for the infant and provide additional protection from infections. Children with HIV infection have additional energy requirements depending on their clinical and nutritional status as discussed previously. These can be met by simple modification of complementary foods for all children, except those with severe acute malnutrition who require therapeutic feeding.

14.5 FOLLOW-UP OF HIV-EXPOSED INFANTS

Normal growth is a sensitive indicator of overall good health of children. Thus, it is important to monitor growth of all children, especially during the first few years of life when the pace of growth is fast. Growth monitoring is even more important for HIV-exposed children given their vulnerability to growth failure. Routine monitoring of weight and length at two or three monthly intervals coupled with appropriate nutritional counseling is imperative to maintaining good health status of these infants.

14.6 ROLE OF MICRONUTRIENT SUPPLEMENTATION

Micronutrient supplementation is shown to reduce child mortality and morbidity related to infectious diseases [76,77]. It is also shown to lead to small but significant increases in length and weight [78,79]. Supplementation is more likely to benefit children living in poor countries, where dietary intake and/or bioavailability of micronutrients are low. Thus, HIV-exposed infants who are at high risk for mortality, infectious diseases, and malnutrition *per se* and who are also more likely to be living under adverse socioeconomic conditions that limit their access to a nutritionally balanced diet, are likely to benefit from them. No robust scientific literature exists regarding benefit of micronutrient supplementation in these infants. Fawzi et al. [80] have shown that high-dose multivitamin supplementation in pregnant women decreased infection-related morbidity and slowed HIV progression. Also, infants of these women were reported to have fewer episodes of diarrhea and better growth [81]. However, further studies by the same group of researchers in Tanzania, in which HIV-exposed infants were given oral high-dose vitamin B, C, and E supplements from 6 to 104 weeks of age, did not show a benefit in terms of decreased mortality or hospitalizations. No benefit was observed in anthropometric parameters in the supplemented group compared with the control group. However, mothers of these infants themselves were also given similar high-dose vitamin supplementation during pregnancy and lactation, which would have given at least some benefit to their infants as well [82,83]. A few other studies on micronutrient supplementation in HIV-exposed or HIV-infected children have also not shown benefits in terms of mortality or gastrointestinal/respiratory morbidity [84–86]; they also have not shown benefits in catch-up growth [87]. More evidence is needed at present to justify routine micronutrient supplementation in these infants.

14.7 ROLE OF NUTRITIONAL SUPPORT SERVICES

For the benefit of advances in research and available guidelines to reach the vulnerable infants, it is critical for the ART centers that provide care to these infants and their parents to also provide various nutritional support services. The most important among these is ongoing nutritional counseling, especially to pregnant and lactating women and children of all ages. Counseling regarding safe young infant feeding practices, whether breastfeeding or RF, and also timely introduction of complementary foods that are locally available and are nutritionally rich, will go a long way in promoting optimum growth. Growth monitoring to facilitate early detection of growth faltering leading to early intervention is another critical service. Other support services include availability of routine immunization, vitamin A and iron supplementation, and medical management and nutritional care of malnourished exposed infants. Provision of food supplements could help improve individual and household food security; it could also lead to improved medication adherence and retention in HIV care and treatment in resource-constrained circumstances [88].

14.8 CHALLENGES IN NUTRITIONAL MANAGEMENT OF EXPOSED INFANTS

The fast pace of scientific research in the field of HIV *per se* and care of HIV-exposed infants in particular have led to development of robust strategies of care that have vastly improved the prospects of HIV-exposed infants. However, there exists confusion in the minds of HIV-infected parents as well as health care practitioners regarding best practices to improve infant survival and health, primarily because of rapidly changing international recommendations that are followed by changes in national guidelines. Slow rollout of updated national guidelines and lag in training and retraining of different levels of health staff have compounded this problem. This has often led to conflicting though well-meaning advice being given by different health care staff to the parents. Thus, the foremost challenge is giving updated, clear, and consistent messages to HIV-infected mothers through trained health care staff and continuing support for optimal feeding of their young infants. Adherence to guidelines for complementary feeding is, in general, poor in resource-constrained nations [89]. The foods are often introduced too early or too late, with little variety, inadequate portions, overdilution, and poor food safety. Thus, growth faltering and incidence of gastrointestinal infections escalate dramatically during the period of introduction of complementary feeding. Providing HIV-exposed infants with nutritionally adequate complementary feeding is even more challenging because of adverse socioeconomic circumstances, and also because these infants may lack a healthy appetite or suffer from other factors affecting their food intake. There is a dearth of high-quality infant feeding counseling material and a shortage of, along with high turnover of, HIV counselors [90]. Yet another challenge is early detection of HIV infection in pregnant women, timely initiation, and continued availability of ART to pregnant women and the exposed infant. Retaining HIV-exposed infants in care until 18 months of age, availability of early infant diagnosis of HIV infection, and timely initiation of ART in infected infants are other challenges.

KEY MESSAGES

1. HIV-exposed infants are vulnerable to malnutrition and have higher morbidity and mortality than unexposed infants.
2. Exclusive breastfeeding during the first 6 months of life followed by timely introduction of complementary feeding is the best feeding option for their healthy survival.
3. HIV-uninfected infants should be breastfed until 12 months of age under cover of maternal ART/ARV prophylaxis.
4. HIV-infected children should continue to breastfeed until the age of 2 years or beyond.
5. Energy needs of HIV-infected children are higher than those of uninfected children—these can be met by home modification of diets for all children except those severely malnourished, who would require therapeutic feeding.
6. Growth monitoring and ongoing availability of nutritional support services are critical to improve survival and health outcomes of HIV-exposed infants.

References

[1] Isanaka S, Duggan C, Fawzi WW. Patterns of postnatal growth in HIV-infected and HIV-exposed children. Nutr Rev 2009;67(6):343–59.

[2] Ram M, Gupte N, Nayak U, Kinikar AA, Khandave M, Shankar AV, SWEN India and BJMC-JHU Clinical Trials Study Team Growth patterns among HIV-exposed infants receiving nevirapine prophylaxis in Pune, India. BMC Infect Dis 2012;12:282. http://dx.doi.org/10.1186/1471-2334-12-282.

[3] Seth A, Chandra J, Gupta R, Kumar P, Aggarwal V, Dutta A. Outcome of HIV exposed infants: experience of a regional pediatric center for HIV in North India. Indian J Pediatr 2012;79(2):188–93. http://dx.doi.org/10.1007/s12098-011-0532-8.

[4] Preidis GA, Mccollum ED, Mwansambo C, Kazembe PN, Schutze GE, Kline MW. Pneumonia and malnutrition are highly predictive of mortality among African children hospitalized with human immunodeficiency virus infection or exposure in the era of antiretroviral therapy. J Pediatr 2011;159:484–9.

[5] Callens SF, Shabani N, Lusiama J, Lelo P, Kitetele F, Colebunders R, et al. Mortality and associated factors after initiation of pediatric antiretroviral treatment in the Democratic Republic of the Congo. Pediatr Infect Dis J 2009;28:35–40.

[6] WHO. Nutrient requirements for people living with HIV. AIDS. Report of a technical consultation, 13–15 May 2003. Geneva, Switzerland: WHO; 2003.

[7] Black RE, Allen LH, Bhutta ZA, for the Maternal and Child undernutrition Group Maternal and child undernutrition: global and regional exposures and health consequences. Lancet 2008;371(9608):243–60.

[8] WHO Collaborative Study Team on the role of Breastfeeding on the Prevention of Infant Mortality. Effect of breastfeeding on infant and child mortality due to infectious diseases in less developed countries: a pooled analysis. Lancet 2000; 355: 451–5.

[9] Ip S, Chung M, Raman G, et al. A summary of the Agency for Healthcare Research and Quality's evidence report on breastfeeding in developed countries. Breastfeed Med 2009;4(Suppl. 1):S17–30.

[10] Black RE, Morris SS, Bryce J. Where and why are 10 million children dying every year? Lancet 2003;361:2226–34.

[11] Horne RS, Parslow PM, Ferens D, Watts AM, Adamson TM. Comparison of evoked arousability in breast and formula fed infants. Arch Dis Child 2004;89:22–5.

[12] Gerstein HC. Cow's milk exposure and type 1 diabetes mellitus. A critical overview of the clinical literature. Diabetes Care 1994;17:13–19.

[13] Armstrong J, Reilly JJ. Child health information team. Breastfeeding and lowering the risk of childhood obesity. Lancet 2002;359:2003–4.

[14] Chulada PC, Arbes Jr SJ, Dunson D, Zeldin DC. Breast-feeding and the prevalence of asthma and wheeze in children: analyses from the Third National Health and Nutrition Examination Survey 1988–1994. J Allergy Clin Immunol 2003;111:328–36.

[15] Bener A, Denic S, Galadari S. Longer breast-feeding and protection against childhood leukaemia and lymphomas. Eur J Cancer 2001;37:234–8.

[16] Filteau S. The HIV-exposed, uninfected African child. Trop Med Int Health 2009;14:276–87.

[17] Landes M, van Lettow M, Chan AK, Mayuni I, Schouten EJ, Bedell RA. Mortality and health outcomes of HIV exposed and unexposed children in a PMTCT cohort in Malawi. PLoS One 2012;7:1–7.

[18] Ndirangu J, Newell ML, Bland RM, Thorne C. Maternal HIV infection associated with small-for-gestational age infants but not preterm births: evidence from rural South Africa. Hum Reprod 2012;27:1846–56.

[19] Onyango-Makambi C, Bagenda D, Mwatha A, et al. Early weaning of HIV exposed uninfeccted infants and risk of serious gastro-enteritis: findings from two perinatal

HIV prevention trials in Kampala, Uganda. J Acquir Immun Defic Syndr 2009 http://dx.doi.org/10.1097/QAI.0b013e3181bdf68e.
[20] Arpadi S, Fawzy A, Aldrovandi GM, Kankasa C, Sinkala M, Mwiya M, et al. Growth faltering due to breastfeeding cessation in uninfected children born to HIV infected mothers in Zambia. Am J Clin Nutr 2009;90:344–53.
[21] Mach O, Lu L, Creek T, et al. Population based study of a wide-spread outbreak of diarrhea associated with increased mortality and malnutrition in Botswana, January–March 2006. Am J Trop Med Hyg 2009;80:812–8.
[22] Gabiano C, Tovo PA, de Martino M, et al. Mother-to-child transmission of human immunodeficiency virus type 1: risk of infection and correlates of transmission. Pediatrics 1992;90:369–74.
[23] de Martino M, Tovo PA, Tozzi AE, et al. HIV-1 transmission through breast-milk: appraisal of risk according to duration of feeding. AIDS 1992;6:991–7.
[24] Dunn DT, Newell ML, Ades AE, Peckham CS. Risk of human immunodeficiency virus type 1 transmission through breastfeeding. Lancet 1992;340:585–8.
[25] AAP Technical Report on Human Milk Breastfeeding and transmission of human immunodeficiency virus type 1 in the United States. Pediatrics 2003;112:1196–205.
[26] Guay LA, Hom DL, Mmiro F, et al. Detection of human immunodeficiency virus type 1 (HIV-1) DNA and p24 antigen in breast milk of HIV-1-infected Ugandan women and vertical transmission. Pediatrics 1996;98:438–44.
[27] Ruff AJ, Coberly J, Halsey NA, et al. Prevalence of HIV-1 DNA and p24 antigen in breast milk and correlation with maternal factors. J Acquir Immune Defic Syndr 1994;7: 68–73.
[28] Coovadia HM, Rollins NC, Bland RM, et al. Mother-to-child transmission of HIV-1 infection during exclusive breastfeeding in the first 6 mo of life: an intervention cohort study. Lancet 2007;369:1107–16.
[29] Iliff PJ, Piwoz EG, Tavengwa NV, Zunguza CD, Marinda ET, Nathoo KJ, et al. Early exclusive breastfeeding reduces the risk of postnatal HIV-1 transmission and increases HIV-free survival. AIDS 2005;19:699–708.
[30] Newell ML, Coovadia H, Cortina-Borja M, et al. Mortality of infected and uninfected infants born to HIV-infected mothers in Africa: a pooled analysis. Lancet 2004;364:1236–43.
[31] Jeffrey BS, Webber L, Mokhondo KR, Erasmus D. Determination of the effectiveness of inactivation of human immunodeficiency virus by Pretoria pasteurization. J Trop Pediatr 2001;47:345–9.
[32] Israel-Ballard K, Chantry C, Dewey K, et al. Viral, nutritional and bacterial safety of flash-heated and Pretoria pasteurized breast milk to prevent mother to child transmission of HIV in resource-poor countries: a pilot study. J Acquir Immune Defic Syndr 2005;40:175–81.
[33] Israel-Ballard K, Abrams BF, Coutsoudis A, et al. Vitamin content of breast milk from HIV-1 infected mothers before and after flash heat treatment. J Acquir Immune Defic Syndr 2008;48:444–9.
[34] Chantry CJ, Israel-Ballard K, Moldoveanu Z, et al. Effect of flash heat treatment on immunoglobulins in breast milk. J Acquir Immune Defic Syndr 2009;51:264–7.
[35] Chantry CJ, Young SL, Rennie W, et al. Feasibility of using flash-heated breastmilk as an infant feeding option for HIV-exposed, uninfected infants after 6 months of age in urban Tanzania. J Acquir Immune Defic Syndr 2012;60(1):43–50.
[36] Mbuya MN, Humphrey JH, Majo F, et al. Heat treatment of expressed breast milk is a feasible option for feeding HIV exposed uninfected children after 6 months of age in rural Zimbabwe. J Nutr 2010;140:1481–8.
[37] Arnold LDW. The cost-effectiveness of using banked donor milk in the neonatal intensive care unit: prevention of necrotizing enterocolitis. J Human Lact 2002;18:172–7.

[38] Arnold L. Global health policies that support the use of banked donor human milk: a human rights issue. Int Breastfeed J 2006;1:26.

[39] Young SL, Mbuya MNN, Chantry CJ, et al. Current knowledge and future research on infant feeding in the context of HIV: basic, clinical, behavioral and programmatic perspectives. Adv Nutr 2011;2:225–43.

[40] Volmink J, Siegfried NL, van der Merwe L, Brocklehurst P. Antiretrovirals for reducing the risk of mother-to-child transmission of HIV infection. Cochrane Database Syst Rev 2007:1. CD003510.

[41] Petra Study Team. Efficacy of three short-course regimens of zidovudine and lamivudine in preventing early and late transmission of HIV-1 from mother to child in Tanzania, South Africa, and Uganda (Petra study): a randomised, double-blind, placebocontrolled trial. Lancet 2002;359:1178–86.

[42] Leroy V, Karon JM, Alioum A, et al. Twenty-four month efficacy of a maternal short-course zidovudine regimen to prevent mother-to-child transmission of HIV-1 in West Africa. AIDS 2002;16:631–41.

[43] Kilewo C, Karlsson K, Massawe A, Lyamuya E, Swai A, Mhalu F, Mitra Study Team Prevention of mother-to-child transmission of HIV-1 through breast-feeding by treating infants prophylactically with lamivudine in Dar esSalaam. Tanzania: the Mitra Study. J Acquir Immune Defic Synd 2008;48:315–23.

[44] Chasela CS, Hudgens MG, Jamieson DJ, et al. Maternal or infant antiretroviral drugs to reduce HIV-1 transmission. N Engl J Med 2010;362:2271–81.

[45] Shapiro R, Hughes M, Ogwu A, et al. A randomized trial comparing highly active antiretroviral therapy regimens for virologic efficacy and the prevention of mother-to-child transmission among breastfeeding women in Botswana (The MmaBana Study). 5th IAS Conference on HIV Pathogenesis Treatment, and Prevention, Cape Town, abstract WELBB101; 2009.

[46] The Kesho Bora Study Group. Triple antiretroviral compared with zidovudine and single-dose nevirapine prophylaxis during pregnancy and breastfeeding for prevention of mother-to-child transmission of HIV-1 (Kesho Bora study): a randomised controlled trial. Lancet Infect Dis 2011;11:171–80.

[47] WHO. New data on the prevention of mother to child transmission of HIV and their policy implications. Conclusions and recommendations. WHO technical consultation on behalf of the UNFPA/ UNICEF/WHO/UNAIDS Inter-agency task team on mother to child transmission of HIV. Geneva, Switzerland; 2000. Geneva WHO 2001, WHO/RHR/01.28.

[48] WHO. Consolidated guidelines on the use of antiretroviral drugs for treating and preventing HIV infection recommendations for a public health approach; 2013.

[49] Horwath T, Madi BC, Luppa IM, et al. Interventions for preventing late post-natal-mother-to-child transmission of HIV. Cochrane Database of Syst Rev 2009:1.

[50] Department of Health, UK. HIV and Infant Feeding: Guidance from the UK Chief Medical Offices' Expert Advisory Group on AIDS, <http://www.dh.gov.uk/en/Publicationsandstatistics/Publications/PublicationsPolicyAndGuidance/DH_4089892>; 2004.

[51] Panel on Treatment of HIV-Infected Pregnant Women and Prevention of Perinatal Transmission. Recommendations for use of antiretroviral drugs in pregnant HIV-1-infected women for maternal health and interventions to reduce perinatal HIV transmission in the United States; 2010 [Cited 2010 December]. Available from: <http://aidsinfo.nih.gov/contentfiles/PerinatalGL.pdf>.

[52] Coutsoudis A, Goga AE, Rollins N, et al. Free formula milk for infants of HIV infected women: blessing or curse. Health Policy Plan 2002;17:154–60.

[53] deWagt A, Clark D. A review of UNICEF experience with the distribution of free infant formula for infants of HIV-infected mothers in Africa. Presented at the LINKAGES Art and Science of Breastfeeding Presentation Series; 2004 [Cited 2010 November].

Available from: <http://www.linkagesproject.org/media/publications/Technical%20 Reports/InfantFormula_UNICEF_Art&Science.pdf>.

[54] Papathakis PC, Rollins NC. Are WHO/UNAIDS/UNICEF-recommended replacement milks for infants of HIV-infected mothers appropriate in the South African context? Bull World Health Organ 2004;82:164–71.

[55] National AIDS Control Organisation, India. Nutrition Guidelines for HIV-Exposed and Infected Children (0–14 Years of Age); 2012.

[56] Townsend CL, Cortina-Borja M, Peckham CS, de Ruiter A, Lyall H, Tookey PA. Low rates of mother-to-child transmission of HIV following effective pregnancy interventions in the United Kingdom and Ireland, 2000–2006. AIDS 2008;22:973–81.

[57] Paul ME, Chantry CJ, Read JS, Frederick MM, Lu M, Pitt J, et al. Morbidity and mortality during the first two years of life among uninfected children born to human immunodeficiency virus type 1-infected women: the women and infants transmission study. Pediatr Infect Dis J 2005;24:46–56.

[58] Kuhn L, Reitz C, Abrams EJ. Breastfeeding and AIDS in the developing world. Curr Opin Pediatr 2009;21:83–93.

[59] Thior I, Lockman S, Smeaton LM, Shapiro RL, Mashi Study Team Breastfeeding plus infant zidovudine prophylaxis for 6 months vs. formula feeding plus infant zidovudine for 1 month to reduce mother-to-child transmission in Botswan: a randomized trial: the MASHI study. JAMA 2006;296:794–805.

[60] Coutsoudis A, Pillay K, Spooner E, et al. Morbidity in children born to women infected with human immunodeficiency virus in South Africa: does mode of feeding matter? Acta Pediatr 2003;92:890–5.

[61] Phadke MA, Gadgil B, Bharucha KE, et al. Replacement fed infants born to HIV-infected mothers in India have a high early postpartum rates of hospitalization. J Nutr 2003;133:3153–7.

[62] Piwoz EG, Humphrey JH, Tavengwa NV, Iliff PJ, Marinda ET, Zunguza CD, et al. The impact of safer breastfeeding practices on postnatal HIV-1 transmission in Zimbabwe. Am J Public Health 2007;97:1249–54.

[63] Coutsoudis A, Pillay K, Spooner E, Kuhn L, Coovadia H. Influence of infant-feeding patterns on early mother-to-child transmission of HIV-1 in Durban, South Africa: a prospective cohort study. South African Vitamin A Study Group. Lancet 1999;354:471–6.

[64] Coovadia HM, Bland RM. Preserving breastfeeding practice through the HIV pandemic. Trop Med Int Health 2007;12:1116–33.

[65] WHO HIV and infant feeding. Guidelines for decision makers. Geneva, Switzerland: WHO; 1998.

[66] WHO Technical Consultation. New data on the prevention of mother-to-child transmission of HIV and their policy implications; 2001 [Cited 2010 December]. Available from: <http://whqlibdoc.who.int/hq/2001/WHO_RHR_01.28.pdf>.

[67] WHO, UNICEF, UNFPA, UNAIDS. HIV and infant feeding: a guide for health-care managers and supervisors. Geneva, Switzerland: WHO; 2003.

[68] Fawzy A, Arpadi S, Kankasa C, Sinkala M, Mwiya M, Thea DM, et al. Early weaning increases diarrhea morbidity and mortality among uninfected children born to HIV-infected mothers in Zambia. J Infect Dis 2011;203:1222–30.

[69] WHO, UNICEF, UNFPA, UNAIDS. HIV and infant feeding: update based on the technical consultation held on behalf of the Inter-agency Team (IATT) on Prevention of HIV Infections in Pregnant Women, Mothers, and Their Infants, Geneva; 2006. Geneva, Switzerland: WHO; 2007.

[70] World Health Organization. Guidelines on HIV and infant feeding 2010: principles and recommendations for infant feeding in the context of HIV and a summary of evidence; 2010.

[71] Seth A. Care of the HIV-exposed child-to breastfeed or not. Indian J Pediatr 2012;79(11):1501–5. 1503.

[72] Miotti PG, Taha TE, Kumwenda NI, et al. HIV transmission through breastfeeding: a study in Malawi. JAMA 1999;282:744–9.
[73] Kuhn L, Aldrovandi GM, Sinkala M, et al. Differential effects of early weaning for HIV free survival of children born to HIV infected mothers by severity of maternal disease. PLoS One 2009;4:e 6059.
[74] Kuhn L, Aldrovandi GM, Sinkala M, et al. Effects of early, abrupt cessation of breastfeeding on HIV-free survival of children in Zambia. N Engl J Med 2008;359:130–41.
[75] Thea DM, Aldrovandi G, Kankasa C, et al. Post-weaning breast milk HIV-1 viral load, blood prolactin levels and breast milk volume. AIDS 2006;20:1539–47.
[76] Bhutta ZA, Ahmed T, Black RE, Cousens S, Dewey K, Giugliani E, et al. What works? Interventions for maternal and child undernutrition and survival. Lancet 2008;371:417–40.
[77] Yakoob MY, Theodoratou E, Jabeen A, Imdad A, Eisele TP, Ferguson J, et al. Preventive zinc supplementation in developing countries: impact on mortality and morbidity due to diarrhea, pneumonia and malaria. BMC Public Health 2011;11(Suppl. 3):S23.
[78] Allen LH, Peerson JM, Olney DK. Provision of multiple rather than two or fewer micronutrients more effectively improves growth and other outcomes in micronutrient-deficient children and adults. J Nutr 2009;139:1022–30.
[79] Ramakrishnan U, Nguyen P, Martorell R. Effects of micronutrients on growth of children under 5 y of age: meta-analyses of single and multiple nutrient interventions. Am J Clin Nutr 2009;89:191–203.
[80] Fawzi WW, Msamanga GI, Spiegelman D, Wei R, Kapiga S, Villamor E, et al. A randomized trial of multivitamin supplements and HIV disease progression and mortality. N Engl J Med 2004;351:23–32.
[81] Villamor E, Saathoff E, Bosch RJ, Hertzmark E, Baylin A, Manji K, et al. Vitamin supplementation of HIV-infected women improves postnatal child growth. Am J Clin Nutr 2005;81:880–8.
[82] Duggan C, Manji KP, Kupka R, et al. Multiple micronutrient supplementation in Tanzanian infants born to HIV-infected mothers: a randomized, double-blind, placebo-controlled clinical trial. Am J Clin Nutr 2012;96:1437–46.
[83] Roland Kupka R, Manji KP, Bosch RJ, et al. Multivitamin supplements have no effect on growth of Tanzanian children born to HIV-infected mothers. J Nutr 2013;143:722–7.
[84] Ndeezi G, Tylleskar T, Ndugwa CM, Tumwine JK. Effect of multiple micronutrient supplementation on survival of HIV-infected children in Uganda: a randomized, controlled trial. J Int AIDS Soc 2010;13:18.
[85] Luabeya KK, Mpontshane N, Mackay M, Ward H, Elson I, Chhagan M, et al. Zinc or multiple micronutrient supplementation to reduce diarrhea and respiratory disease in South African children: a randomized controlled trial. PLoS One 2007;2:e541.
[86] Chhagan MK, Van den Broeck J, Luabeya KK, Mpontshane N, Tucker KL, Bennish ML. Effect of micronutrient supplementation on diarrhoeal disease among stunted children in rural South Africa. Eur J Clin Nutr 2009;63:850–7.
[87] Filteau S, Baisley K, Chisenga M, the CIGNIS Study Team Provision of micronutrient-fortified food from 6 months of age does not permit HIV-exposed uninfected Zambian children to catch up in growth to HIV-unexposed children: a randomized controlled trial. J Acquir Immune Defic Syndr 2011;56:166–75.
[88] Rosen S, Fox MP, Gill CJ. Patient retention in antiretroviral therapy programs in sub-Saharan Africa: a systematic review. PLoS Med 2007;4:e298.
[89] Dewey KG, Adu-Afarwuah S. Systematic review of the efficacy and effectiveness of complementary feeding interventions in developing countries. Matern Child Nutr 2008;4:24–85.
[90] Connell J, Zurn P, Stilwell B, Awases M, Braichet JM. Sub-Saharan Africa: beyond the health worker migration crisis? Soc Sci Med 2007;64:1876–91.

CHAPTER

15

HIV-Positive Patients Respond to Dietary Supplementation with Cysteine or Glutamine

Roberto Carlos Burini[1], *Fernando Moreto*[1] *and Yong-Ming Yu*[2]

[1]Centre for Nutritional and Physical Exercise Metabolism, Department of Public Health, Botucatu Medical School, Sao Paulo State University—UNESP, Botucatu, SP, Brazil, [2]Massachusetts General Hospital, Department of Surgery, Shriners Burns Hospital, Harvard Medical School, Boston, MA, USA

15.1 HIV–HOST CELL INTERACTIONS

Viral infections are becoming more common around the world. People living in the poorest countries represent the most infected population because of their unhygienic food conditions, illiteracy, and lack of basic health care. Acquired immunodeficiency syndrome (AIDS) is a disease of the human immune system caused by a pathogen, human immunodeficiency virus (HIV). This leads to the onset of a clinical condition that is characterized by progressive reduction of the efficacy of the immune system, with the host becoming susceptible to opportunistic infections or cancer appearance [1]. AIDS is the consequence of HIV infection and is one of the most dreaded infectious diseases causing mortality in individuals. This pandemic is caused by the HIV-1 and HIV-2 groups of cytopathic viruses [2].

In most viruses, DNA is transcribed into RNA, and then RNA is translated into protein. However, retrovirus (such as HIV) is a single-stranded RNA virus that stores its nucleic acid in the form of an mRNA genome

Health of HIV Infected People, Volume 2.
DOI: http://dx.doi.org/10.1016/B978-0-12-800767-9.00015-7

(including the 5′ cap and 3′ poly A tail) and targets a host cell as an obligate parasite [3,4]. The CD4$^+$ T-helper cells that form important components of the immune system are the main targets of the HIV virus [2]. With its specific protease, the HIV-1 uses glycoprotein (gp120) to enter host cells (T cells and monocytes). Once inside, there are two other important proteins for its development, the HIV-1 transactivation protein (Tat) and the p24 antigenic proteins required to form the viral coat [5]. Once replicated, the virus can be either flushed out of the cell or removed together with the whole cell by phagocytes. Cytotoxic T lymphocytes (CTLs) and natural killer (NK) cells can eradicate virus-infected target cells via the apoptosis process.

The survival of HIV inside the CD4$^+$ lymphocytes will depend on cells properly signaling pathways. Hence, nuclear factor kappa B (NF-kB) is necessary for viral replication and also for activation of many of the immune system's inflammatory cytokines. One of these cytokines is tumor necrosis factor alpha (TNF-alpha), which, when activated, can suppress the apoptosis process inside the cell using different signaling pathways. In turn, these pathways stimulate the expression of antiapoptotic genes such as IAP, BCL-2, and BCL-XL and TNF receptor (TNFR)-associated factors that do not allow the activation of caspase family proteins.

15.1.1 Cell-Born Free Radicals

The virus–host cell contact, installation, replication, proliferation, and dissemination are accompanied by metabolic changes resulting in prooxidant activities with higher free-radical production. A free radical is defined as any atom (e.g., oxygen, nitrogen) with at least one unpaired electron in the outermost shell and is capable of independent existence. A free radical is easily formed when a covalent bond between chemical entities is broken and one electron remains with each newly formed atom. When free radicals "steal" an electron from a surrounding compound or molecule, a new free radical is formed in its place. In turn, the newly formed radical then returns to its ground state by stealing electrons with antiparallel spins from cellular structures or molecules. Thus, the chain reaction continues and the free radicals keep changing the nonradicals into new free radicals. There are many types of radicals, but those of most concern in biological systems are derived from oxygen and are known collectively as reactive oxygen species (ROS). Oxygen has two unpaired electrons in separated orbitals in its outer shell. This electronic structure makes oxygen especially susceptible to radical formation.

ROS are mostly produced in the electron transport chains in mitochondria, peroxisomes, endoplasmic reticulum (ER), and in nuclear and plasma membranes in aerobic cell metabolism. However, the formation of ROS may trigger different unfavorable reactions such as the damage of DNA, proteins, and polysaccharides, alteration of immune function, enhancing apoptosis, and modification of critical aspects of redox-dependent metabolism. Therefore, ROS has been considered as "friend" as well as "foe" of the cell.

ROS has been described as (oxi-reduction-dependent) secondary messengers and regulators playing an important role in cell signaling and regulating hormone action, growth factors, cytokines, transcription, apoptosis, ion transport, immunomodulation, and neural modulation [1]. Therefore, ROS influences a number of different molecular processes, including the apoptotic, antiapoptotic, and pro-apoptotic expression of a number of genes. They lend fundamental aid to the normal functioning of the body's immune system and proliferate T cells that provide immunological defense (adaptive immunity) [6,7]. However, when the same ROS are produced by activated neutrophils and macrophages, they destroy microbes/viruses and neighboring cells via oxidative bursts [8]. Hence, cells respond to the ROS they produce according to different parameters such as intensity, duration, and amount. Once more, ROS can be distinctly beneficial and deleterious for the host cell [2].

The intracellular redox environment must be more reducing than the oxidative environment to maintain optimal cell function [5]. However, ROS are typically produced in all types of cells during normal metabolic processes and serve as important messengers in cell signaling and various signal transduction pathways. Then, the ROS produced inside cells are maintained by complex intracellular regulatory systems that maintain ROS neutralized by antioxidant defense systems, including enzymes, free-radical scavengers, and metal chelates. Consequently, oxidative stress is defined as the imbalance between the oxidant and antioxidant systems.

15.1.2 HIV-Induced ROS

The redox status of humans may be influenced by HIV-1 infection or treatment of such patients with anti-HIV-1 regimen [5]. After entering a cell, a virus disturbs the cell's normal functioning by using the cell's machinery to replicate itself. This, in turn, leads to an imbalance in the cell's ROS system. Hence, for the virus, the physiological role played by ROS is important because viruses depend on the biosynthetic mechanisms of their host cells as intracellular parasites [2]. However, many host mechanisms have been shown or are suspected to contribute to the pathogenesis of viral infections, such as ROS and cytokines.

The available evidence indicates that free radicals play a complex role in different viral diseases, beginning with their influence on the host cell's metabolism and viral replication and extending to their desired inactivation effects on viruses and less desired toxic effects on host tissues [2]. Hence, oxidative stress may contribute to different stages of the viral life cycle, including viral replication and its consequences such as inflammatory response and decreased immune cell proliferation [2,5].

The effect of ROS on the host's immune response is an important factor of viral pathogenesis and mutation. The toxicity and reactivity of ROS, which are produced in excess amounts by the overreactions of immune responses against the organs or tissues in which viruses replicate, may explain the tissue injury mechanisms observed in the different viral diseases involving immunological interactions [2].

Current studies of ROS are based on the lethal effects of ROS in various diseases such as cancer, HIV, hepatitis, and diabetes. In the case of bacterial and viral infections, ROS are produced by phagocytes to generate the respiratory burst resulting from the NADPH oxidase activity. The discovery of "respiratory bursts" revealed that ROS are only produced by phagocyte cells to protect against microbial invasions and are thus considered toxic molecules [2]. Hence, ROS can be considered part of the defense system against viral/bacterial infections. Therefore, the effect of ROS on the cellular functions depends on the amount of ROS and how much time the cell has been exposed to ROS. The ROS produced by the virus-infected cell must be specific and also produced in limited amounts, because they can destroy the cell for which they are generated in addition to the cell's neighboring surroundings during highly inflammatory reactions.

The antioxidant defense mechanism comprises two components: (1) enzymatic components, including catalases, superoxide dismutase (SOD), and glutathione (GSH) peroxidase (GPx) and (2) nonenzymatic components, including vitamin C, vitamin E, carotenoids, GSH, and flavonoids, among others. Various reviews and research papers have indicated the role and mechanism of both enzymatic and nonenzymatic components in protecting against oxidative stress. Changes to the body's antioxidant defense system, in relation to SOD, ascorbic acid, selenium, carotenoids, and GSH, have been reported in various tissues of RNA virus–infected patients [2].

15.1.3 HIV-Induced Oxidative Stress

Oxidative stress has been found to occur in various viral infections by enhancing viral replication [2]. The role of oxidants in viral diseases is more complex because it includes metabolic regulations for host metabolisms and viral replication. A number of different additional host mechanisms have been shown or are suspected to contribute to the pathogenesis of viral infections, including excessive cytokine, lipid peroxidation, lipid mediator release, and compliment activation [9]. The role of oxidative stress in disease progression has been shown to be more complicated in HIV-infected individuals receiving HAART compared with those who remain untreated [10].

There is clear evidence that oxidative stress may contribute to several aspects of HIV disease, including viral replication, inflammatory response, and decreased immune cell proliferation [5]. An increase in oxidative stress may also play an important role in the genesis of cellular DNA damage, resulting in HIV-associated malignancies and disease progression [11].

HIV-1 uses glycoprotein (gp120) to enter host cells (T cells and monocytes), and it is described that gp120 increases oxidative stress through GSH and lipid peroxidation [12,13]. It is important because infected monocytes can cross the blood–brain barrier (BBB) and finally replicate in astrocytes and microglia [14]. In addition, it has been shown that HIV-1 induces ROS production (oxidative stress) in astrocytes and microglia [12,15], and that gp120 can directly induce apoptosis in neurons [16]. Oxidative stress is involved in the pathology of HIV-associated neurocognitive disorders [17].

Most virus-induced ROS generation is linked to the activation of different signaling molecules and transcription factors such as NF-kB, STAT (STAT1, STAT3), and JAK (JAK2) [2]. The nuclear transcription factor NF-kB, which is necessary for viral replication, is activated when oxidative stress is present. The other role of NF-kB is to activate many of the immune system's inflammatory cytokines. When the TNF-alpha pathway is activated, it can also suppress the apoptosis process inside the cell using different signaling pathways, which in turn stimulates the expression of antiapoptotic genes such as IAP, BCL-2, and BCL-XL and TNFR-associated factors that do not allow the activation of caspase family proteins. The NF-kB signaling pathway has been proven to be important in cell death studies. Although a P53-mediated cell death requires the activation of the NF-kB signaling pathway, the activation of NF-kB by P53 is quite different because it requires MEKi (MEK inhibitor) and pp90rsk [18]. Research performed on the Epstein Bar virus has shown that NF-kB plays an important role in virus-mediated cell death compared with other signaling pathways [19,20].

Mitochondria is the major source of ROS production and consequently is the major target of the ROS produced inside a cell. These ROS mostly target the mtDNA due to its lack of protective histones and its proximity to the electron transport chain, which is the main center of ATP production in mitochondria. Mitochondrial DNA encodes 13 polypeptides, 2 ribosomal RNA, and 22 tRNA. All of these by-products of mtDNA are essential components in electron transport chains for the generation of ATP via the oxidative phosphorylation process. ATP generation requires proteins from both the nuclear genome and mitochondria. Therefore, the production of ATP through the oxidative phosphorylation process in mitochondria also generates ROS that can damage the mtDNA, membrane lipid permeability, release of cytochrome C into the cytosol, and activation of the key effector protease caspase-3 via proteolytic cleavage that ultimately results in the mitochondrial-mediated apoptosis pathway [21].

In the case of mitochondrial dysfunction, when released into cytoplasm, cytochrome C interacts with the apoptotic release factor (Apaf1) to initiate apoptosis (the mitochondrial-mediated apoptosis pathway). The pro-apoptotic gene Bax from the BCL family can cause mitochondria to release cytochrome C directly [22]. Along with other members of the BCL-2 family, Bax has the ability to create ion channels on the outer membrane of mitochondria, through which cytochrome C is released easily into the cytoplasm. Although how ROS act on mitochondria to release cytochrome C remains unknown, the ROS could cause membrane protein loss [22,23], which can allow pore formation and the release of cytochrome C into cytoplasm, activating the cell death mechanism [2].

It is currently believed that the oxidation of proteins in ER, which is associated with protein folding, is responsible for the generation of ROS that cause oxidative stress. ER is mainly responsible for protein folding and assembly. It also acts as a primary storage house of calcium, which is required for the proper folding of proteins [24]. Any change in the normal function of ER results in the accumulation of misfolded and unfolded proteins, and changes in calcium homeostasis cause ER stress that finally leads to apoptosis [25]. This oxidative stress results in the leakage of calcium from ER lumen into cytoplasm [26]. Therefore, increasing calcium concentration in the cytoplasm causes calcium entry into mitochondria and nuclei [25]. In mitochondria, calcium causes the activation of mitochondrial metabolism that can switch from a physiological beneficial process to a cell death signal, whereas in nuclei calcium modulates gene transcription and nucleases that control cell death. Moreover, it had experimentally shown that increased levels of calcium in the cytoplasm are not necessarily toxic if the calcium uptake by mitochondria is inhibited. Therefore, this indicates that mitochondria are important targets for switching normal calcium signaling to signals for cell death during severe oxidative stress [2].

The imbalances of calcium inside and outside the cell cause the cell to undergo a programmed death. AIDS, which is characterized by a decrease in the CD4 lymphocytes, is currently believed to be the main culprit of this apoptosis. The imbalance in the ROS seems to contribute to the progression of AIDS in different ways, including the apoptosis of CD4 cells and the functioning of other immune system components [2].

Apoptosis, the process of programmed cell death, involves a sequence of events that lead to various morphological changes in a cell, including cell shrinkage, changes to the cell membrane such as the loss of membrane asymmetry and attachment, nuclear fragmentation, chromatin condensation, and genomic DNA fragmentation. Apoptosis has a key role in the pathogenesis of many diseases, including cancer, inflammation, and neurodegenerative diseases. The process of programmed cell death is controlled by different ranges of cell signaling pathways originating either the external from surroundings of a cell (extrinsic inducers) or from within the cell itself (intrinsic inducers). Extrinsic inducers include heat, radiations, toxins [27], nitric oxide [28], and hormones. They must either pass into the cell or interact with the specific receptors present on the cell membrane to initiate the specific signal transduction pathway inside. This action leads the cell to undergo apoptosis. Thus, any external or internal disturbance in the signal transduction pathways within a cell, such as heat, radiation, viral infection, lack of nutrients, or an increase in calcium concentration, leads the cell to undergo continuous proliferation or necrosis [2].

CTLs and NK cells can eradicate virus-infected target cells via the apoptosis process through the perforin/granzyme pathway. Three different families of pattern recognition receptors, toll-like (TLRs), nod-like (NLRRs), and retinoid acid-inducible gene I (RIG-I)-like, initiate innate immunity to the inborn host response to common pathogens such as viruses, bacteria, and fungi. These receptors recognize and bind pathogen-associated molecular patterns (PAMPs), such as viral DNA and RNA, or bacterial and fungal cell wall components. PAMP-receptor binding activates the innate immune response, initiates downstream signaling, and induces expression of inflammatory cytokines as well as the type I interferon response. The innate immune system attracts immune cells to the site of infection and activates the adaptive immune response. Dysregulation of innate immune processes can lead to widespread infection, sepsis, and immune deficiencies.

Another important apoptosis-related host defense mechanism involves CTL and recognizes and kills target cells by sending signals through cell surface death receptors. Death receptors are a special type of receptor belonging to the tumor necrosis family. They contain specific homologous amino acid sequences in their cytoplasmic tails, referred to as the death domain (DD). The most well-studied death receptors include CD95/FAS and TNFRI, although additional death receptors such as DR3, DR4, and DR5 have been examined. In addition to killing virus-infected cells, death receptors aid in killing mature T cells at the end of immune responses [2].

In the case of FAS-mediated apoptosis, the interaction between the receptor and legend needs the help of adaptor proteins to signal the target cell to undergo the apoptosis process. The interaction between the two cells results in a clustering of intracellular DDs on the target cell. However, to be effective, this activates the FADD adaptor protein within the target cell. In addition to interacting with the receptor, the FADD also contains a caspase-recruiting domain (CARD) that is responsible for activating the caspases (caspase-8). On oligomerization, the caspase-8 activates itself and the cascade of caspases (caspase-3) to begin the apoptosis process. TNFR1-type and DR3-type death receptors require FADD in addition to the TNFR-associated DD (TRADD) adaptor protein. TNFR1-mediated and DR3-mediated cell deaths rarely occur unless protein synthesis is inhibited.

Different kinds of cellular components may help regulate apoptosis; until now, more than 139,000 research articles have been published in relation to the molecules involved in the activation of intrinsic and extrinsic apoptotic pathways such as BCL-2, TNF, NF-kB, and p53 [27]. Caspases are the 30- to 60-kD apo enzymes inside cells. They are made continuously and activated by proteolytic processing either autocatalytically or in a cascade by enzymes with similar characteristics [29]. This indicates that the apoptosis process is highly conserved.

In the case of cell injury where the injured cell swells and bursts, the cells leak their contents out and attract different immune cells such as local and blood-borne phagocytes by engaging in an unwanted inflammatory response [30]. The respiratory burst is accompanied by increased resting oxygen consumption for the ROS production. Nearby phagocytes are prevented from engulfing the dead cell, which in turn results in the formation of dead tissue.

AIDS is the terminal phase of HIV infection and is reported to be associated with excessive production of ROS (termed as oxidants) causing oxidative stress, which may augment further the rate of viral replication in an individual. The presence of oxidative stress challenges the cellular systems. Their responses may create conditions that are favorable for the replication of not only HIV but also different types of other viruses [5]. Oxidative stress always plays a dominant pathogenic role in HIV. Reactive intermediates such as peroxide and free radicals can be very damaging to many parts of cells such as proteins, lipids, and DNA. Severe oxidative stress via RNA virus infections can contribute to several aspects of viral disease pathogenesis, including apoptosis, loss of immune function, viral replication, organelle function, inflammatory response, and loss of body weight.

15.1.4 HIV Antioxidant Defenses

Oxidative stress is a critical mechanism in the progression of AIDS. It has been observed that perturbations in antioxidant defense systems and, consequently, redox imbalance are present in many tissues of HIV-infected patients [5].

The cellular defense response to oxidative stress includes induction of detoxifying enzymes and antioxidant enzymes. The transcription of these genes is stimulated by the binding of the nuclear factor erythroid 2–related factor (Nrf2) to the antioxidant response elements (ARE) within the promoter of these (enzyme) genes. Inactive Nrf2 is retained in the cytoplasm by association with an actin-binding protein, Keap1. On exposure of cells to oxidative stress, Nrf2 is phosphorylated in response to the protein kinase C, phosphatidylinositol 3-kinase, and MAP kinase pathways. After phosphorylation, Nrf2 translocates to the nucleus, binds AREs, and transactivates detoxifying enzymes (GSH *S*-transferase, cytochrome P450) and antioxidant enzymes (SOD, GPx, NAD(P)H quinone oxidoreductase, heme oxygenase).

The virus and lymphocytes use hydrogen peroxide (H_2O_2) to signal their survival and function. H_2O_2 is generated near the cell membrane, where lymphocytes establish contact with mitogens, viruses, and other activation agents [31]. The generated H_2O_2 is rapidly inactivated by local peroxidases, mostly by GPx, resulting in oxidized GSH (GSSG), which is converted back to reduced GSH by the enzyme GSH reductase (GR) to maintain the reduced intracellular status [32].

The ROS produced during the normal metabolic process vanish in the body's antioxidant pools such as catalases, GPx, and SOD. Patients suffering from HIV infection have exhibited decreased SOD levels and activity. Antioxidant enzyme catalase activity increases as AIDS progresses in HIV-infected patients. The level of GPx in RBCs and plasma also decreases. This clearly shows that the body's antioxidant system becomes weaker as HIV progresses.

15.2 GLUTATHIONE

GSH is a major component involved in the control and maintenance of cellular redox state and cellular homeostasis. GSH is also important in an array of cellular functions such as protein synthesis, transport across membranes, receptor action, and cell growth. GSH also plays an important role [33] in activating vitamin C and vitamin E. It scavenges singlet oxygen and hydroxyl radicals, detoxifies hydrogen, and lipid peroxide, and is a cofactor in several detoxifying enzymes [2].

Consider the case of GSH, which acts as a redox buffer inside a cell [33]. GSSG represents the oxidized form of GSH inside a cell. Therefore, measuring the ratio of GSH to GSSG can provide a good indication of the oxidative stress [34,35].

GSH is found in almost every cell compartment, including the cytosol. When a cell is treated with GSH, it is readily taken by the mitochondria against the concentration gradient. Mitochondria are the major source of ROS production inside a cell, and its most important component of antioxidant defense is the GSH (reduced GSH). Although there is no proof that GSH biosynthesis occurs inside mitochondria, these organelles have their own distinct GSH polls [23].

Utilization of molecular oxygen during oxidative catabolism of biomolecules in mitochondria generates ROS, which are reduced to hydrogen peroxide. It is converted into water and oxygen by GPx (selenium-dependent) or catalase. This oxygen helps oxidize two molecules of reduced GSH to one molecule of oxidized glutathione (GSSG). The GSSG is further reduced to two molecules of GSH by catalytic action of (vitamin B2–dependent) GR using NADPH + H, which in turn gets converted into NADP. The HIV-1 infection or application of anti-HIV-1 regimen by HIV-1–infected patients may negatively influence the levels and functions of these three key antioxidative enzymes [5].

The GSH inside the nucleus helps maintain the redox of sulfhydryl proteins, which are important for repair and expression. The reversible thiolation of proteins is known to regulate several metabolic processes, including enzyme activity, signal transduction, and gene expression through redox-sensitive nuclear transcription factors such as AP-1, NF-kB, and p53 protein [36]. These proteins are related either to the cell inflammatory (AP-1 and NF-kB) or genome (p53) responses to aggression or to the virus survival. In fact, DNA-binding activity of transcription factors often involves critical cysteine (Cys) residues, and the maintenance of these residues in a reduced form, at least in the nuclear compartment, is necessary. AP-1 is a transcription factor whose DNA-binding activity can be diminished if Cys-252 is oxidized similarly to p53, which contains 12 Cys residues in its amino acid sequence, and oxidation of some of these inhibits p53 function [37].

The molecular mechanism of how GSH modulates cell proliferation remains largely speculative. A key mechanism for the role of GSH in DNA synthesis relates to the maintenance of reduced glutaredoxin or thioredoxin, which is required for the activity of ribonucleotide reductase, the rate-limiting enzyme in DNA synthesis [37].

As a natural antioxidant, GSH scavenges peroxide species and its deficiency leads to the generation of enormous levels of oxidative stress that damage and kill otherwise healthy cells [38]. The decreased levels of GSH cause reduction in the number and activities of macrophages, CD4, CD8, and CTLs. Low levels of GSH have been shown to play a role in the apoptosis of $CD4^+$ T cells, which is the major pathology of the HIV infection, therefore signifying the importance of GSH [39].

The presence of sufficient concentrations of cellular GSH protects cells from any bacterial, viral, and fungal infections. The infection is subsequently flushed out from the system by normal means, which reduces viral load. GSH may cause intervention at different steps of HIV-1 replication and inhibits the expression of p24 antigenic proteins of HIV-1 required to form the viral coat [5].

15.2.1 GSH Deficiency in HIV Patients

AIDS-associated deficiency of GSH may be to efflux of GSH disulfide from cells due to viral infection. Tat protein produced by HIV-1 significantly decreases GSH levels, which are associated with free-radical injury to immune system components such as T-helper lymphocytes cells [5].

The lack of specific trace elements in diets such as minerals and vitamins adversely influences the redox status of the body. For example, low selenium intake reduces production of selenoproteins and GSH. In addition, malnutrition has been shown to be associated with the acceleration in production of ROS in HIV-1–infected individuals. The extent of adverse effects of ROS induced by anti-HIV-1 compounds may be mitigated by application of different vitamins (A, E, C), proper nutrition (proteins), antioxidants (Cys, GSH), and whey protein, which is able to supply precursors for the synthesis of GSH to people living with HIV/AIDS [5].

The Kupfer cells, liver macrophages attached to the endothelium, are normally involved in phagocytosis of pathogens and degradation of antigens. The anti-HIV-1 drugs adversely influence the liver function and immunity of the body by producing free radicals. The level of the antioxidant system of the liver including the GSH biochemical pathways involved in xenobiotic metabolism is also depleted. It is reported that the reduction in GSH level less than 80% due to acute oxidative stress in cells may lead to the death of cells [5].

Compromised levels of GSH in HIV-infected individuals are due to decreased levels of GSH-synthetic enzymes, as demonstrated by Morris et al. [39], who analyzed the levels of enzymes responsible for the synthesis of GSH such as GSH synthase (GS), glutamate–cysteine ligase-catalytic subunit (GCLC), and GR and showed they were significantly reduced in the red blood cells isolated from individuals with HIV infection. Additionally, it was shown that this reduction correlated with the decreased levels of intracellular GSH. Furthermore, the same group had shown that the GSH levels in plasma and peripheral blood mononuclear cells of HIV-positive individuals were also compromised [40,41].

HIV-positive individuals have increased levels of TGF-beta in their plasma and macrophage supernatants, and TGF-beta is known to block the production of GCLC, which leads to decreased GSH synthesis [40]. In addition, HIV-1 Tat increases free-radical production and also decreases the amount of GSH through the modulation of its biosynthetic enzymes [42]. Therefore, marked increases in oxidative stress along with increased levels of TGF-beta lead to the compromised levels of GSH synthesis enzymes [39].

Nrf2 regulates the expression of antioxidant and phase II–metabolizing enzymes by activating ARE, thereby protecting cells and tissues from oxidative stress. Nrf2 gene binding to ARE results in the upregulation of GSH synthesis enzymes such as GCLC, GCLM, and GR [39].

15.3 NUTRITION INTERVENTIONS IN ANTIOXIDANTS

A decrease in antioxidants indicates the weakening of the immune system, because immune cells require more antioxidants to maintain their function and integrity [2]. In fact, low plasma or serum levels of vitamins A, E, B6, B12, and C; carotenoids; selenium; and zinc are common in many HIV-infected populations. They all have some antioxidant hole in the host. Therefore, this may contribute to the pathogenesis of the HIV infection via increased oxidative stress and compromised immunity. The levels of GSH, Cys, vitamin C, and SOD are also decreased, and the oxidative products, malonyldialdehyde, and hydroxynonenal levels are elevated in patients infected with HIV-1 [2].

Malnutrition impairs not only the optimal cellular functions but also the body's immune system by inducing a significant decrease in the count of macrophages and lymphocytes, particularly the NK cells [5]. Consequently, undernourishment and micronutrient deficiencies significantly contribute to augment oxidative stress, immunosuppression, and acceleration of HIV-1 replication and depletion of CD4 T-cell count in HIV-1 infected individuals. Deficiencies of micronutrients are more pronounced in HIV-1–positive subjects with CD4 counts less than 200 cell/μL. Hence, serum levels of micronutrients decrease sharply because of HIV-1 infection or because of increase in the severity of the viral infection [43].

The $CD4^+$ T-helper cells that form important components of the immune system are the main targets of the HIV virus. The virus production decreases because approximately 5% of the T cells are destroyed and replaced each day via the apoptotic process. This, in turn, leads to decreases in zinc and vitamin E (antioxidants). The decrease in zinc results in the inhibition of intracellular virus replication [26], and the selenium decrease indicates the progression of HIV toward AIDS [2].

HIV-2 infection is slow compared with HIV-1 infection [2]. These viruses have the highest mutation rates among every living creature [3,4]. The anti-HIV-1 regimen comprising mainly two viral enzymes such as reverse-transcriptase and protease as viable targets helps AIDS patients to live longer, but their chemotherapy fails mainly because of the emergence of drug-resistant mutants under selection pressure of these compounds and partly because of their side effects. The toxicity induced by the anti-HIV-1 regimen includes the potential to produce ROS, which cause damage to different organs of the patients.

Studying the oxidative stress in HIV-infected patients has opened new doors for cellular ROS researchers to use antioxidants as novel drugs to decrease HIV-1 pathogenesis in humans. Nutrition makes the most significant contribution to the body's antioxidant defense system. It is widely believed that diet-derived antioxidants play a role in the prevention of human diseases. These antioxidants work in a coordinated manner, where a deficiency in one may affect the efficiency of another [2].

15.3.1 Increasing GSH Production

Patients with HIV infection present low GSH. On infusion of GSH at a constant rate, the increment in plasma GSH was significantly larger in the HIV-infected patients than controls. The input of GSH into the circulation and the clearance were significantly lower in patients with HIV infection. During infusion of GSH, the concentration of Cys in peripheral blood mononuclear cells of the HIV-infected patients increased significantly. Nevertheless, intracellular GSH did not increase. Thus, the consumption of GSH is not increased in HIV infection; rather, it is suggested that GSH in patients is low because of a decreased systemic synthesis of GSH [44].

Cell GSH levels can be controlled either by its synthesis or by its removal. GSH biosynthesis can be controlled either by its enzymes or by its constituent amino acids. GSH is synthesized in the cell by the sequential actions of gamma-glutamylcysteine synthase (GCS), GS, GCLC, and GR in a series of six-enzyme-catalyzed reactions [45]. The Nrf2 regulates the expression of antioxidant metabolizing enzymes by activating ARE and thereby protects cells and tissues from oxidative stress. Nrf2 gene binding to ARE results in the upregulation of GSH synthesis enzymes such as GCLC, GCLM, and GR [39]. New findings argue that HIV-1–related proteins downregulate Nrf2 expression and/or activity within the alveolar epithelium, which in turn impairs antioxidant defenses and barrier function. Furthermore, it is suggested that activating the Nrf2/ARE pathway with the dietary supplement sulforaphane could increase antioxidant defenses and lung health in HIV-1–infected individuals [46]. Under normal physiological conditions, the rate of GSH synthesis is largely determined by GCL activity and Cys availability. Cys is normally derived from diet (protein breakdown and in liver) from Met via trans-sulfuration (conversion of Hcy to Cys) [47].

In vivo studies have shown that when healthy adults are fed diets either deficient in sulfur amino acids or containing reduced amounts of total protein, GSH turnover is suppressed. Moreover, the flux of nonessential amino acids, such as glutamate, Cys, and glycine, consists of its release from protein breakdown and from *de novo* synthesis. Thus, it seems that GSH deficiency is, in large part, due to decreased synthesis secondary to a decreased supply of the precursor amino acids [48,49].

Under normal physiological conditions, the rate of sulfur-containing amino acids plays a role in determining the flux of Cys and GSH synthesis. In stressed and inflammatory states, sulfur amino acids metabolism adapts to meet the increased requirements for Cys as a rate-limiting substrate for GSH. Therefore, Cys is now widely recognized as a conditionally essential (or indispensible) sulfur amino acid. It plays a key role in the metabolic pathways involving Met, Tau, and GSH, and it may help fight chronic inflammation by boosting antioxidant status [50]. Storage of Cys is another important function of GSH because Cys is extremely unstable extracellularly and rapidly auto-oxidizes to cystine in a process that produces potentially toxic oxygen-free radicals [37].

Plasma GSH arises largely from the liver. Intracellularly, the majority of GSH is found in the cytosol (90%), whereas mitochondria contains nearly 10% and the ER contains a very small percentage [47]. The content of GSH in mammalian cells is dynamically maintained by the gamma-glutamyl cycle, using GSH as a substrate for transpeptidases. Tissues that present low transpeptidase activity (e.g., liver, pancreas, and muscle) export GSH through the blood to cells that have high transpeptidase activity, such as kidney [51]. GS(SG)H is effluxed by cells through gamma glutamyl–mediated metabolism, allowing a "GSH-cycle" to take place. In normal conditions, the GSH predominates over the GSSG form, with the ratio GSH/GSSG exceeding 100 in a normal resting cell. The ratio decreases to values between 10 and 1 in oxidative stress [52]. In extreme conditions of oxidative stress, the ability of the cell to reduce GSSG to GSH may be less, inducing the accumulation of GSSG within the cytosol. To avoid a shift in the redox equilibrium, the GSSG can be actively transported out of the cell or react with protein sulfydryl groups and form mixed disulfides [37].

The gamma glutamyl cycle allows GSH to be the main source of Cys. In this cycle, GSH is released from the cell and the ecto-enzyme gamma glutamyl transfers the gamma glutamyl moiety of GSH to an amino acid (the best acceptor being Cys), forming gamma glutamyl amino acid and cysteinyl glycine [53]. Cysteinyl glycine is broken-down by dipeptidase to generate Cys and Gly. Once inside the cell, the majority of Cys is incorporated into GSH, with some being incorporated into protein and some degraded into sulfate and Tau. The gamma glutamyl amino acid (glutamine [Gln]) can be transported back into the cell and, once inside, can be converted to Glu and used for GSH synthesis [37].

Cys can be endogenously synthesized from the Met-transmethylation/trans-sulfuration pathway. In fact, the GSH synthesis pathway is one of the five major biochemical pathways of the methionine metabolism. GSH synthesis is preceded by transmethylation/remethylation pathway (through folate/B12-dependent reactions) and trans-sulfuration pathway (through vitamin B6–dependent reactions). Hcy is formed from transmethylation of Met to *S*-adenosyl-methionine (SAM), and Hcy is mostly remethylated to Met and minorly trans-sulfurated to Cys, which can be further incorporated to protein or GSH or metabolized to Tau [54].

The trans-sulfuration pathway is sensitive to pro-oxidants and antioxidants, which enhance or diminish Hcy flux [55]. However, trans-sulfuration pathway provides the amount of Cys required to synthesize the cellular redox-controlling molecules like GSH and Tau, which protect the molecular constituents of cells against RS-induced damage [54].

In the presence of high Cys levels, cystathionine is directed into the GSH and Tau synthesis pathways. Thus, Cys levels are considered the limited step in liver GSH synthesis (major source of plasma GSH). Approximately half of the Cys used for GSH anabolism is derived from Met that was synthesized from the trans-sulfuration pathway. However, half of the circulating Cys is derived from GSH breakdown [54].

15.3.2 Interventions with Exogenous Amino Acids

Among the agents tested are lipoic acid, cysteamine, and 2-oxothiazolidine 4-carboxylate, but improving Cys availability is the most extensively studied approach for enhancing the cell GSH pool. There are some known natural as well as synthetic compounds such as *N*-acetyl cysteine (NAC) that act as safe antidotes against free-radical species. For example, NAC may act as an antidote for Cys/GSH deficiency as well as for four major interdependent redox couples, GSH/GSSG, NADPH/NADP, NADH/NAD, and reduced thioredoxin (TRX(SH)2/oxidized thioredoxin (TRX(S-S), and then interact to regulate the redox environment in the cellular milieu [5].

Oral L-glutamine also increases plasma GSH in healthy subjects and patients [51,56–58]. Gln is the preferential substrate of rapidly dividing cells such as enterocytes and immune cells; therefore, its supplying is associated with less infectious complications in critically ill patients [59].

15.3.2.1 Methodological Design

As published elsewhere [56], a randomized controlled supplementation study was conducted in an HIV-positive group composed of 12 patients (6 men and 6 women; 22–45 years old) who had been diagnosed clinically and in the laboratory by viral load and CD4þ and CD8þ lymphocyte counts. All patients had been undergoing highly active antiretroviral treatment for at least 1 year, receiving one HIV protease inhibitor (PI) (indinavir 800 mg twice daily, $n = 10$; or ritonavir 600 mg twice daily, $n = 11$) in combination with two nucleoside analogs (zidovudine 250 mg plus lamivudine 150 mg twice daily, $n = 11$; or lamivudine 150 mg plus stavudine 40 mg twice daily, $n = 1$). The exclusion criteria were the presence of any renal or liver failure and the ingestion of GSH precursors or any form of vitamin B. The healthy control group consisted of 20 adults (10 men and 10 women; 20–59 years old) who were negative for HIV and clinically healthy. At baseline, all selected subjects underwent an anthropometric assessment and had fasting blood drawn to analyze markers for glomerular filtration (creatinine and urea) and hepatocyte injury marker (gamma-glutamyl transpeptidase), nutritional variables (albumin, calcium, folate, and vitamin B12), glucose, lipids (triacylglycerols and cholesterol fractions), uric acid, folate, and vitamin B12. After a baseline assessment, the two groups were randomly assigned to different dietary supplements (NAC 1g/day or Gln 20g/day) with their usual diet as the baseline and washout in a crossover design. All dietary supplements were administered throughout the consecutive 7-day period, preceded and followed by fasting blood sampling for the amino acids and GSH quantifications [56].

15.3.2.2 NAC Results

The GSH and free amino acids were used as metabolic markers, either isolated or assembled to designate thiol-antioxidant capacity (GSH:GSSG ratio) [60], remethylation of Hcy (Met:Hcy ratio) [61], or trans-sulfuration of Hcy (Hcy:Cys ratio) all in situations of either usual diet (Do) or NAC-supplemented diet under fasting [54].

The HIV-positive group presented lower levels of amino acids (Met, Hcy, and Cys), similar remethylation (Met:Hcy ratio), and lower trans-sulfuration (Hcy:Cys ratio) in association with lower GSH concentrations and lower antioxidant capacity (GSH:GSSG ratio) than controls. Even though the GSH was increased, the antioxidant capacity continued to be below that of controls [54].

The prevalence of HHcy in HIV-positive patients has been reported to be between 12.3% and 35% [62]. In the study, the prevalence (>10 μmol/L) was 65% in controls and 50% in HIV-positive patients. High levels of Hcy have been correlated with nutritional deficiency, antiretroviral therapies, and the presence of HIV-positive comorbidities [62–64].

The main removal of synthesized Hcy is by Met synthase converting 5-methylene tetrahydrofolate (the methyl donor) to tetrahydrofolate in a folate/vitamin B12–dependent reaction. In our data, the HIV-positive group showed lower folate and similar vitamin B12 levels than non-HIV-positive controls [56]. The study showed the Met:Hcy ratio (remethylation marker) with similar results between groups in both diets without (2.56 × 2.06) or with (2.29 × 2.11) NAC supplementation. Therefore, it seems that the clearance of Hcy in this case was normal by the remethylation pathway, even considering the lower plasma folate state [54].

However, when compared with the usual diet, the presence of NAC resulted in Hcy 3.11 increased higher in HIV-positive patients than in the healthy control group [65]. In healthy humans, a spared effect of dietary Cys on Met oxidation [66] has been described that, in the present case, would overcharge the already compromised remethylation clearance of

Hcy. In this study, the NAC supplementation normalized not only Met but also Hcy and GSH in association with normal remethylation and reduced trans-sulfuration. Despite normalized GSH, the antioxidant capacity continued to be lower than that of controls [54].

Muller et al. [67] found lower Met concentrations in HIV-positive patients than in control individuals, as we did. The Met metabolism-derived polyamines (putrescine, spermine, and spermidine) present in all living cells have been implicated in the replication of some viruses, and elevated levels of these polyamines have been found in lymphocytes of patients infected with HIV-1. Nevertheless, the effect of HIV infection on polyamine pools in cell culture was not significant [68]. In our study, the HIV-positive plasma levels of Met were comparable with that of the non-HIV-positive group only in the presence of NAC supplementation [54].

Half of the cell Cys is provided by the trans-sulfuration pathway; another half comes from GSH breakdown [69]. The increase of Hcy:Cys ratio (*de novo* Cys synthesis index) higher than that of controls in both diets, that is, absence (0.04×0.08) and presence (0.03×0.05) of NAC, suggested higher flux of Hcy through the trans-sulfuration pathway in HIV-positive patients, resulting in normal GSH values under NAC supplementation. These occurred despite not achieving normal (control) values for Cys [54].

Our patients were on stable HAART for more than 1 year, and these treatments have been associated with significantly higher plasma Hcy fasting levels in HIV-positive children [61] and also in fasting adults after 6 months of ART [70]. Surprisingly, no significant association was found between Hcy levels and the use of ART by Guaraldi et al. [64]. Additionally, plasma Hcy was not associated with HIV serostatus or use of ART in a cross-sectional study that found 16.9% of HHcy (>10 μmol/L) in HIV-infected individuals ($n = 249$) and 13.4% of HHcy in noninfected ($n = 127$) individuals [71]. In the study, the prevalence was 50% and 65%, respectively [54].

By refining the cutoff for males (>15 μmol/L) and females (>13 μmol/L), Uccelli et al. [72] found a prevalence of 28.6% in a sample of 98 HIV-positive patients. However, no significant correlations were observed between HHcy and length of exposure to HAART. In two articles [71,72], the reduced availability of folate was raised as a confounding factor in the association between HHcy and ART. In fact, before the advent of HAART, 20% and 10% of HIV-infected patients had low vitamin B12 and red blood cell folate concentrations, respectively; now, the prevalence of low vitamin B12 is significantly lower in patients receiving HAART (8.7% versus 27%); 22.5% with low vitamin B12 and 51.4% with low folate had HHcy (>17.5 μmol/L). In that case, treatment with folic acid and vitamin B12 normalized HHcy [73]. The Hcy levels in blood are a sensitive indicator of folate and vitamin B12 deficiencies, and plasma HCy can be lowered with B vitamin supplementation [74].

HIV-positive comorbidities also have been associated with high HCy. In a cross-sectional study, Roca et al. [63] found 37% of HIV-positive individuals with HHcy, and the increased levels were associated with the presence of coinfections such as hepatitis C virus.

Patients on PI treatment showed significantly higher plasma Hcy and lower Met:Hcy ratios compared with patients using other ART [61]. This publication contrasted with another published previously [75] that denied differences in the levels of Hcy (Hcy >15 μmol/L; HIV-positive: 16.4% and HIV-negative: 12.9%) regardless of the presence of HIV, AIDS, or the use of ART. However, Hcy was significantly higher in patients with metabolic syndrome and lipodystrophy [64], pointing out the pivotal role of hyper-adiposity as a comorbidity of the HIV treatment. Hcy has been correlated with values of blood pressure, waist circumference, waist/hip ratio, visceral adipose tissue, total lean body mass, HDL cholesterol, triglycerides, apolipoproteins A1 and B, HOMA-IR, and creatinine [64].

Lipodystrophy is more related to PIs than ART. High peroxide levels were found in patients receiving PI regimens [76], and higher lipid and protein oxidation were found in HIV-positive individuals with lipodystrophy syndrome [77]. In human adipocytes, PIs and ART (except ampenavir, atazanavir, and abacavir) increased ROS production, monocyte chemoattractant protein (MCP-1), and IL-6 release [78]. Hcy accumulation and synthesis of pro-inflammatory molecules by macrophages are common findings of the trans-sulfuration deficiencies leading to lower cystathionase beta-synthase activity, elevated Hcy levels, and associated elevated risk of blood clots and atherosclerosis [79]. In endothelial cells, chronic HAART exposure increased oxidative stress and induced mononuclear cell recruitment. HAART has been associated with significant side effects such as diabetes, atherosclerosis, and cardiovascular complications [80].

15.3.2.3 *Gln Results*

The HIV-positive patients were matched with healthy controls by age, BMI, and plasma concentrations of albumin and vitamin B12. Their plasma levels of folate and all but Hcy amino acids and GSH levels were lower than those of controls [56]. After 1 week of Gln supplementation, the HIV-positive group had increased GSH (71.4%) and its precursor amino acids Gly (27.2%), Glu (13.7%), and Cys (10.8%). However, only Met, Hcy, Gly, and GSH reached the levels of the controls [51].

The plasma concentration of Glu after Gln supplementation increased 3.4% in controls and decreased 1.0% in HIV-positive patients. Ser also decreased (25.1% more than controls), whereas Gly (21.8%), Tau (14.4%), and GSH (47.9%) increased higher than that of controls. Therefore, after Gln supplementation both groups presented similar plasma ratio for Tau/Cys, suggesting low influence on the Cys–Tau pathway. However, the HIV-positive group presented a higher ratio of Gly/Glu and lower ratios of Ser/Gly and Ser/Cys, clearly showing the effects of Gln prioritizing Gly formation rather than Ser and Glu [51].

The increased concentration of GSH found after Gln supplement is the result of the increased source of its precursors either by higher protein catabolism or by increased *de novo* synthesis. The higher protein breakdown could be excluded because it has been described that Gln administration promotes an increase in lean body mass even in HIV infection [57]. Instead, the increased *de novo* synthesis could be why Gly increased 21.8% after Gln supplementation. However, decreased *de novo* synthesis would be the case for Glu and Ser. Glu is formed from deamination of Gln (by glutaminase) and further deaminated to α-ketoglutarate (2-oxoglutarate) by glutamate dehydrogenase [51]. Gln supplementation resulted in higher Gln plasma levels in the controls (18.7%) and the HIV-positive (19.6%) group. However, this similarity was not seen for the Glu levels found, which were 60% for controls and only 13.7% for the patients. Thus, the HIV-positive group showed a lack of response of plasma Glu to the Gln supplementation. Besides fueling the Krebs cycle (with α-ketoglutarate), Glu also participates in biosynthetic processes of other amino acids such as Orn (and Arg), Pro, Gln, and Ser. Ser is the main precursor of Gly, another GSH component. Actually, among the GSH precursors Gly was the only amino acid achieving the control values after the Gln supplementation [51].

In the Gly–Ser cycle and GSH pathway, the major contribution to whole-body Gly flux is the whole-body protein breakdown [81]. Pathways utilizing Gly are serine, GSH, protein synthesis, and gluconeogenesis [82].

Gly and Ser are interchangeable through mitochondrial and cytosolic serine hydroxymethyltransferase (SHMT). These reactions account for approximately 41% of whole-body Gly flux [83]. The mitochondrial glycine clearance system (GCS) accounts for 22% of the whole-body Gly flux [84]. The GCS cleaves Gly to CO_2, ammonia, and a 1-carbon unit in the methylene state reacting with folate as 5,10-methylenetetrahydrofolate. SHMT reversibly transfers a 1-carbon group from 5,10-methylenetetrahydrofolate to Gly forming tetrahydrofolate and Ser. The rate of Ser synthesis is as high as the rate of Gly cleavage [83]. The incorporation of GCS-derived 1-carbon units enters serine synthesis, but the other 40% enters other aspects of 1-carbon metabolism, including nucleoside synthesis, homocysteine remethylation, and *S*-adenosyl methionine-dependent methylation reactions [84]. Gly is the major substrate in Ser synthesis and Ser is the major 1-carbon source for homocysteine remethylation [85]. However, it is considered that GCS produces 1-carbon units as 5,10-methylenetetrahydrofolate at a higher rate (~20 times) that needed for Hcy remethylation (to Met) and, thus, for methylation demand [82]. Thus, nearly all GCS-derived 1-carbon units are consumed in Ser synthesis, whereas a much smaller percentage enters all other reactions of 1-carbon metabolism [86].

In the study, the plasma concentrations of Met and Hcy were similar in both groups under both diets, which means preserved transmethylation/remethylation reactions. Interestingly, the remethylation reaction of Hcy to Met is folate-dependent [85] and its plasma level was found to be lower in the HIV-positive group than in the control group [56].

Besides remethylation reaction (folate/vitamin B12–dependent) to Met, Hcy can be metabolized to cystathionine by trans-sulfuration reactions (vitamin B6–dependent) consuming Ser and resulting in Cys as the end product [54]. In the present study, different from Gly and Ser, Cys levels were minimally affected by the Gln supplementation of HIV-positive patients [51]. Increased Gly concentration has been described during low vitamin B6 status and slower trans-sulfuration reactions to maintain Ser synthesis [84]. This probably would not be the present case if Gln supplementation did not significantly affect Hcy and Cys levels or maintain Ser levels [51].

15.3.2.4 Conclusion

It appears that NAC supplementation led to some plasma increase of Cys, which slowed the trans-sulfuration pathway, sparing homocysteine (which increased significantly) and serine. The existing serine was then diverted from the Cys to the glycine pathway [54], which was consumed with the spared Cys (from NAC) to normalize GSH levels [51].

The Gln-induced GSH increase and its normalization were probably achieved by generating glycine (from glutamic acid) and sparing serine to form Cys (from homocysteine), with all three (glutamic acid, glycine, and Cys) together generating GSH [51,54].

Thus, the NAC and Gln, through different mechanisms, were able to supply substrates to increase GSH levels. NAC acted by sparing Hcy and Cys, whereas Gln acted by replenishing the Gly pool. Normalized GSH was unable to restore Cys or glutamic acid concentrations to the normal control level, and neither of the two supplements had significant effects on the GSSG/GSH ratio, indicating a need for an additional supplement (perhaps riboflavin) [56].

Acknowledgments

Special thanks to the Brazilian Research Funding FAPESP (financial support) and CNPq (RCB fellowship).

References

[1] Biesinger T, Kimata JT. HIV-1 transmission, replication fitness and disease progression. Virology (Auckl) 2008;2008(1):49–63.

[2] Reshi ML, Su YC, Hong JR. RNA viruses: ROS-mediated cell death. Int J Cell Biol 2014 2014:467452. http://dx.doi.org/10.1155/2014/467452.

[3] Duffy S, Shackelton LA, Holmes EC. Rates of evolutionary change in viruses: patterns and determinants. Nat Rev Genet 2008;9(4):267–76. http://dx.doi.org/10.1038/nrg2323.
[4] Garcia-Villada L, Drake JW. The three faces of riboviral spontaneous mutation: spectrum, mode of genome replication, and mutation rate. PLoS Genet 2012;8(7):e1002832. http://dx.doi.org/10.1371/journal.pgen.1002832.
[5] Sharma B. Oxidative stress in HIV patients receiving antiretroviral therapy. Curr HIV Res 2014;12(1):13–21.
[6] Devadas S, Zaritskaya L, Rhee SG, Oberley L, Williams MS. Discrete generation of superoxide and hydrogen peroxide by T cell receptor stimulation: selective regulation of mitogen-activated protein kinase activation and fas ligand expression. J Exp Med 2002;195(1):59–70.
[7] Hildeman DA. Regulation of T-cell apoptosis by reactive oxygen species. Free Radic Biol Med 2004;36(12):1496–504. http://dx.doi.org/10.1016/j.freeradbiomed.2004.03.023.
[8] Fang FC. Antimicrobial actions of reactive oxygen species. MBio 2011;2(5). http://dx.doi.org/10.1128/mBio.00141-11.
[9] Peterhans E. Oxidants and antioxidants in viral diseases: disease mechanisms and metabolic regulation. J Nutr 1997;127(Suppl. 5):962S–965SS.
[10] Sundaram M, Saghayam S, Priya B, Venkatesh KK, Balakrishnan P, Shankar EM, et al. Changes in antioxidant profile among HIV-infected individuals on generic highly active antiretroviral therapy in southern India. Int J Infect Dis 2008;12(6):e61–6. http://dx.doi.org/10.1016/j.ijid.2008.04.004.
[11] Chitapanarux T, Tienboon P, Pojchamarnwiputh S, Leelarungrayub D. Open-labeled pilot study of cysteine-rich whey protein isolate supplementation for nonalcoholic steatohepatitis patients. J Gastroenterol Hepatol 2009;24(6):1045–50. http://dx.doi.org/10.1111/j.1440-1746.2009.05865.x.
[12] Reddy PV, Gandhi N, Samikkannu T, Saiyed Z, Agudelo M, Yndart A, et al. HIV-1 gp120 induces antioxidant response element-mediated expression in primary astrocytes: role in HIV associated neurocognitive disorder. Neurochem Int 2012;61(5):807–14. http://dx.doi.org/10.1016/j.neuint.2011.06.011.
[13] Silverstein PS, Shah A, Gupte R, Liu X, Piepho RW, Kumar S, et al. Methamphetamine toxicity and its implications during HIV-1 infection. J Neurovirol 2011;17(5):401–15. http://dx.doi.org/10.1007/s13365-011-0043-4.
[14] Kaul M, Zheng J, Okamoto S, Gendelman HE, Lipton SA. HIV-1 infection and AIDS: consequences for the central nervous system. Cell Death Differ 2005;12(Suppl. 1):878–92. http://dx.doi.org/10.1038/sj.cdd.4401623.
[15] Carroll-Anzinger D, Kumar A, Adarichev V, Kashanchi F, Al-Harthi L. Human immunodeficiency virus-restricted replication in astrocytes and the ability of gamma interferon to modulate this restriction are regulated by a downstream effector of the Wnt signaling pathway. J Virol 2007;81(11):5864–71. http://dx.doi.org/10.1128/JVI.02234-06.
[16] Ronaldson PT, Bendayan R. HIV-1 viral envelope glycoprotein gp120 produces oxidative stress and regulates the functional expression of multidrug resistance protein-1 (Mrp1) in glial cells. J Neurochem 2008;106(3):1298–313. http://dx.doi.org/10.1111/j.1471-4159.2008.05479.x.
[17] Dasuri K, Zhang L, Keller JN. Oxidative stress, neurodegeneration, and the balance of protein degradation and protein synthesis. Free Radic Biol Med 2013;62:170–85. http://dx.doi.org/10.1016/j.freeradbiomed.2012.09.016.
[18] Ryan KM, Ernst MK, Rice NR, Vousden KH. Role of NF-kappaB in p53-mediated programmed cell death. Nature 2000;404(6780):892–7. http://dx.doi.org/10.1038/35009130.
[19] Feuillard J, Schuhmacher M, Kohanna S, Asso-Bonnet M, Ledeur F, Joubert-Caron R, et al. Inducible loss of NF-kappaB activity is associated with apoptosis and Bcl-2 down-regulation in Epstein–Barr virus-transformed B lymphocytes. Blood 2000;95(6):2068–75.

[20] Cahir-McFarland ED, Davidson DM, Schauer SL, Duong J, Kieff E. NF-kappa B inhibition causes spontaneous apoptosis in Epstein–Barr virus-transformed lymphoblastoid cells. Proc Natl Acad Sci USA 2000;97(11):6055–60. http://dx.doi.org/10.1073/pnas.100119497.

[21] Chrobot AM, Szaflarska-Szczepanik A, Drewa G. Antioxidant defense in children with chronic viral hepatitis B and C. Med Sci Monit 2000;6(4):713–8.

[22] Reed DJ. Mitochondrial glutathione and chemically induced stress including ethanol. Drug Metab Rev 2004;36(3–4):569–82. http://dx.doi.org/10.1081/DMR-200033449.

[23] Hengartner MO. The biochemistry of apoptosis. Nature 2000;407(6805):770–6. http://dx.doi.org/10.1038/35037710.

[24] Hong JR. Betanodavirus: mitochondrial disruption and necrotic cell death. World J Virol 2013;2(1):1–5. http://dx.doi.org/10.5501/wjv.v2.i1.1.

[25] Malhotra JD, Kaufman RJ. Endoplasmic reticulum stress and oxidative stress: a vicious cycle or a double-edged sword? Antioxid Redox Signal 2007;9(12):2277–93. http://dx.doi.org/10.1089/ars.2007.1782.

[26] Gorlach A, Klappa P, Kietzmann T. The endoplasmic reticulum: folding, calcium homeostasis, signaling, and redox control. Antioxid Redox Signal 2006;8(9–10):1391–418. http://dx.doi.org/10.1089/ars.2006.8.1391.

[27] Popov SG, Villasmil R, Bernardi J, Grene E, Cardwell J, Wu A, et al. Lethal toxin of bacillus anthracis causes apoptosis of macrophages. Biochem Biophys Res Commun 2002;293(1):349–55. http://dx.doi.org/10.1016/S0006-291X(02)00227-9.

[28] Brune B. Nitric oxide: NO apoptosis or turning it ON? Cell Death Differ 2003;10(8):864–9. http://dx.doi.org/10.1038/sj.cdd.4401261.

[29] Barber GN. Host defense, viruses and apoptosis. Cell Death Differ 2001;8(2):113–26. http://dx.doi.org/10.1038/sj.cdd.4400823.

[30] Proskuryakov SY, Konoplyannikov AG, Gabai VL. Necrosis: a specific form of programmed cell death? Exp Cell Res 2003;283(1):1–16.

[31] Pitts OM. Con a cytotoxicity: a model for the study of key signaling steps leading to lymphocyte apoptosis in AIDS? Med Hypotheses 1995;45(3):311–5.

[32] Meister A. Glutathione metabolism and its selective modification. J Biol Chem 1988;263(33):17205–17208.

[33] Masella R, Di Benedetto R, Vari R, Filesi C, Giovannini C. Novel mechanisms of natural antioxidant compounds in biological systems: involvement of glutathione and glutathione-related enzymes. J Nutr Biochem 2005;16(10):577–86. http://dx.doi.org/10.1016/j.jnutbio.2005.05.013.

[34] Nogueira CW, Zeni G, Rocha JB. Organoselenium and organotellurium compounds: toxicology and pharmacology. Chem Rev 2004;104(12):6255–85. http://dx.doi.org/10.1021/cr0406559.

[35] Jones DP, Carlson JL, Mody VC, Cai J, Lynn MJ, Sternberg P. Redox state of glutathione in human plasma. Free Radic Biol Med 2000;28(4):625–35.

[36] Townsend DM, Tew KD, Tapiero H. The importance of glutathione in human disease. Biomed Pharmacother 2003;57(3–4):145–55.

[37] Traverso N, Ricciarelli R, Nitti M, Marengo B, Furfaro AL, Pronzato MA, et al. Role of glutathione in cancer progression and chemoresistance. Oxid Med Cell Longev 2013;2013. http://dx.doi.org/10.1155/2013/972913.

[38] Bounous G. Whey protein concentrate (WPC) and glutathione modulation in cancer treatment. Anticancer Res 2000;20(6C):4785–92.

[39] Morris D, Ly J, Chi PT, Daliva J, Nguyen T, Soofer C, et al. Glutathione synthesis is compromised in erythrocytes from individuals with HIV. Front Pharmacol 2014;5:73. http://dx.doi.org/10.3389/fphar.2014.00073.

[40] Morris D, Guerra C, Donohue C, Oh H, Khurasany M, Venketaraman V. Unveiling the mechanisms for decreased glutathione in individuals with HIV infection. Clin Dev Immunol 2012;2012. http://dx.doi.org/10.1155/2012/734125.

[41] Morris D, Guerra C, Khurasany M, Guilford F, Saviola B, Huang Y, et al. Glutathione supplementation improves macrophage functions in HIV. J Interferon Cytokine Res 2013;33(5):270–9. http://dx.doi.org/10.1089/jir.2012.0103.
[42] Choi J, Liu RM, Kundu RK, Sangiorgi F, Wu W, Maxson R, et al. Molecular mechanism of decreased glutathione content in human immunodeficiency virus type 1 Tat-transgenic mice. J Biol Chem 2000;275(5):3693–8.
[43] Bilbis LS, Idowu DB, Saidu Y, Lawal M, Njoku CH. Serum levels of antioxidant vitamins and mineral elements of human immunodeficiency virus positive subjects in Sokoto, Nigeria. Ann Afr Med 2010;9(4):235–9. http://dx.doi.org/10.4103/1596-3519.70963.
[44] Helbling B, von Overbeck J, Lauterburg BH. Decreased release of glutathione into the systemic circulation of patients with HIV infection. Eur J Clin Invest 1996;26(1): 38–44.
[45] Balendiran GK, Dabur R, Fraser D. The role of glutathione in cancer. Cell Biochem Funct 2004;22(6):343–52. http://dx.doi.org/10.1002/cbf.1149.
[46] Fan X, Staitieh BS, Jensen JS, Mould KJ, Greenberg JA, Joshi PC, et al. Activating the Nrf2-mediated antioxidant response element restores barrier function in the alveolar epithelium of HIV-1 transgenic rats. Am J Physiol Lung Cell Mol Physiol 2013;305(3):L267–77. http://dx.doi.org/10.1152/ajplung.00288.2012.
[47] Lu SC. Regulation of glutathione synthesis. Mol Aspects Med 2009;30(1–2):42–59. http://dx.doi.org/10.1016/j.mam.2008.05.005.
[48] Lyons J, Rauh-Pfeiffer A, Yu YM, Lu XM, Zurakowski D, Tompkins RG, et al. Blood glutathione synthesis rates in healthy adults receiving a sulfur amino acid-free diet. Proc Natl Acad Sci USA 2000;97(10):5071–6. http://dx.doi.org/10.1073/pnas.090083297.
[49] Jackson AA, Gibson NR, Lu Y, Jahoor F. Synthesis of erythrocyte glutathione in healthy adults consuming the safe amount of dietary protein. Am J Clin Nutr 2004;80(1):101–7.
[50] Ben-Baruch A. The multifaceted roles of chemokines in malignancy. Cancer Metastasis Rev 2006;25(3):357–71. http://dx.doi.org/10.1007/s10555-006-9003-5.
[51] Burini RC, Borges-Santos MD, Moreto F, Yu YM. Plasma antioxidants and glutamine supplementation in HIV. Rajendram R, Preedy VR, Patel VB, editors. Glutamine in clinical nutrition. Springer; 2015.
[52] Abdalla MY. Glutathione as potential target for cancer therapy: more or less is good? Jordan. J Biol Sci 2011;4(3):6.
[53] Tamba M, Quintiliani M. Kinetic studies of reactions involved in hydrogen transfer from glutathione to carbohydrate radicals. Radiat Phys Chem 1984;23:5.
[54] Burini RC, Moreto F, Borges-Santos MD, Yu YM. Plasma homocysteine and thiol redox states in HIV+ patients. McCully KS, editor. Homocysteine: biosynthesis and health implications. Hauppauge, NY: Nova Science Publishers; 2013. p. 14.
[55] Zou CG, Banerjee R. Tumor necrosis factor-alpha-induced targeted proteolysis of cystathionine beta-synthase modulates redox homeostasis. J Biol Chem 2003;278(19):16802–16808. http://dx.doi.org/10.1074/jbc.M212376200 M212376200[pii].
[56] Borges-Santos MD, Moreto F, Pereira PC, Ming-Yu Y, Burini RC. Plasma glutathione of HIV(+) patients responded positively and differently to dietary supplementation with cysteine or glutamine. Nutrition 2012;28(7–8):753–6. doi:S0899-9007(11)00377-7[pii]. http://dx.doi.org/10.1016/j.nut.2011.10.014.
[57] Patrick L. Nutrients and HIV: part three—*N*-acetylcysteine, alpha-lipoic acid, L-glutamine, and L-carnitine. Altern Med Rev 2000;5(4):290–305.
[58] Valencia E, Marin A, Hardy G. Impact of oral L-glutamine on glutathione, glutamine, and glutamate blood levels in volunteers. Nutrition 2002;18(5):367–70.
[59] Dechelotte P, Hasselmann M, Cynober L, Allaouchiche B, Coeffier M, Hecketsweiler B, et al. L-alanyl-L-glutamine dipeptide-supplemented total parenteral nutrition reduces infectious complications and glucose intolerance in critically ill patients: the French controlled, randomized, double-blind, multicenter study. Crit Care Med 2006;34(3): 598–604. http://dx.doi.org/10.1097/01.CCM.0000201004.30750.D1.

[60] Fraternale A, Paoletti MF, Casabianca A, Nencioni L, Garaci E, Palamara AT, et al. GSH and analogs in antiviral therapy. Mol Aspects Med 2009;30(1–2):99–110. http://dx.doi.org/10.1016/j.mam.2008.09.001.
[61] Vilaseca MA, Sierra C, Colome C, Artuch R, Valls C, Munoz-Almagro C, et al. Hyperhomocysteinaemia and folate deficiency in human immunodeficiency virus-infected children. Eur J Clin Invest 2001;31(11):992–8.
[62] Bernasconi E, Uhr M, Magenta L, Ranno A, Telenti A. Homocysteinaemia in HIV-infected patients treated with highly active antiretroviral therapy. AIDS 2001;15(8):1081–2.
[63] Roca B, Bennasar M, Ferrero JA, del Monte MC, Resino E. Hepatitis C virus co-infection and sexual risk behaviour are associated with a high homocysteine serum level in HIV-infected patients. Swiss Med Wkly 2012;141:w13323. http://dx.doi.org/10.4414/smw.2011.13323 2011;141:w13323[pii]smw-13323[pii].
[64] Guaraldi G, Ventura P, Garlassi E, Orlando G, Squillace N, Nardini G, et al. Hyperhomocysteinaemia in HIV-infected patients: determinants of variability and correlations with predictors of cardiovascular disease. HIV Med 2009;10(1):28–34. http://dx.doi.org/10.1111/j.1468-1293.2008.00649.x HIV649[pii].
[65] Burini RC, Borges-Santos MD, Moreto F, Ming-Yu Y. The failure of methionine load to restore plasma values of cysteine in HIV+ patients with oral *N*-acetylcysteine-induced glutathione-normal levels ESPEN 2012. Barcelona, Spain: Clinical Nutrition; 2012. p. 1.
[66] Fukagawa NK, Yu YM, Young VR. Methionine and cysteine kinetics at different intakes of methionine and cysteine in elderly men and women. Am J Clin Nutr 1998;68(2):380–8.
[67] Muller F, Svardal AM, Aukrust P, Berge RK, Ueland PM, Froland SS. Elevated plasma concentration of reduced homocysteine in patients with human immunodeficiency virus infection. Am J Clin Nutr 1996;63(2):242–8.
[68] White EL, Rose LM, Allan PW, Buckheit Jr. RW, Shannon WM, Secrist III. JA. Polyamine pools in HIV-infected cells. J Acquir Immune Defic Syndr Hum Retrovirol 1998;17(2):101–3.
[69] Fukagawa NK, Ajami AM, Young VR. Plasma methionine and cysteine kinetics in response to an intravenous glutathione infusion in adult humans. Am J Physiol 1996;270(2 Pt 1):E209–14.
[70] Coria-Ramirez E, Cisneros LN, Trevino-Perez S, Ibarra-Gonzalez I, Casillas-Rodriguez J, Majluf-Cruz A. Effect of highly active antiretroviral therapy on homocysteine plasma concentrations in HIV-1-infected patients. J Acquir Immune Defic Syndr 2010;54(5):477–81. http://dx.doi.org/10.1097/QAI.0b013e3181d91088.
[71] Raiszadeh F, Hoover DR, Lee I, Shi Q, Anastos K, Gao W, et al. Plasma homocysteine is not associated with HIV serostatus or antiretroviral therapy in women. J Acquir Immune Defic Syndr 2009;51(2):175–8. http://dx.doi.org/10.1097/QAI.0b013e3181a42bdf.
[72] Uccelli MC, Torti C, Lapadula G, Labate L, Cologni G, Tirelli V, et al. Influence of folate serum concentration on plasma homocysteine levels in HIV-positive patients exposed to protease inhibitors undergoing HAART. Ann Nutr Metab 2006;50(3):247–52. doi:91682[pii]. http://dx.doi.org/10.1159/000091682.
[73] Remacha AF, Cadafalch J, Sarda P, Barcelo M, Fuster M. Vitamin B-12 metabolism in HIV-infected patients in the age of highly active antiretroviral therapy: role of homocysteine in assessing vitamin B-12 status. Am J Clin Nutr 2003;77(2):420–4.
[74] Homocysteine Lowering Trialists' Collaboration Dose-dependent effects of folic acid on blood concentrations of homocysteine: a meta-analysis of the randomized trials. Am J Clin Nutr 2005;82(4):806–12. doi:82/4/806[pii].
[75] de Larranaga G, Alonso B, Puga L, Benetucci J. Plasma homocysteine in human immunodeficiency virus infected patient. Medicina (B Aires) 2003;63(5):393–8.
[76] Masia M, Padilla S, Bernal E, Almenar MV, Molina J, Hernandez I, et al. Influence of antiretroviral therapy on oxidative stress and cardiovascular risk: a prospective cross-sectional study in HIV-infected patients. Clin Ther 2007;29(7):1448–55. doi:S0149-2918(07)00217-2[pii]. http://dx.doi.org/10.1016/j.clinthera.2007.07.025.

[77] Vassimon HS, Deminice R, Machado AA, Monteiro JP, Jordao AA. The association of lipodystrophy and oxidative stress biomarkers in HIV-infected men. Curr HIV Res 2010;8(5):364–9. doi:ABS-78[pii].

[78] Lagathu C, Eustace B, Prot M, Frantz D, Gu Y, Bastard JP, et al. Some HIV antiretrovirals increase oxidative stress and alter chemokine, cytokine or adiponectin production in human adipocytes and macrophages. Antivir Ther 2007;12(4):489–500.

[79] Weiss N, Heydrick S, Zhang YY, Bierl C, Cap A, Loscalzo J. Cellular redox state and endothelial dysfunction in mildly hyperhomocysteinemic cystathionine beta-synthase-deficient mice. Arterioscler Thromb Vasc Biol 2002;22(1):34–41.

[80] Mondal D, Pradhan L, Ali M, Agrawal KC. HAART drugs induce oxidative stress in human endothelial cells and increase endothelial recruitment of mononuclear cells: exacerbation by inflammatory cytokines and amelioration by antioxidants. Cardiovasc Toxicol 2004;4(3):287–302. doi:CT:4:3:287[pii].

[81] Gibson NR, Jahoor F, Ware L, Jackson AA. Endogenous glycine and tyrosine production is maintained in adults consuming a marginal-protein diet. Am J Clin Nutr 2002;75(3):511–8.

[82] Lamers Y, Williamson J, Theriaque DW, Shuster JJ, Gilbert LR, Keeling C, et al. Production of 1-carbon units from glycine is extensive in healthy men and women. J Nutr 2009;139(4):666–71. http://dx.doi.org/10.3945/jn.108.103580 [pii].

[83] Lamers Y, Williamson J, Gilbert LR, Stacpoole PW, Gregory III. JF. Glycine turnover and decarboxylation rate quantified in healthy men and women using primed, constant infusions of [1,2-(13)C2]glycine and [(2)H3]leucine. J Nutr 2007;137(12):2647–52. doi:137/12/2647 [pii].

[84] Lamers Y, Williamson J, Ralat M, Quinlivan EP, Gilbert LR, Keeling C, et al. Moderate dietary vitamin B-6 restriction raises plasma glycine and cystathionine concentrations while minimally affecting the rates of glycine turnover and glycine cleavage in healthy men and women. J Nutr 2009;139(3):452–60. http://dx.doi.org/10.3945/jn.108.099184 [pii].

[85] Bailey LB, Gregory III. JF. Folate metabolism and requirements. J Nutr 1999;129(4):779–82.

[86] Robinson K, Arheart K, Refsum H, Brattstrom L, Boers G, Ueland P, et al. Low circulating folate and vitamin B6 concentrations: risk factors for stroke, peripheral vascular disease, and coronary artery disease. European COMAC group. Circulation 1998;97(5):437–43.

CHAPTER

16

Micronutrients in HIV Infection Without HAART: A Focus on Resource-Limited Settings

Marilia Rita Pinzone, Bruno Cacopardo and Giuseppe Nunnari

Department of Clinical and Molecular Biomedicine, Division of Infectious Diseases, University of Catania, Catania, Italy

16.1 INTRODUCTION

Globally, an estimated 35.3 million people were living with human immunodeficiency virus (HIV) infection in 2012. More than 95% of HIV infections are in developing countries. Sub-Saharan Africa is the most severely affected area, where approximately two-thirds of HIV-positive individuals live [1]. Micronutrients deficiencies are common in HIV-infected adults and children, especially in resource-limited settings where diet is often inadequate to guarantee the recommended daily requirements [2]. Several studies have reported micronutrient deficiencies to be associated with increased morbidity and mortality in HIV-positive subjects.

In this chapter, we briefly review the main findings of observational studies and randomized controlled trials (RCTs) evaluating the impact of serum micronutrient levels (particularly vitamins A, D, C, E, B6, B12, folic acid, zinc, selenium, iron, and multiple supplements) on clinical outcomes of HIV-infected patients living in resource-limited settings. Moreover, we report on studies assessing the possible role of micronutrient supplementation as an adjunct treatment for children and adults with HIV infection.

Health of HIV Infected People, Volume 2.
DOI: http://dx.doi.org/10.1016/B978-0-12-800767-9.00016-9

16.2 VITAMIN A

Vitamin A is a fat-soluble vitamin acquired from the diet as *all-trans*-retinol, retinyl esters, or β-carotene. *All-trans*-retinol is esterified by the enzyme lecithin:retinol acyltransferase (LCAT) to retinyl esters and stored primarily in liver stellate cells. *All-trans*-retinol and β-carotene are oxidized to *all-trans*-retinal by alcohol dehydrogenases or short chain dehydrogenase reductases. *All-trans*-retinal is then oxidized to *all-trans*-retinoic acid through an irreversible reaction catalyzed by retinal dehydrogenases (RALDHs). Another metabolite, *9-cis*-retinoic acid, can be formed either by spontaneous isomerization of *all-trans*-retinoic acid or through oxidation of *9-cis*-retinal by RALDH. Retinal is required for rhodopsin formation and vision, whereas retinoic acid acts as a hormone, binding to retinoic acid receptors (RARs). Two families of receptors interact with vitamin A: the RAR family, which can bind *all-trans*-retinoic acid and *9-cis*-retinoic acid, and the retinoic acid X receptor (RXR) family, which can bind only *9-cis*-retinoic acid [3].

Vitamin A metabolites have a role in the immune system that extends to innate and adaptive immune responses. It has been shown to maintain epithelial barriers, to activate acute phase responses, to promote monocyte differentiation, to increase natural killer cell (NKC) cytotoxicity, and to improve neutrophil function. Moreover, vitamin A has been reported to modulate antigen presentation by exerting direct effects on dendritic cells (DCs), to enhance T-cell count (particularly of $CD4^+$ T cells), to support immune tolerance, and to potentiate antibody responses to tetanus toxoid and measles vaccines [4–6].

Observational studies in HIV-infected cohorts have shown low vitamin A levels to be associated with the risk of HIV clinical progression and mortality [7,8]. However, RCTs have failed to demonstrate an association between vitamin A and/or β-carotene supplementation and HIV progression [9–11]. In one trial in Kenya, 400 HIV-positive women were randomized to receive 10,000 IU of vitamin A daily for 6 weeks or placebo [11]. No differences between the two groups were observed regarding either HIV viral load or CD4/CD8 T-cell count. Other RCTs in Tanzania [10] and South Africa [9] confirmed that vitamin A with or without β-carotene supplementation had no beneficial effect on viro-immunological parameters.

The results of studies evaluating the relationship between vitamin A levels and HIV horizontal transmission have been equivocal. In a nested case–control study of sexually active adult women in Rwanda, the investigators compared the baseline levels of various nutrients in 45 women who seroconverted during the 24-month study period with those of 74 women who remained seronegative throughout the study. The authors did not find any differences in baseline serum levels of vitamin A, carotenoids, and vitamin E [12]. Similar results were observed in another nested case–control study in Tanzania [13]. In India, Mehendale et al. [14] reported that individuals with β-carotene concentration less than 0.075 mmol/L were 21-times more likely to acquire HIV infection than those with higher β-carotene levels. Opposing results were published by MacDonald et al. [15], who evaluated the risk of seroconversion in men with concurrent genital ulcers in Kenya. They found that seroconversion was independently associated with a retinol level more than 20 mg/dL (hazard ratio [HR], 2.43; 95% confidence interval (CI), 1.25–4.7).

In observational studies, low serum retinol levels during pregnancy have been associated with increased neonatal mortality, higher HIV DNA concentration in milk, and increased risk of vertical transmission [16–18]. Several trials evaluated whether maternal vitamin A supplementation was able to reduce mother-to-child transmission (MTCT) of HIV, with disappointing results [19,20]. In South Africa and Malawi, no effect on MTCT was observed among mothers receiving antenatal supplementation with vitamin A, whereas in Tanzania daily supplementation with vitamin A and β-carotene throughout pregnancy and lactation was associated with a 38% increase in the risk of MTCT [21,22]. Vitamin A/β-carotene supplementation was also associated with a significant increase in viral shedding in vaginal secretions. In a large trial performed in Zimbabwe by the ZVITAMBO Study Group, the authors investigated the effect of a single large dose of vitamin A given at delivery to HIV-positive women and/or their infants [23]; 4,495 HIV-positive mothers were enrolled in the study. Vitamin A supplementation did not increase breastfeeding-associated MTCT of HIV. Neither maternal nor neonatal vitamin A supplementation was associated with decreased child mortality at 24 months. However, the authors reported that the impact of vitamin A supplementation on mortality significantly varied according to the time when the children were infected with HIV. In fact, they found that neonatal vitamin A supplementation reduced mortality by 28% among infants who were infected during the late intrauterine/intrapartum/early postnatal period, that is, HIV-exposed infants who were polymerase chain reaction (PCR)-negative for HIV at baseline and PCR-positive at 6 weeks. On the contrary, vitamin A supplementation, either maternal or neonatal, was associated with a twofold increased risk of death among HIV-exposed infants who were PCR-negative at 6 weeks; 40% of children negative at 6 weeks who died were PCR-positive before death and therefore became infected during breastfeeding. A possible explanation for these findings is that priming with vitamin A might have favored HIV replication in the subgroup of children who became infected during the postnatal period, hastening their progression to death. This hypothesis is supported by *in vitro* studies showing that monocyte pretreatment with retinol acid before HIV infection may increase viral production [24,25]. On the contrary, HIV transcription is inhibited when HIV-infected cells are treated with retinol acid [25–28]. These data are in keeping with clinical studies reporting decreased mortality and morbidity in HIV-positive children receiving vitamin A supplements [29–31]. In Uganda, HIV-positive children receiving vitamin A supplements were found to have a lower risk of mortality compared with those receiving placebo (relative risk [RR], 0.54; 95% CI, 0.3–0.98) [30]. In another trial in Tanzania, periodic supplementation with vitamin A resulted in a significant reduction in mortality and morbidity among HIV-infected children [29]. Vitamin A supplements decreased all-cause mortality by 63% (RR, 0.37; 95% CI, 0.14–0.95) and was associated with increased short-term growth. After 4 months of supplementation, there was a mean increase in height of 2.8 cm (95% CI, 1–4.6) of HIV-infected supplemented children younger than 18 months of age. Moreover, the investigators reported a nonsignificant reduction in the risk of respiratory tract infections (RR, 0.54; 95% CI, 0.24–1.2) and severe diarrhea (RR, 1.55; 95% CI, 0.75–3.17). AIDS-related deaths decreased by 68% and diarrhea-related deaths decreased by 92%. In South Africa, a placebo-controlled trial of children born to HIV-positive women reported that vitamin A supplementation reduced morbidity associated with diarrhea by 50% (odds ratio [OR], 0.51; 95% CI, 0.27–0.99) [31]. In a recent meta-analysis, vitamin A was confirmed to reduce mortality in HIV-positive children by 50% (RR, 0.5; 95% CI, 0.31–0.79), whereas no benefits could be demonstrated in adults [32].

16.3 VITAMIN D

Vitamin D is a fat-soluble compound whose major production occurs in the skin, where the photochemical action of UVB light is able to transform the precursor 7-dehydrocholesterol to previtamin D, which is, in turn, converted to vitamin D through a nonenzymatic thermal isomerization. Vitamin D is then metabolized in the liver to 25-hydroxyvitamin D (25OHD) by 25α-hydroxylase; 25OHD is subsequently converted to the biologically active compound 1,25-dihydroxyvitamin D (1,25$(OH)_2$D) by 1α-hydroxylase (or CYP27B1). Although 1α-hydroxylase is predominantly expressed in the kidney, several extrarenal tissues and cells, like monocytes/macrophages, are also able to convert 25OHD to 1,25$(OH)_2$D. A catabolic pathway involving 24α-hydroxylase (CYP24A1) is responsible for 25OHD and 1,25$(OH)_2$D hydroxylation to inactive metabolites, named 24,25$(OH)_2$D and 1,24,29 5$(OH)_3$D, respectively [33,34]. Vitamin D is not only a key regulator of calcium homeostasis but also an important mediator of both innate and adaptive immune responses [35,36]. In fact, vitamin D receptor (VDR) is expressed on DCs and macrophages, T cells, and B cells, and its signaling pathway has been associated with anti-inflammatory and antimicrobial effects. Vitamin D downregulates the production of pro-inflammatory cytokines, including tumor necrosis factor-alpha (TNF-α) and interferon-gamma. Furthermore, it induces the production of antimicrobial peptides, such as defensins and cathelicidin, an antimicrobial peptide capable of killing intracellular pathogens such as *Mycobacterium tuberculosis*. 1,25$(OH)_2$D was shown to inhibit HIV replication *in vitro* on primary human monocytes/macrophages, although it enhanced HIV replication on promonocytic cell line U937 [34].

A growing amount of data suggest that vitamin D deficiency is highly prevalent in the setting of HIV infection, with up to 80–90% of individuals having low vitamin D levels in some cohorts [37–39]. However, hypovitaminosis D seems to be common in the general population, and the majority of studies including a control group of HIV-uninfected subjects have found no differences in vitamin D levels by HIV status. As for the general population, older age, winter season, female sex, dark skin pigmentation, and low vitamin D dietary intake are risk factors for vitamin D deficiency [34]. Some studies have suggested an association between exposure to certain antiretroviral drugs and low vitamin D levels. In particular, initiation of an efavirenz (EFV)-based regimen has been associated with a significant decline in vitamin D levels after 6–12 months in comparison with a non-EFV–based one [40]. A possible explanation is that EFV is able to induce 24α-hydroxylase, leading to the inactivation of 25OHD and 1,25$(OH)_2$D [41]. These findings have been confirmed by other research groups in the past few years [42,43]. *In vitro* studies suggested that protease inhibitors (PIs) may lower vitamin D levels by inhibiting 1α-hydroxylase, although clinical studies have not shown a consistent association between exposure to PIs and hypovitaminosis D [44]. Tenofovir may indirectly affect vitamin D metabolism, because it may cause proximal renal tubular dysfunction, leading to hypophosphatemia. Hypophosphatemia may induce a compensatory increase in 1α-hydroxylase to enhance gut absorption of phosphate.

Observational studies have associated low vitamin D levels with increased risk of cardiovascular disease, bone disease, and overall mortality [34]. In Tanzania, the prevalence of low vitamin D levels (<20 ng/mL) was 44% in a cohort of 1,100 adults starting highly active antiretroviral therapy (HAART). The HR for mortality was 2 (95% CI, 1.19–3.37; $P = 0.009$) among subjects with vitamin D levels less than 20 ng/mL versus those with levels more than 30 ng/mL over 24 months [45]. In another study, low vitamin D levels (<32 ng/mL) were associated with increased risk of HIV clinical progression (incidence rate ratio [IRR], 1.25; 95% CI, 1.05–1.5) in a cohort of 884 HIV-positive pregnant women who were followed-up for a median of 69.5 months. Moreover, women in the highest quintile of vitamin D levels had a 42% lower risk of all-cause mortality as compared with those in the lowest quintile (RR, 0.58; 95% CI, 0.4–0.84). Low vitamin D levels were also associated with increased risk of developing severe anemia (RR, 1.46; 95% CI, 1.09–1.96) [46]. In the same cohort, low vitamin D levels were associated with an increased risk of wasting (HR, 1.43; 95% CI, 1.03–1.99), acute upper respiratory infections (HR, 1.27; 95% CI, 1.04–1.54), and thrush (HR, 2.74; 95% CI, 1.29–5.83) in the first 2 years of follow-up [47]. Studies evaluating the association between hypovitaminosis D and the risk of MTCT of HIV have reported conflicting results. In the aforementioned Tanzanian cohort of HIV-positive pregnant women [46,47], 39% of subjects had vitamin D levels less than 32 ng/mL. Mehta et al. [48] found low maternal vitamin D levels to be associated with a 50% higher risk of MTCT of HIV at 6 weeks, a twofold higher risk of MTCT through breastfeeding among children who were HIV-uninfected at 6 weeks, and a 46% higher overall risk of HIV infection. The incidence of HIV infection by 24 months of age was 46% higher in the group with low vitamin D levels than in the group with sufficient vitamin D levels. A 61% increase in the risk of dying during the first 24 months of follow-up was described among children born to women with low vitamin D levels. The investigators found no association between maternal vitamin D levels and the risk of low birth weight, preterm birth, and small-for-gestational-age status [48]. On the contrary, another study performed in India did not find any significant association between maternal vitamin D levels and MTCT of HIV (adjusted OR, 0.66; 95% CI, 0.3–1.45) [49]. There are few data on the efficacy and safety of vitamin D supplementation in HIV-infected subjects living in resource-limited settings. Wejse et al. [50] evaluated the effect of periodic vitamin D supplements (100,000 IU cholecalciferol at baseline, 5 months, and 8 months) in addition to antitubercular treatment in 365 adults in Guinea-Bissau, 131 of whom were HIV-positive. For both the whole cohort and the HIV-infected subgroup, vitamin D supplementation did not improve the clinical severity of tuberculosis (TB) and had no effect on 12-month mortality (HR, 1.8; 95% CI, 0.8–4.1).

Taken together, these data suggest that there is insufficient evidence to recommend universal vitamin D supplementation among HIV-infected subjects. Findings coming from observation studies need to be assessed in the setting of large RCTs and, if found to be effective, vitamin D supplementation may represent a helpful adjunct therapy to improve the quality of life of adults and children with HIV infection.

16.4 VITAMINS E AND C

Vitamin E is a lipid-soluble compound with potent antioxidant functions. The term vitamin E refers to a group of molecules including four tocopherols (α, β, γ, δ) and four tocotrienols (α, β, γ, δ). Vitamin E is also involved in host immune functions, because it is responsible for improving delayed-type hypersensitivity skin response, neutrophil phagocytosis, interleukin (IL)-2 production, lymphocyte proliferation, and antibody response to T-cell-dependent vaccines; moreover, it reduces the production of inflammatory cytokines, such as TNF-α and IL-6 [51,52]. Vitamin C, also known as ascorbic acid, is a water-soluble vitamin and an essential cofactor in several enzymatic reactions, for example, in the biosynthesis of collagen, carnitine, and catecholamines. Vitamin C is also a potent antioxidant and participates in redox recycling of other antioxidants, including vitamin E. Vitamin C exerts immunomodulatory functions, including improvement of T-cell and B-cell proliferative responses and reduction of pro-inflammatory cytokine levels [53,54].

In HIV-infected cells, oxidative stress is an important cause of cell death. In fact, reactive oxygen species (ROS) may trigger cell apoptosis and enhance HIV replication [55,56]. Pro-inflammatory cytokines, especially TNF-α, favor free radical release by immune cells, which is responsible for cellular damage, apoptosis, and further activation of viral replication through the induction of nuclear factor kappa light-chain enhancer of activated B cells (NF-κB) [57]. Antioxidants, such as vitamin E, may reduce NF-κB activity in HIV-infected cells. In fact, α-tocopheryl acetate has been shown to block NF-κB activation in HIV-infected cell cultures, probably by inhibiting free radical production in the mitochondria. Moreover, α-tocopheryl succinate has been found to completely inhibit NF-κB binding [58]. Similarly, vitamin C has been reported to inhibit NF-kB activation and T-cell pathways of apoptosis via multiple pathways, including the upregulation of the antiapoptotic B cell lymphoma-2 [59–61]. Vitamin C in combination with *N*-acetylcysteine, but not vitamin C alone, was reported to reduce lipopolysaccharide-induced activation of $CD4^+$ T cells from patients with untreated asymptomatic HIV infection [62].

In vivo studies have shown hypovitaminosis E to be common among HIV-infected people and to be associated with increased oxidative stress [63,64]. In the Multicenter AIDS Cohort Study, the investigators reported that higher vitamin E serum levels were associated with reduced risk of HIV progression [65]. A small RCT evaluated the effects of daily supplementation of 800 IU vitamin E and 1,000 mg vitamin C for 3 months in 49 HIV-positive subjects [64]. Compared with the placebo arm, subjects receiving supplementation had decreased oxidative stress and a trend toward a reduction of the viral load. No differences in morbidity were reported between the two groups. However, it was a short-term study that was performed before HAART became widely available. As a consequence, these findings should be confirmed in larger studies that include patients receiving the current standard of care for HIV infection.

16.5 VITAMIN B6, VITAMIN B12, AND FOLIC ACID

Vitamin B6, vitamin B12, and vitamin B9 (also known as folic acid) are water-soluble compounds that belong to the vitamin B complex. Vitamin

B6 is known to increase lymphocyte and antibody production, cell-mediated toxicity, and delayed-type hypersensitivity responses. Vitamin B12 has been implicated in the promotion of humoral responses, whereas folic acid improves neutrophil phagocytosis and activity [66,67]. Low levels of vitamins B6 and B12 have been reported in HIV-positive cohorts, whereas the evidence for folate deficiency has been less consistent [63,68–70]. Vitamin B12 deficiency has been associated with altered immunological and neurological functions, including increased mortality, $CD4^+$ T-cell decline, increased zidovudine-associated bone marrow toxicity, and increased peripheral neuropathy and myelopathy [71–74]. Low vitamin B6 levels have been linked to a reduced response of lymphocytes to mitogens and decreased NKT cytotoxicity [75].

In a longitudinal study, Saah and coworkers [76] examined the association between serum levels of vitamins B6, B12, and folate and the risk of clinical progression to AIDS in 310 men participating in the Baltimore Multicenter AIDS Cohort Study; the men were followed-up for 9 years. At baseline, 11% of subjects had vitamin B6 deficiency, 12% had low vitamin B12 levels, and 8% had low serum folate. Compared with normal vitamin B12 levels, low vitamin B12 levels (<120 ρmol/L) were found to independently predict shorter AIDS-free time (4 versus 8 years respectively; $P = 0.004$), but not $CD4^+$ T-cell decline. The authors reported the risk of clinical progression to AIDS to be 87% higher among subjects with vitamin B12 deficiency (adjusted RR, 1.89; 95% CI, 1.15–3.1), even after correcting for baseline $CD4^+$ T-cell count. On the contrary, low serum levels of vitamin B6 and folate were not associated with either AIDS diagnosis or $CD4^+$ T-cell decline over time. Chatterjee et al. [77] found no association between vitamin B12 status and mortality and morbidity in a cohort of 529 children born to HIV-positive mothers in Tanzania. In Uganda, a cross-sectional study found that 37% of 204 HAART-naive adults had suboptimal vitamin B12 levels, whereas 10% had vitamin B12 deficiency [78]. Suboptimal vitamin B12 levels were associated with longer duration of HIV infection, higher mean corpuscular volume, irritable mood, and higher rate of $CD4^+$ T-cell decline among individuals eligible for HAART. However, given the study design, causality could not be established. Further prospective research is needed to shed more light on the role of vitamin B12 and its possible use as adjunct therapy in HIV-infected individuals.

16.6 ZINC

Zinc is an essential trace element and a component of more than 200 mammalian metallo-enzymes. Zinc has important antioxidant and immunomodulatory functions [79]. In fact, zinc deficiency leads to increased susceptibility to infections, including malaria, diarrhea, and pneumonia. Zinc deficiency has been associated with decreased serum levels of IL-2 and thymulin, a zinc-dependent thymic peptide whose activity is important for the maturation and differentiation of thymocytes [80,81]. Moreover, zinc deficiency may impair T-cell proliferation and cytolytic activity. Zinc stimulates water and electrolytes absorption from the intestinal mucosa and it increases the concentration of enterocyte brush-border enzymes [82]; it also exerts anti-inflammatory activities, through the inhibition of the NF-κB pathway and may inhibit TNF-α-induced cell death [83]. The HIV protease enzyme, which is essential for the production of new viral particles, can be inhibited by high zinc concentration [84]. In addition, zinc cellular levels affect HIV integration into the host genome. In fact, zinc binds to the HIV integrase enzyme via "zinc finger protein" structures and seems to be necessary for its optimal enzymatic activity [85].

Observational studies conducted in HIV-positive cohorts have failed to show a consistent association between zinc serum levels/zinc dietary intake and HIV clinical outcomes. Some authors reported low zinc levels to be linked to disease progression [86], decreased $CD4^+$ T-cell count, and increased mortality [86,87]. However, other studies have found no association between zinc intake and time to clinical progression to AIDS [88], with one study reporting self-prescribed zinc consumption above the recommended dietary allowance (RDA) to be associated with faster HIV progression and lower survival [89,90]. In one trial in Tanzania, 400 pregnant Tanzanian women were randomized to receive daily zinc supplements (25 mg) or placebo in addition to multivitamin supplements during pregnancy and up to 6 weeks after delivery [91]. Zinc supplementation had no effect on fetal and neonatal mortality, duration of pregnancy, birth weight, MTCT of HIV, maternal T-cell counts, and HIV viral load. Hemoglobin concentrations increased between baseline and 6 weeks postpartum in both groups, but the increase in hemoglobin as well as packed cell volume and red blood cell count were significantly lower in the zinc group compared with the placebo arm. In a recent RCT, the investigators randomized 52 children older than 6 months starting HAART to receive daily 20 mg zinc supplementation or placebo for 24 weeks [92]. There was no difference between the two arms in $CD4^+$ percentage increase, viral load reduction, anthropometric indices, and morbidity. In a safety trial in South Africa, 96 children aged 6–60 months were randomized to receive a daily dose of 10 mg zinc sulfate or placebo for 6 months [93]. HIV viral load, $CD4^+$ percentage, and hemoglobin levels were similar in the two arms. Of importance, reduced diarrheal morbidity was observed in the group of children receiving zinc supplementation compared with placebo (7.4 versus 14.5%, respectively; $P = 0.001$). In Peru, a 2-week course of 100 mg of elemental zinc daily to adults with diarrhea had no effect on the persistence and severity of diarrhea [94]. In a study performed in the United States that included only subjects with low plasma zinc levels, zinc supplementation was associated with reduced risk of diarrhea (OR, 0.4; 95% CI, 0.18–0.99) and reduced risk of immunologic failure (RR, 0.24; 95% CI, 0.1–0.56), defined as a decrease in $CD4^+$ T-cell count less than 200 cells/μL. No differences in mortality after 18 months were reported between the two arms [95].

Zinc supplementation seems to reduce diarrhea-associated morbidity and to have no adverse effects on HIV clinical progression; however, several questions remain to be answered. There is a need for larger, well-designed trials to determine the influence of treatment dose and duration and to assess how zinc supplements may affect HIV viral load, mortality, MTCT, fetal, and child outcomes.

16.7 SELENIUM

Selenium is an essential constituent of the enzyme glutathione peroxidase, a key mediator of the antioxidant system, other peroxidase enzymes, and iodothyronine deiodinase. Selenium deficiency has been linked to immune dysfunction, inadequate phagocytosis and antibody production, and impaired NKT and $CD8^+$ cytotoxic activity. In addition, selenium deficiency lowers glutathione peroxidase activity, which may lead to increased $CD4^+$ T-cell apoptosis [96]. In HIV infection, ROS have been shown to upregulate viral replication, mainly through the NF-κB and activator protein 1 as intermediates [97], whereas antioxidants, including selenoproteins, may inhibit viral activation [98]. Interestingly, HIV itself has been reported to produce a selenium-based homolog of glutathione peroxidase [99]. The virus has been postulated to accelerate selenium depletion in HIV-infected lymphocytes, favoring its own replication by decreasing glutathione peroxidase availability. *In vitro* studies have shown reduced induction of HIV replication in chronically infected T-lymphocyte and monocytic cell lines supplemented with selenium prior to exposure to TNF-α. The suppressive effect of selenium supplementation was not observed in acute HIV infection of T lymphocytes and monocytes in the absence of exogenous TNF-α, whereas selenium was found to suppress the enhancing effect of TNF-α on HIV replication in acutely infected human monocytes, but not in T lymphocytes [100,101].

Observational studies have reported a relationship between selenium deficiency and HIV progression and mortality in adults and children [102–104]. A prospective cohort study in Rwanda found that low serum selenium status was associated with increased risk of developing dilated cardiomyopathy in HIV-infected subjects [105]. On the contrary, in Tanzania higher selenium levels were associated with increased risk of HIV genital shedding [106]. Some studies have shown low maternal serum selenium concentrations to be related to adverse pregnancy outcomes, including child mortality, risk of HIV transmission through the intrapartum route [104], and poor weight gain during pregnancy [107].

Few RCTs have evaluated this association with conflicting results. Two small RCTs in the United States found selenium supplementation to be associated with reduced hospitalization rates [108], decreased HIV viral load, and better $CD4^+$ T-cell recovery [109]. Only one trial evaluated the effect of selenium supplementation in sub-Saharan Africa. In Tanzania, Kupka et al. [110] randomized 915 HAART-naive women to receive selenium supplements or placebo during pregnancy and until 6 months postpartum. Selenium supplementation was not associated with delayed maternal HIV progression or improved pregnancy outcomes; however, in the selenium group, maternal diarrheal morbidity was reduced by 40% (RR, 0.6; 95% CI, 0.42–0.84). Overall child mortality was not different between the two groups, although a reduction in child mortality at 6 weeks was described (RR, 0.43; 95% CI, 0.19–0.99) in the supplemented group [111]. Several factors may have contributed to the lack of effect of selenium supplementation on maternal and neonatal outcomes. First, all the patients were receiving high-dose multivitamin supplements, which may have limited selenium effect. Second, selenium deficiency was not highly prevalent in the study population. Third, although the study participants were primarily asymptomatic at baseline and the majority of them were HAART-naive, it may be hypothesized that selenium supplementation could have a more significant impact on patients with advanced HIV disease or receiving HAART. With the increase in HAART coverage in sub-Saharan Africa, there is a need for further trials evaluating the safety and efficacy of selenium supplementation in this setting.

16.8 IRON

Iron deficiency is the most common nutritional cause of anemia worldwide, affecting approximately 50% of women and children in developing countries [112]. There is a significant overlap between areas where iron deficiency and HIV infection are both highly prevalent. Anemia affects up to 90% of pediatric patients with HIV infection in resource-limited settings. Iron deficiency has been described in more than 50% of HIV-positive children and has been associated with the severity of HIV infection [113].

In Malawi [114], 209 children aged 6–59 months with moderate anemia were randomized to receive elemental iron and multivitamins or multivitamins alone for 3 months. Participants were followed-up for 6 months. The investigators found that iron supplementation was associated with greater increase in hemoglobin concentrations (adjusted mean difference [aMD], 0.6; 95% CI, 0.06–1.13; $P = 0.03$) and reduced risk of anemia persisting for up to 6 months of follow-up (adjusted prevalence ratio, 0.59;

95% CI, 0.38–0.92; $P = 0.02$). Children receiving iron had a better $CD4^+$ percentage response at 3 months (aMD, 6; 95% CI, 1.84–10.16; $P = 0.005$) but an increased incidence of malaria at 3 months (incidence rate 78.1 versus 36; aIRR, 2.68; 95% CI, 1.08–6.63; $P = 0.03$) and 6 months (incidence rate 120.2 versus 71.7; aIRR, 1.8; 95% CI, 1.04–3.16; $P = 0.04$). Of interest, iron supplementation was associated with increased incidence of malaria in children older than 24 months but not in children aged 6–24 months, which is unexpected considering that younger children are at increased risk for severe malaria because of immature immune responses. A possible explanation could be iron deficiency–associated protection from malaria, because iron deficiency was almost threefold more frequent in children aged 6–24 months than in children aged older than 24 months, although in subgroup analysis no difference in the incidence of malaria was observed between children who were iron-deficient and those who were not. An alternative explanation could be that younger children were more likely to sleep under bed nets, which were strongly associated with protection from malaria. Moreover, the association between iron supplementation and malaria was observed only among children who were not receiving HAART. This observation may be due to a direct antiparasitic activity of certain antiretroviral drugs, such as PIs, or to a prolongation of the half-life of antimalarial medications in children treated for malaria [115,116]. This study shed some light on the effects of iron supplementation in HIV-infected children living in a malaria-endemic area. However, it could not determine the true effect of iron supplementation on all-cause sick visits, hospitalizations, and progression to AIDS, and it was not adequately powered to address mortality. Larger studies are needed to provide a better understanding of the association between iron supplementation and malaria in HIV-infected children.

In adults with HIV infection, anemia is highly prevalent and associated with increased morbidity and mortality. However, some *in vitro* experiments and observational studies have raised the concern that iron supplementation may have detrimental effects in HIV-infected subjects, leading to accelerated clinical progression and decreased survival [117–122]. In a small study enrolling HIV-positive patients with thalassemia major, those who were treated with inadequate doses compared with optimal doses of desferrioxamine, an iron chelating agent, had faster progression of HIV disease [121]. Analogously, patients with high serum ferritin levels experienced a faster progression of HIV disease [123]. Patients receiving prophylaxis against *Pneumocystis carinii* pneumonia with a dapsone/iron supplement (60 mg) were found to have lower survival in comparison with those receiving aerosolized pentamidine [119], whereas administration of dapsone alone was not associated with higher mortality rates [124]. A possible explanation is related to NF-κB, which is involved in viral replication, whose activity is affected by the cellular redox state

[117]. As a consequence, in the presence of excessive cellular iron, which is a strong pro-oxidant, HIV replication could be enhanced [125]. In a study on polymorphisms of hemoglobin-binding haptoglobin, a plasma antioxidant, the haptoglobin 2-2 phenotype, which has a relatively weaker hemoglobin-binding capacity, was associated with higher iron stores and decreased survival in a cohort of 653 HIV-positive subjects [122]. Moreover, a retrospective study of bone marrow macrophage iron in HIV-positive adults in the pre-HAART era found that high iron stores were associated with a shorter survival [120]. Prospective studies have not confirmed the association between iron and HIV progression. In the United States, a trial involving 320 HIV-negative and 138 HIV-positive female drug users (36% on HAART) with hepatitis C infection reported that daily supplementation with 18 mg of iron reduced anemia at 6 months and had no impact on plasma HIV viral load [126]. Analogously, in a *post hoc* analysis of 45 HAART-naive HIV-infected adults in Kenya who participated in a larger study of nonanemic subjects ($n = 181$), low-dose iron supplementation (60 mg twice weekly for 4 months) did not increase HIV viral load [127].

This brief overview of available studies suggests that there is a lot of uncertainty about the use of iron supplements in HIV-infected individuals. Good-quality evidence is lacking and RCTs are urgently needed to examine the safety and efficacy of iron supplementation in the clinical setting of HIV infection.

16.9 MULTIPLE SUPPLEMENTS

Some RCTs have evaluated the effect of multiple supplements in HIV-infected patients. In Tanzania [10], 1,078 HIV-infected pregnant women were randomized to receive either daily vitamin A supplements, multivitamins (thiamine, riboflavin, niacin, vitamins B6, B12, C, E, and folic acid in doses up to 22-times the RDA), both, or neither. At delivery, women in the vitamin A groups received an additional oral dose of vitamin A, whereas those in non-vitamin A groups received a placebo. In addition, all women received iron and folate supplementation daily and chloroquine as malaria prophylaxis weekly. The authors found no association between the administration of either multivitamins (RR, 0.95; 95% CI, 0.73–1.24) or vitamin A (RR, 1.06; 95% CI, 0.81–1.39) and the risk of HIV transmission or survival at 6 weeks postpartum. A beneficial effect of multivitamins, but not vitamin A, on birth weight was observed among children who were HIV-negative at birth. The administration of multivitamins, but not vitamin A, was found to decrease the risk of fetal death by 39% (RR, 0.61; 95% CI, 0.39–0.94) [22]. Multivitamin supplements, but not vitamin A, were also associated with a significant increase in T-cell counts in women [128]. Multivitamins had no impact on the risk of overall vertical

HIV transmission, whereas vitamin A/β-carotene increased the risk of transmission by 38%. In multivitamin-supplemented women with low immunological or nutritional status, the authors reported a significant reduction in the risk of child mortality by 24 months of age [21]. Women receiving multivitamins had a 30% reduction in the risk of progression to WHO stage IV or AIDS-related death (RR, 0.71; 95% CI, 0.51–0.98). Multivitamins significantly reduced oral and gastrointestinal manifestations of HIV disease such as oral thrush, oral ulcers, as well as the incidence of reported fatigue, rash, and acute upper respiratory infections [10]. Moreover, multivitamins reduced the risk of maternal wasting [129]. In Kenya, 400 HAART-naive nonpregnant women received multivitamins and selenium or placebo for 6 weeks [130]. Supplementation resulted in a significantly higher $CD4^+$ (+23 cells/μL; $P = 0.03$) and $CD8^+$ T-cell counts (+74 cells/μL; $P = 0.005$) compared with placebo, whereas no differences in HIV viral load were observed. Interestingly, the investigators found that the odds of detection of vaginal HIV-infected cells was 2.5-fold higher ($P = 0.001$) and the quantity of HIV RNA in vaginal secretions was 0.37 log copies/swab higher ($P = 0.004$) among women who received micronutrients in comparison with placebo.

In Thailand, one trial evaluated the effect of daily micronutrient supplementation (vitamin A, β-carotene, vitamins D, E, K, C, B1, B2, B6, B12, folate, iron, zinc, and selenium) versus placebo for 48 weeks in 481 HIV-infected adults. The authors did not find any association between supplementation and $CD4^+$ T-cell count or HIV viral load. However, a reduction in mortality was reported in the intervention group, which was significant only among subjects with a baseline $CD4^+$ T-cell count less than 100 cells/μL (HR, 0.26; 95% CI, 0.07–0.97) [131]. In Zambia, the investigators randomized 141 HIV-positive HAART-naive patients with persistent diarrhea to albendazole *plus* vitamins A, C, E, selenium, and zinc or to albendazole *plus* placebo for 2 weeks. Supplementation was not associated with significant effects on $CD4^+$ T-cell count or any clinical markers of illness severity [8]. The study had a short duration, which may have limited the potential benefits of supplementation. In another trial [132], the effects of multiple supplements on diarrhea were evaluated in a Zambian community that included 161 HIV-positive subjects. The intervention arm received vitamins A, B, C, D, E, zinc, copper, selenium, iodine, and folic acid at a dose similar to the RDA for an average of 3.3 years. No differences in $CD4^+$ T-cell count, anthropometric measures, and incidence of diarrhea were observed between the two arms. However, a 75% lower mortality was reported in the supplemented group.

Some studies evaluated the effects of multiple supplements in patients with TB, including subgroups with HIV coinfection. In a Tanzanian study with a two-by-two factorial design, 499 patients initiating treatment of pulmonary TB, 213 of whom were coinfected with HIV, were randomized to receive an 8-month course of high-dose multivitamins with or without zinc [133]. The authors found that neither multivitamins alone nor zinc alone affected mortality and viro-immunological parameters. On the contrary, mortality was reduced by 71% (RR, 0.29; 95% CI, 0.1–0.8) in the group receiving multivitamins and zinc. In another trial of 1,402 Malawian patients with pulmonary TB, 829 of whom were HIV-positive, the investigators reported no differences in mortality between HIV-infected patients receiving daily multiple supplements including zinc and those receiving placebo for 24 months [134]. Finally, Villamor et al. [135] randomized 887 Tanzanian adults with TB, 471 of whom were coinfected with HIV, to receive 8 months of high-dose multiple micronutrient supplement (without zinc) or placebo at TB therapy initiation. HIV-positive patients were not on HAART. Mortality, viral load, $CD4^+$ T-cell count, and HIV disease progression were similar between the supplemented and the placebo group. Among HIV-positive patients whose TB cultures had become negative by 1 month after the initiation of treatment, micronutrients decreased the risk of a recurrence during the remaining duration of treatment by 63% (95% CI, 8–85%; $P = 0.02$). Among HIV-infected patients assigned to the supplementation group, recurrences 8 months after treatment initiation were 34% less common but did not reach statistical significance (95% CI, −67% to 31%). Micronutrients significantly decreased the incidence of peripheral neuropathy (57%; 95% CI, 41–69%), irrespective of HIV status.

A recent meta-analysis of six RCTs [10,131–135] evaluated the impact of multiple micronutrient supplementation on mortality and morbidity of HIV-infected adults living in developing countries [136]. The authors found a nonsignificant reduction in mortality and morbidity in subjects receiving supplementation (RR, 0.9; 95% CI, 0.8–1.02). However, sensitivity analysis revealed that micronutrient supplementation decreased mortality and morbidity of patients infected with HIV alone (RR, 0.75; 95% CI, 0.58–0.95) but had no favorable effects on patients coinfected with HIV and TB (RR, 0.97; 95% CI, 0.84–1.11). Coinfection with TB is likely to induce more severe immune dysfunctions and greater oxidative stress, which may not be reverted by micronutrient supplementation. Considering that TB and HIV epidemics largely overlap, these findings suggest the need for future research specifically evaluating the nutritional needs of individuals with HIV/TB coinfection.

16.10 CONCLUSIONS

Overall, our evidence review suggests that daily supplementation with multiple micronutrients is safe in HIV-infected subjects and may be associated with certain beneficial effects. For some micronutrients, especially vitamin A and iron, the safety of supplementation has been questioned.

In particular, maternal vitamin A supplementation has been associated with increased risk of HIV vertical transmission in one RCT, leading the authors to raise some concern about the use of universal maternal postpartum vitamin A supplements in countries with a high prevalence of HIV infection. However, there is evidence to indicate that vitamin A supplementation reduces mortality and morbidity of HIV-infected children. Analogously, zinc supplementation may help reduce diarrheal morbidity in children living with HIV in resource-limited settings [32].

Available trials generally used different combinations and doses of nutritional interventions, making it difficult to compare outcomes across studies. Future research should try to identify the most appropriate dosage of micronutrients. Studies assessing the effects of micronutrient supplementation often have a small sample size, resulting in limited statistical power, and a short follow-up, which does not allow proper assessment of the long-term effects of micronutrients. Future studies should better-evaluate the baseline immunological and nutritional status of participants, as well as the presence of coinfections, such as TB, which may significantly affect the clinical outcomes of RCTs of micronutrient supplementation. In addition, the special needs of children, pregnant women, and lactating women also require careful evaluation.

In conclusion, in resource-limited countries where the burden of HIV and malnutrition is still dramatic, poor nutritional status leads to decreased quality of life and increased HIV-associated mortality and morbidity. In this setting, micronutrient supplementation may represent a complementary intervention in the care of HIV-infected patients for whom wider access to HAART remains the mainstay to improve health and reduce the risk of HIV transmission.

References

[1] UNAIDS Global report 2013. Available at: <www.unaids.org/en/resources/campaigns/globalreport2013/globalreport/>.

[2] Nunnari G, Coco C, Pinzone MR, Pavone P, Berretta M, Di Rosa M, et al. The role of micronutrients in the diet of HIV-1-infected individuals. Front Biosci (Elite Ed) 2012;4:2442–56.

[3] Mora JR, Iwata M, von Andrian UH. Vitamin effects on the immune system: vitamins A and D take centre stage. Nat Rev Immunol 2008;8(9):685–98.

[4] Coutsoudis A, Kiepiela P, Coovadia HM, Broughton M. Vitamin A supplementation enhances specific IgG antibody levels and total lymphocyte numbers while improving morbidity in measles. Pediatr Infect Dis J 1992;11(3):203–9.

[5] Semba RD. The role of vitamin A and related retinoids in immune function. Nutr Rev 1998;56(1 Pt. 2):S38–48.

[6] Semba RD, Muhilal Scott AL, Natadisastra G, Wirasasmita S, Mele L, et al. Depressed immune response to tetanus in children with vitamin A deficiency. J Nutr 1992;122(1):101–7.

[7] Visser ME, Maartens G, Kossew G, Hussey GD. Plasma vitamin A and zinc levels in HIV-infected adults in Cape Town, South Africa. Br J Nutr 2003;89(4):475–82.
[8] Kelly P, Musonda R, Kafwembe E, Kaetano L, Keane E, Farthing M. Micronutrient supplementation in the AIDS diarrhoea-wasting syndrome in Zambia: a randomized controlled trial. AIDS 1999;13(4):495–500.
[9] Coutsoudis A, Moodley D, Pillay K, Harrigan R, Stone C, Moodley J, et al. Effects of vitamin A supplementation on viral load in HIV-1-infected pregnant women. J Acquir Immune Defic Syndr Hum Retrovirol 1997;15(1):86–7.
[10] Fawzi WW, Msamanga GI, Spiegelman D, Wei R, Kapiga S, Villamor E, et al. A randomized trial of multivitamin supplements and HIV disease progression and mortality. N Engl J Med 2004;351(1):23–32.
[11] Baeten JM, McClelland RS, Overbaugh J, Richardson BA, Emery S, Lavreys L, et al. Vitamin A supplementation and human immunodeficiency virus type 1 shedding in women: results of a randomized clinical trial. J Infect Dis 2002;185(8):1187–91.
[12] Moore PS, Allen S, Sowell AL, Van de Perre P, Huff DL, Serufilira A, et al. Role of nutritional status and weight loss in HIV seroconversion among Rwandan women. J Acquir Immune Defic Syndr 1993;6(6):611–6.
[13] Villamor E, Kapiga SH, Fawzi WW. Vitamin A serostatus and heterosexual transmission of HIV: case–control study in Tanzania and review of the evidence. Int J Vitam Nutr Res 2006;76(2):81–5.
[14] Mehendale SM, Shepherd ME, Brookmeyer RS, Semba RD, Divekar AD, Gangakhedkar RR, et al. Low carotenoid concentration and the risk of HIV seroconversion in Pune, India. J Acquir Immune Defic Syndr 2001;26(4):352–9.
[15] MacDonald KS, Malonza I, Chen DK, Nagelkerke NJ, Nasio JM, Ndinya-Achola J, et al. Vitamin A and risk of HIV-1 seroconversion among Kenyan men with genital ulcers. AIDS 2001;15(5):635–9.
[16] Semba RD, Miotti PG, Chiphangwi JD, Saah AJ, Canner JK, Dallabetta GA, et al. Maternal vitamin A deficiency and mother-to-child transmission of HIV-1. Lancet 1994;343(8913):1593–7.
[17] Greenberg BL, Semba RD, Vink PE, Farley JJ, Sivapalasingam M, Steketee RW, et al. Vitamin A deficiency and maternal–infant transmission of HIV in two metropolitan areas in the United States. AIDS 1997;11(3):325–32.
[18] Nduati RW, John GC, Richardson BA, Overbaugh J, Welch M, Ndinya-Achola J, et al. Human immunodeficiency virus type 1–infected cells in breast milk: association with immunosuppression and vitamin A deficiency. J Infect Dis 1995;172(6):1461–8.
[19] Coutsoudis A, Pillay K, Spooner E, Kuhn L, Coovadia HM. Randomized trial testing the effect of vitamin A supplementation on pregnancy outcomes and early mother-to-child HIV-1 transmission in Durban, South Africa. AIDS 1999;13(12):1517–24.
[20] Kumwenda N, Miotti PG, Taha TE, Broadhead R, Biggar RJ, Jackson JB, et al. Antenatal vitamin A supplementation increases birth weight and decreases anemia among infants born to human immunodeficiency virus–infected women in Malawi. Clin Infect Dis 2002;35(5):618–24.
[21] Fawzi WW, Msamanga GI, Hunter D, Renjifo B, Antelman G, Bang H, et al. Randomized trial of vitamin supplements in relation to transmission of HIV-1 through breastfeeding and early child mortality. AIDS 2002;16(14):1935–44.
[22] Fawzi WW, Msamanga G, Hunter D, Urassa E, Renjifo B, Mwakagile D, et al. Randomized trial of vitamin supplements in relation to vertical transmission of HIV-1 in Tanzania. J Acquir Immune Defic Syndr 2000;23(3):246–54.
[23] Humphrey JH, Iliff PJ, Marinda ET, Mutasa K, Moulton LH, Chidawanyika H, ZVITAMBO Study Group Effects of a single large dose of vitamin A, given during the postpartum period to HIV-positive women and their infants, on child HIV infection, HIV-free survival, and mortality. J Infect Dis 2006;193(6):860–71. [Erratum in: J Infect Dis 2008; 197(10): 1485].

[24] Turpin JA, Vargo M, Meltzer MS. Enhanced HIV-1 replication in retinoid-treated monocytes: retinoid effects mediated through mechanisms related to cell differentiation and to a direct transcriptional action on viral gene expression. J Immunol 1992;148(8):2539–46.
[25] Poli G, Kinter AL, Justement JS, Bressler P, Kehrl JH, Fauci AS. Retinoic acid mimics transforming growth factor b in the regulation of human immunodeficiency virus expression in monocytic cells. Proc Natl Acad Sci USA 1992;89(7):2689–93.
[26] Towers G, Harris J, Lang G, Collins MK, Latchman DS. Retinoic acid inhibits both the basal activity and phorbol ester-mediated activation of the HIV long terminal repeat promoter. AIDS 1995;9(2):129–36.
[27] Maciaszek JW, Coniglio SJ, Talmage DA, Viglianti GA. Retinoid-induced repression of human immunodeficiency virus type 1 core promoter activity inhibits virus replication. J Virol 1998;72(7):5862–9.
[28] Kiefer HL, Hanley TM, Marcello JE, Karthik AG, Viglianti GA. Retinoic acid inhibition of chromatin remodeling at the human immunodeficiency virus type 1 promoter. J Biol Chem 2004;279(42):43604–613.
[29] Fawzi WW, Mbise RL, Hertzmark E, Fataki MR, Herrera MG, Ndossi G, et al. A randomized trial of vitamin A supplements in relation to mortality among human immunodeficiency virus-infected and uninfected children in Tanzania. Pediatr Infect Dis J 1999;18(2):127–33.
[30] Semba RD, Ndugwa C, Perry RT, Clark TD, Jackson JB, Melikian G, et al. Effect of periodic vitamin A supplementation on mortality and morbidity of human immunodeficiency virus-infected children in Uganda: controlled clinical trial. Nutrition 2005;21(1):25–31.
[31] Coutsoudis A, Bobat RA, Coovadia HM, Kuhn L, Tsai W-Y, Stein ZA. The effects of vitamin A supplementation on the morbidity of children born to HIV-infected women. Am J Public Health 1995;85(8):1076–81.
[32] Irlam JH, Visser MME, Rollins NN, Siegfried N. Micronutrient supplementation in children and adults with HIV infection. Cochrane Database Syst Rev 2010:12. CD003650.
[33] Di Rosa M, Malaguarnera L, Nicolosi A, Sanfilippo C, Mazzarino C, Pavone P, et al. Vitamin D3: an ever green molecule. Front Biosci (Schol Ed) 2013;5:247–60.
[34] Pinzone MR, Di Rosa M, Malaguarnera M, Madeddu G, Focà E, Ceccarelli G, et al. Vitamin D deficiency in HIV infection: an underestimated and undertreated epidemic. Eur Rev Med Pharmacol Sci 2013;17(9):1218–32.
[35] Di Rosa M, Malaguarnera G, De Gregorio C, Palumbo M, Nunnari G, Malaguarnera L. Immuno-modulatory effects of vitamin D3 in human monocyte and macrophages. Cell Immunol 2012;280(1):36–43.
[36] Pinzone MR, Di Rosa M, Celesia BM, Condorelli F, Malaguarnera M, Madeddu G, et al. LPS and HIV gp120 modulate monocyte/macrophage CYP27B1 and CYP24A1 expression leading to vitamin D consumption and hypovitaminosis D in HIV-infected individuals. Eur Rev Med Pharmacol Sci 2013;17(14):1938–50.
[37] Dao CN, Patel P, Overton ET, Rhame F, Pals SL, Johnson C, the Study to Understand the Natural History of HIV and AIDS in the Era of Effective Therapy (SUN) Investigators Low vitamin D among HIV-infected adults: prevalence of and risk factors for low vitamin D levels in a cohort of HIV-infected adults and comparison to prevalence among adults in the US general population. Clin Infect Dis 2011;52(3):396–405.
[38] Viard JP, Souberbielle JC, Kirk O, Reekie J, Knysz B, Losso M, for the EuroSIDA Study Group Vitamin D and clinical disease progression in HIV infection: results from the EuroSIDA study. AIDS 2011;25(10):1305–15.
[39] Yin MT, Lu D, Cremers S, Tien PC, Cohen MH, Shi Q, et al. Short-term bone loss in HIV-infected premenopausal women. J Acquir Immune Defic Syndr 2010;53(2): 202–8.

[40] Brown T, McComsey G. Association between initiation of antiretroviral therapy with efavirenz and decreases in 25-hydroxyvitamin D. Antivir Ther 2010;15(3):425–9.
[41] Hariparsad N, Nallani SC, Sane RS, Buckley DJ, Buckley AR, Desai PB. Induction of CYP3A4 by efavirenz in primary human hepatocytes: comparison with rifampin and phenobarbital. J Clin Pharmacol 2004;44(11):1273–81.
[42] Welz T, Childs K, Ibrahim F, Poulton M, Taylor CB, Moniz CF, et al. Efavirenz is associated with severe vitamin D deficiency and increased alkaline phosphatase. AIDS 2010;24(12):1923–8.
[43] Fux CA, Baumann S, Furrer H, Mueller NJ. Is lower serum 25-hydroxy vitamin D associated with efavirenz or the non-nucleoside reverse transcriptase inhibitor class? AIDS 2011;25(6):876–8.
[44] Cozzolino M, Vidal M, Arcidiacono MV, Tebas P, Yarasheski KE, Dusso AS. HIV protease inhibitors impair vitamin D bioactivation to 1,25-dihydroxyvitamin D. AIDS 2003;17(4):513–20.
[45] Sudfeld CR, Wang M, Aboud S, Giovannucci EL, Mugusi FM, Fawzi WW. Vitamin D and HIV progression among Tanzanian adults initiating antiretroviral therapy. PLoS One 2012;7(6):e40036.
[46] Mehta S, Giovannucci E, Mugusi FM, Spiegelman D, Aboud S, Hertzmark E, et al. Vitamin D status of HIV-infected women and its association with HIV disease progression, anemia, and mortality. PLoS One 2010;5(1):e877.
[47] Mehta S, Mugusi FM, Spiegelman D, Villamor E, Finkelstein JL, Hertzmark E, et al. Vitamin D status and its association with morbidity including wasting and opportunistic illnesses in HIV-infected women in Tanzania. AIDS Patient Care STDS 2011;25(10):579–85.
[48] Mehta S, Hunter DJ, Mugusi FM, Spiegelman D, Manji KP, Giovannucci EL, et al. Perinatal outcomes, including mother-to-child transmission of HIV, and child mortality and their association with maternal vitamin D status in Tanzania. J Infect Dis 2009;200(7):1022–30.
[49] Mave V, Shere D, Gupte N, Suryavanshi N, Kulkarni V, Patil S, SWEN India and Byramjee-Jeejeebhoy Medical College Clinical Trials Unit Study Team Vitamin D deficiency is common among HIV-infected breastfeeding mothers in Pune, India, but is not associated with mother-to-child HIV transmission. HIV Clin Trials 2012;13(5):278–83.
[50] Wejse C, Gomes VF, Rabna P, Gustafson P, Aaby P, Lisse IM, et al. Vitamin D as supplementary treatment for tuberculosis, a double-blind, randomized, placebo-controlled trial. Am J Respir Crit Care Med 2009;179(9):843–50.
[51] Wang Y, Huang DS, Wood S, Watson RR. Modulation of immune function and cytokine production by various levels of vitamin E supplementation during murine AIDS. Immunopharmacology 1995;29(3):225–33.
[52] Meydani SN, Meydani M, Blumberg JB, Leka LS, Siber G, Loszewski R, et al. Vitamin E supplementation and *in vivo* immune response in healthy elderly subjects. A randomized controlled trial. JAMA 1997;277(17):1380–6.
[53] Bendich A. Antioxidant vitamins and immune responses. In: Chandra R, editor. Nutrition and immunology. New York, NY: Liss; 1988. pp. 125–47.
[54] Hemila H. Vitamin C and infectious diseases. In: Pacler L, Fuchs J, editors. Vitamin C in health and disease. New York, NY: Marcel Dekker; 1997. pp. 471–504.
[55] Baruchel S, Wainberg MA. The role of oxidative stress in disease progression in individuals infected by the human immunodeficiency virus. J Leukoc Biol 1992;52(1):111–4.
[56] Matsuyama T, Kobayashi N, Yamamoto N. Cytokines and HIV infection: Is AIDS a tumor necrosis factor disease? AIDS 1991;5(12):1405–7.
[57] Duh EJ, Maury WJ, Folks TM, Fauci AS, Rabson AB. Tumor necrosis factor alpha activates human immunodeficiency virus type 1 through induction of nuclear factor binding to the NF-kB sites in the long terminal repeat. Proc Natl Acad Sci USA 1989;86(15):5974–8.

[58] Packer L, Suzuki Y. Vitamin E and alphalipoate: role in antioxidant recycling and activation of the NF-kB transcription factor. Mol Aspects Med 1993;14(3):229–39.

[59] Bowie AG, O'Neill LA. Vitamin C inhibits NF-κB activation by TNF via the activation of p38 mitogen-activated protein kinase. J Immunol 2000;165(12):180–8.

[60] Perez-Cruz I, Carcamo JM, Golde DW. Vitamin C inhibits FAS-induced apoptosis in monocytes and U937 cells. Blood 2003;102(1):336–43.

[61] Saitoh Y, Ouchida R, Kayasuga A, Miwa N. Antiapoptotic defense of bcl-2 gene against hydroperoxide-induced cytotoxicity together with suppressed lipid peroxidation, enhanced ascorbate uptake, and upregulated Bcl-2 protein. J Cell Biochem 2003;89(2):321–34.

[62] Mburu S, Marnewick JL, Abayomi A, Ipp H. Modulation of LPS-induced CD4+ T-cell activation and apoptosis by antioxidants in untreated asymptomatic HIV infected participants: an *in vitro* study. Clin Dev Immunol 2013;2013:631063.

[63] Beach RS, Mantero-Atienza E, Shor-Posner G, Javier JJ, Szapocznik J, Morgan R, et al. Specific nutrient abnormalities in asymptomatic HIV-1 infection. AIDS 1992;6(7):701–8.

[64] Allard JP, Aghdassi E, Chau J, Tam C, Kovacs CM, Salit IE, et al. Effects of vitamin E and C supplementation on oxidative stress and viral load in HIV-infected subjects. AIDS 1998;12(13):1653–9.

[65] Tang AM, Graham NM, Semba RD, Saah AJ. Association between serum vitamin A and E levels and HIV-1 disease progression. AIDS 1997;11(5):613–20.

[66] Meydani SN, Ribaya-Mercado JD, Russell RM, Sahyoun N, Morrow FD, Gershoff SN. Vitamin B-6 deficiency impairs interleukin 2 production and lymphocyte proliferation in elderly adults. Am J Clin Nutr 1991;53(5):1275–80.

[67] Bendich A, Cohen M. B vitamins: effects on specific and nonspecific immune responses. Chandra R, editor. Nutrition and immunology. New York, NY: Liss; 1988. pp. 101–23.

[68] Burkes RL, Cohen H, Krailo M, Sinow RM, Carmel R. Low serum cobalamin levels occur frequently in the acquired immune deficiency syndrome and related disorders. Eur J Haematol 1987;38(2):141–7.

[69] Herbert V, Jacobson J, Shevchuk O, Fong W, Stopler T, Castellar L, et al. Vitamin B12, folate and lithium in AIDS. Clin Res 1989;37(2):594A.

[70] Coodley GO, Coodley MK, Nelson HD, Loveless MO. Micronutrient concentrations in the HIV wasting syndrome. AIDS 1993;7(12):1595–600.

[71] Herzlich BC, Ranginwala M, Nawabi I, Herbert V. Synergy of inhibition of DNA synthesis in human bone marrow by azidothymidine plus deficiency of folate and/or vitamin B12? Am J Hematol 1990;33(3):177–83.

[72] Baum MK, Shor-Posner G, Lu Y, Rosner B, Sauberlich HE, Fletcher MA, et al. Micronutrients and HIV-1 disease progression. AIDS 1995;9(9):1051–6.

[73] Kieburtz KD, Giang DW, Schiffer RB, Vakil N. Abnormal vitamin B12 metabolism in human immunodeficiency virus infection. Association with neurological dysfunction. Arch Neurol 1991;48(3):312–4.

[74] Remacha AF, Riera A, Cadafalch J, Gimferrer E. Vitamin B12 abnormalities in HIV-infected patients. Eur J Haematol 1991;47(1):60–4.

[75] Baum MK, Mantero-Atienza E, Shor-Posner G, Fletcher MA, Morgan R, Eisdorfer C, et al. Association of vitamin B6 status with parameters of immune function in early HIV-1 infection. J Acquir Immune Defic Syndr 1991;4(11):1122–32.

[76] Tang AM, Graham NMH, Chandra RK, Saah AJ. Low serum vitamin B-12 concentrations are associated with faster human immunodeficiency virus type 1 (HIV-1) disease progression. J Nutr 1997;127(2):345–51.

[77] Chatterjee A, Bosch RJ, Hunter DJ, Manji K, Msamanga GI, Fawzi WW. Vitamin A and vitamin B-12 concentrations in relation to mortality and morbidity among children born to HIV-infected women. J Trop Pediatr 2010;56(1):27–35.

[78] Semeere AS, Nakanjako D, Ddungu H, Kambugu A, Manabe YC, Colebunders R. Suboptimal vitamin B-12 levels among ART-naïve HIV-positive individuals in an urban cohort in Uganda. PLoS One 2012;7(7):e40072.
[79] Prasad AS. Clinical, immunological, anti-inflammatory and antioxidant roles of zinc. Exp Gerontol 2008;43(5):370–7.
[80] Beck FW, Prasad AS, Kaplan J, Fitzgerald JT, Brewer GJ. Changes in cytokine production and T cell subpopulations in experimentally induced zinc-deficient humans. Am J Physiol 1997;272(6):E1002–7.
[81] Prasad AS, Meftah S, Abdallah J, Kaplan J, Brewer GJ, Bach JF, et al. Serum thymulin in human zinc deficiency. J Clin Invest 1988;82(4):1202–10.
[82] Hoque KM, Binder HJ. Zinc in the treatment of acute diarrhea: current status and assessment. Gastroenterology 2006;130(7):2201–5.
[83] Fleiger D, Reithmuller G, Ziegler-Heitbrock HWL. Zn^{2+} inhibits both tumor necrosis factor-mediated DNA fragmentation and cytolysis. Int J Cancer 1989;44(2):315–9.
[84] Zhang Z, Reardon IM, Hui JO, O'Connell KL, Poorman RA, Tomasselli AG, et al. Zinc inhibition of renin and the protease from human immunodeficiency virus type 1. Biochemistry 1991;30(36):8717–21.
[85] Zheng R, Jenkins TM, Craigie R. Zinc folds the N-terminal domain of HIV-1 integrase, promotes multimerization, and enhances catalytic activity. Proc Natl Acad Sci USA 1996;93(24):13659–64.
[86] Graham NM, Sorensen D, Odaka N, Brookmeyer R, Chan D, Willett WC, et al. Relationship of serum copper and zinc levels to HIV-1 seropositivity and progression to AIDS. J Acquir Immune Defic Syndr 1991;4(10):976–80.
[87] Baum MK, Campa A, Lai S, Lai H, Page JB. Zinc status in human immunodeficiency virus type 1 infection and illicit drug use. Clin Infect Dis 2003;37(S2):S117–23.
[88] Abrams B, Duncan D, Hertz-Picciotto I. A prospective study of dietary intake and acquired immune deficiency syndrome in HIV-seropositive homosexual men. J Acquir Immune Defic Syndr 1993;6(8):949–58.
[89] Tang AM, Graham NM, Kirby AJ, McCall LD, Willett WC, Saah AJ. Dietary micronutrient intake and risk of progression to acquired immunodeficiency syndrome (AIDS) in human immuno-deficiency virus type 1 (HIV-1)-infected homosexual men. Am J Epidemiol 1993;138(11):937–51.
[90] Tang AM, Graham NM, Saah AJ. Effects of micronutrient intake on survival in human immunodeficiency virus type 1 infection. Am J Epidemiol 1996;143(12):1244–56.
[91] Fawzi WW, Villamor E, Msamanga GI, Antelman G, Aboud S, Urassa W, et al. Trial of zinc supplements in relation to pregnancy outcomes, hematologic indicators, and T cell counts among HIV-1-infected women in Tanzania. Am J Clin Nutr 2005;81(1):161–7.
[92] Lodha R, Shah N, Mohari N, Mukherjee A, Vajpayee M, Singh R, et al. Immunologic effect of zinc supplementation in HIV-infected children receiving highly active antiretroviral therapy: a randomized, double-blind, placebo-controlled trial. J Acquir Immune Defic Syndr 2014;66(4):386–92.
[93] Bobat R, Coovadia H, Stephen C, Naidoo KL, McKerrow N, Black RE, et al. Safety and efficacy of zinc supplementation for children with HIV-1 infection in South Africa: a randomised double-blind placebo controlled trial. Lancet 2005;366(9500):1862–7.
[94] Carcamo C, Hooton T, Weiss NS, Gilman R, Wener MH, Chavez V, et al. Randomized controlled trial of zinc supplementation for persistent diarrhea in adults with HIV-1 infection. J Acquir Immune Defic Syndr 2006;43(2):197–201.
[95] Baum MK, Lai S, Sales S, Page JB, Campa A. Randomized, controlled clinical trial of zinc supplementation to prevent immunological failure in HIV-infected adults. Clin Infect Dis 2010;50(12):1653–60.
[96] Kiremidjian-Schumacher L, Stotzky G. Selenium and immune responses. Environ Res 1987;42(2):277–303.

[97] Poli G, Fauci AS. The effect of cytokines and pharmacological agents on chronic HIV infection. AIDS Res Hum Retroviruses 1992;8(2):191–7.

[98] Sappey C, Legrand-Poels S, Best-Belpomme M, Favier A, Rentier B, Piette J. Stimulation of glutathione peroxidase activity decreases HIV type 1 activation after oxidative stress. AIDS Res Hum Retroviruses 1994;10(11):1451–61.

[99] Taylor EW, Nadimpalli RG, Ramanathan CS. Genomic structures of viral agents in relation to the biosynthesis of selenoproteins. Biol Trace Elem Res 1997;56(1):63–91.

[100] Romero-Alvira D, Roche E. The keys of oxidative stress in acquired immune deficiency syndrome apoptosis. Med Hypotheses 1998;51(2):169–73.

[101] Hori K, Hatfield D, Maldarelli F, Lee BJ, Clouse KA. Selenium supplementation suppresses tumor necrosis factor alpha-induced human immunodeficiency virus type 1 replication *in vitro*. AIDS Res Hum Retroviruses 1997;13(15):1325–32.

[102] Baum MK, Shor-Posner G, Lai S, Zhang G, Lai H, Fletcher MA, et al. High risk of HIV-related mortality is associated with selenium deficiency. J Acquir Immune Defic Syndr Hum Retrovirol 1997;15(5):370–4.

[103] Kupka R, Msamanga GI, Spiegelman D, Morris S, Mugusi F, Hunter DJ, et al. Selenium status is associated with accelerated HIV disease progression among HIV-1-infected pregnant women. J Nutr 2004;134(10):2556–60.

[104] Kupka R, Garland M, Msamanga GI, Spiegelman D, Hunter D, Fawzi WW. Selenium status, pregnancy outcomes and mother-to-child transmission of HIV-1. J Acquir Immune Defic Syndr 2005;39(2):203–10.

[105] Twagirumukiza M, Nkeramihigo E, Seminega B, Gasakure E, Boccara F, Barbaro G. Prevalence of dilated cardiomyopathy in HIV-infected African patients not receiving HAART: a multicenter, observational, prospective, cohort study in Rwanda. Curr HIV Res 2007;5(1):129–37.

[106] Kupka R, Msamanga GI, Xu C, Anderson D, Hunter D, Fawzi WW. Relationship between plasma selenium levels and lower genital tract levels of HIV-1 RNA and interleukin 1-B. Eur J Clin Nutr 2007;61(4):542–7.

[107] Villamor E, Msamanga G, Spiegelman D, Peterson KE, Antelman G, Fawzi WW. Pattern and predictors of weight gain during pregnancy among HIV-1-infected women from Tanzania. J Acquir Immune Defic Syndr 2003;32(5):560–9.

[108] Burbano X, Miguez-Burbano MJ, McCollister K, Zhang G, Rodriguez A, Ruiz P, et al. Impact of a selenium chemoprevention clinical trial on hospital admissions of HIV-infected participants. HIV Clin Trials 2002;3(6):483–91.

[109] Hurwitz BE, Klaus JR, Llabre MM, Gonzalez A, Lawrence PJ, Maher KJ, et al. Suppression of human immunodeficiency virus type 1 viral load with selenium supplementation: a randomized controlled trial. Arch Intern Med 2007;167(2):148–54.

[110] Kupka R, Mugusi F, Aboud S, Msamanga GI, Finkelstein JL, Spiegelman D, et al. Randomized, double-blind, placebo-controlled trial of selenium supplements among HIV-infected pregnant women in Tanzania: effects on maternal and child outcomes. Am J Clin Nutr 2008;87(6):1802–8.

[111] Kupka R, Mugusi F, Aboud S, Hertzmark E, Spiegelman D, Fawzi WW. Effect of selenium supplements on hemoglobin and morbidity among HIV-infected Tanzanian women. Clin Infect Dis 2009;48(10):1475–8.

[112] UNICEF/WHO/UNU. Iron deficiency anaemic—assessment, prevention, and control. A guide for programme Managers. Available at: <http://www.who.int/nutrition/publications/en/ida_assessment_prevention_control.pdf>; 2001.

[113] Adetifa I, Okomo U. Iron supplementation for reducing morbidity and mortality in children with HIV. Cochrane Database Syst Rev 2009:1. CD006736.

[114] Esan MO, van Hensbroek MB, Nkhoma E, Musicha C, White SA, Ter Kuile FO, et al. Iron supplementation in HIV-infected Malawian children with anemia: a double-blind, randomized, controlled trial. Clin Infect Dis 2013;57(11):1626–34.

[115] Nsanzabana C, Rosenthal PJ. *In vitro* activity of antiretroviral drugs against plasmodium falciparum. Antimicrob Agents Chemother 2011;55(11):5073–7.
[116] Achan J, Kakuru A, Ikilezi G, Ruel T, Clark TD, Nsanzabana C, et al. Antiretroviral agents and prevention of malaria in HIV-infected Ugandan children. N Engl J Med 2012;367(22):2110–8.
[117] Boelaert JR, Weinberg GA, Weinberg ED. Altered iron metabolism in HIV infection: mechanisms, possible consequences, and proposals for management. Infect Agents Dis 1996;5(1):36–46.
[118] Savarino A, Pescarmona GP, Boelaert JR. Iron metabolism and HIV infection:reciprocal interactions with potentially harmful consequences? Cell Biochem Funct 1999;17(4):279–87.
[119] Salmon-Ceron D, Fontbonne A, Saba J. Lower survival in AIDS patients receiving dapsone compared with aerosolized pentamidine for secondary prophylaxis of *Pneumocystis carinii* pneumonia. J Infect Dis 1995;172(3):656–64.
[120] De Monye C, Karcher DS, Boelaert JR, Gordeux VR. Bone marrow macrophage iron grade and survival of HIVseropositive patients. AIDS 1999;13(3):375–80.
[121] Costagliola DG, Montalembert M, Lefrere JJ, Briand C, Rebulla P, Baruchel S, et al. Dose of deferroxamine and evolution of HIV-1 infection in thalassaemic patients. Br J Haematol 1994;87(4):849–52.
[122] Delanghe JR, Langlois MR, Boelaert JR, Van Acker J, Van Wanzeele F, van der Groen G, et al. Haptoglobin polymorphism, iron metabolism and mortality in HIV infection. AIDS 1998;12(9):1027–32.
[123] Sahli Y, Castagliola D, Rebulla P, Dessi C, Karagiorga M, Lena-Russo D, et al. Serum ferritin, desferrioxamine, and evolution of HIV-1 infection in thalassemic patients. J Acquir Immune Defic Syndr Hum Retrovirol 1998;18(5):473–8.
[124] Bozzette SA, Finkelstein DM, Spector SA, Frame P, Powderly WG, He W, et al. Randomized trial of three antipneumocystis agents in patients with advanced human immunodeficiency virus infection. NIAID AIDS clinical trials group. N Engl J Med 1995;332(11):693–9.
[125] Georgiou NA, van der Bruggen T, Oudshoorn M, Nottet HS, Marx JJ, van Asbeck BS. Inhibition of human immunodeficiency virus type 1 replication in human mononuclear blood cells by the iron chelators deferoxime, deferiprone, and bleomycin. J Infect Dis 2000;181(2):484–90.
[126] Semba RD, Ricketts EP, Mehta S, Netski D, Thomas D, Kirk G, et al. Effect of micronutrients and iron supplementation on hemoglobin, iron status, and plasma hepatitis C and HIV RNA levels in female injection drug users: a controlled clinical trial. J Acquir Immune Defic Syndr 2007;45(3):298–303.
[127] Olsen A, Mwaniki D, Krarup H, Friis H. Low-dose iron supplementation does not increase HIV-1 load. J Acquir Immune Defic Syndr 2004;36(1):637–8.
[128] Fawzi WW, Msamanga GI, Spiegelman D, Urassa EJ, McGrath N, Mwakagile D, et al. Randomised trial of effects of vitamin supplements on pregnancy outcomes and T cell counts in HIV-1-infected women in Tanzania. Lancet 1998;351(9114):1477–82.
[129] Villamor E, Fawzi WW. Effects of vitamin a supplementation on immune responses and correlation with clinical outcomes. Clin Microbiol Rev 2005;18(3):446–64.
[130] McClelland RS, Baeten JM, Overbaugh J, Richardson BA, Mandaliya K, Emery S, et al. Micronutrient supplementation increases genital tract shedding of HIV-1 in women: results of a randomized trial. J Acquir Immune Defic Syndr 2004;37(5):1657–63.
[131] Jiamton S, Pepin J, Suttent R, Filteau S, Mahakkanukrauh B, Hanshaoworakul W, et al. A randomized trial of the impact of multiple micronutrient supplementation on mortality among HIV-infected individuals living in Bangkok. AIDS 2003;17(17):2461–9.
[132] Kelly P, Katubulushi M, Todd J, Banda R, Yambayamba V, Fwoloshi M, et al. Micronutrient supplementation has limited effects on intestinal infectious disease

and mortality in a Zambian population of mixed HIV status: a cluster randomized trial. Am J Clin Nutr 2008;88(4):1010–7.

[133] Range N, Changalucha J, Krarup H, Magnussen P, Andersen AB, Friis H. The effect of multi-vitamin/mineral supplementation on mortality during treatment of pulmonary tuberculosis: a randomised two-by-two factorial trial in Mwanza, Tanzania. Br J Nutr 2006;95(4):762–70.

[134] Semba RD, Kumwenda J, Zijlstra E, Ricks MO, van Lettow M, Whalen C, et al. Micronutrient supplements and mortality of HIV-infected adults with pulmonary TB: a controlled clinical trial. Int J Tuberc Lung Dis 2007;11(8):854–9.

[135] Villamor E, Mugusi F, Urassa W, Bosch RJ, Saathoff E, Matsumoto K, et al. A trial of the effect of micronutrient supplementation on treatment outcome, T cell counts, morbidity, and mortality in adults with pulmonary tuberculosis. J Infect Dis 2008;197(11):1499–505.

[136] Jiang S, He J, Zhao X, Li H. The effect of multiple micronutrient supplementation on mortality and morbidity of HIV-infected adults: a meta-analysis of randomized controlled trials. J Nutr Sci Vitaminol 2012;58(2):105–12.

SECTION III

EXERCISE AND BEHAVIORAL LIFESTYLE CHANGES IN THE PREVENTION AND TREATMENT OF HIV/AIDS NUTRITIONAL CHANGES

CHAPTER

17

Exercise and Management of Body Weight in Older People Living with HIV

Anella Yahiaoui and Joachim G. Voss

University of Washington, School of Nursing, Biobehavioral Nursing and Health Systems, Seattle, WA, USA

17.1 INTRODUCTION

In 2015, of the 1.1 million people living with HIV (PLWH) in the United States, approximately 50% will be age 50 years or older [1]. This cohort of older people living with HIV (OPLWH) has been HIV-infected for up to two to three decades, has experienced many medication regimens, and survived what was previously deemed a deadly disease. The advent of antiretroviral therapy (ART) has been instrumental in increasing the longevity of people living with the virus, which ultimately transformed the once deadly disease into a manageable chronic illness. However, ARTs also have a number of side effects and symptoms that often impact an individual's physical and psychological functioning and quality of life [2]. Table 17.1 illustrates the effect of various ARTs on lipid levels.

Because PLWH live longer with their disease, they experience the onset of age-related chronic conditions, such as cardiovascular disease (CD), cancer, metabolic effects, and physical declines such as pulmonary, muscle, and cognitive functions, with decreasing strength and increases in body weight and sedentary behavior [4]. Today, we have substantial knowledge that HIV infection may alter the biology of aging so that individuals may experience premature manifestations associated with aging,

Health of HIV Infected People, Volume 2.
DOI: http://dx.doi.org/10.1016/B978-0-12-800767-9.00017-0

TABLE 17.1 Lipid–Drug Interaction

Antiretroviral	Total cholesterol	LDL-C	HDL-C	Triglycerides
PIS				
Lopinavir	++	++	⇔/−	+++
Atazanavir	+	⇔/+	⇔/−	⇔
Fosamprenavir	+	+	⇔/−	++
Saquinavir	++	++	⇔/−	+
NRTIS				
Tenofovir	⇔/+	⇔/ +	⇔/ +	⇔/+
Abacavir	⇔/+	+	+	+
Lamivudine	⇔	⇔	⇔	⇔
Zidovudine	+	+	+	++
Stavudine	++	++	+	++
NNRTIS				
Efavirenz	+	+	+	+
Nevirapine	+	+	++	⇔/+

Source: Feeney and Mallon [3].

such as immunoscenesence, and higher rates of metabolic syndrome and obesity [5,6]. Furthermore, virus and drug-induced metabolic effects in OPLWH can drastically change an individual's body weight, which may be further exacerbated by ART medications.

Providers, patients, and the advertising industry agree on one fact: increasing the time to perform daily and weekly physical activity is a major factor in maintaining body weight, improving body composition, and strengthening cardiovascular fitness. A number of research studies have demonstrated that increasing physical activity has positive influences on the prevention and management of chronic illnesses in the younger HIV population [7–13]. Studies have shown that moderate exercise can improve immune functions, improve cardiovascular fitness, lower type 2 diabetes (T2D) incidence, and lower incidence of developing metabolic syndrome [6,14–17]. However, we know little about the effects of aerobic and resistance exercise in OPLWH on body composition, obesity, dyslipidemia, glucose uptake, insulin resistance, metabolic syndrome, and diabetes.

17.2 BACKGROUND

17.2.1 Body Composition

Excess body weight has been found to cause a number of physical changes that have detrimental long-term effects. As more calories are added to a person's diet that can be burned in a 24-hour period, the body tries to store these extra calories in the form of fat in the abdominal subcutaneous fat [18]. In times of food scarcity, those deposits would be beneficial and used to provide the body with energy and sustenance.

PLWH have unique challenges with ARTs and their effects of altering fat metabolism. More than 50% of HIV-infected patients experience abnormal fat redistribution when using ARTs [19–21]. The disorder, known as lipodystrophy syndrome, results from the redistribution of adipose tissue from the periphery to central deposits. This leads to atrophy of subcutaneous tissue (in the arms and legs) and hypertrophy of visceral tissue with accumulation of fat in the neck and shoulders, known as "buffalo hump" [22]. The pathophysiologic mechanisms that cause body fat changes in HIV also lead to changes in cellular metabolism, which result in ectopic visceral fat deposition [23,24]. Evidence shows distinct transcriptional and metabolic differences between visceral and subcutaneous fat [25,26] and suggests that visceral fat may be resistant to the wasting effect of nucleoside reverse-transcriptase inhibitors (NRTIs) and protease inhibitors (PIs).

A study by Samaras et al. [27] found that inflammatory markers may lead to an increase in body composition abnormalities. The authors examined circulating inflammatory molecules in treated HIV-infected men versus insulin-resistant obese men and found that C-reactive protein (CRP) levels were similar between the two groups, with higher CRP in HIV-treated participants with lipoatrophy. Furthermore, HIV-treated subjects with higher CRP also had significantly higher total cholesterol, visceral adipose tissue, and intramyocellular lipid than the insulin-resistant obese men, despite having lower body fat and body mass index (BMI).

Research has shown that newer combination ART medications have attenuated many of the metabolic challenges experienced with older drugs [28], but problems continue to arise, posing a higher risk of comorbidities and frailty in OPLWH [29]. The occurrence of some treatment-related toxicities such as lipodystrophy have not shown a particularly significant improvement over time. A 2001 study by Hadigan et al. [30] tested various metabolic variables in PLWH with and without lipodystrophy compared with age- and BMI-matched HIV-negative controls also with and without lipodystrophy. The authors reported that PLWH with lipodystrophy were far more likely than the control subjects to have impaired glucose tolerance (IGT) (52% versus 5.2%), fasting insulin levels more than 18 μU/mL (26.5% versus 6.1%), triglyceride levels more than 200 mg/dL

(57.1% versus 8.9%), and HDL levels less than 35 mg/dL (45.7% versus 16.9%). Interestingly, there was no difference in results for insulin, cholesterol, triglyceride, and LDL between PLWH with no lipodystrophy and control subjects. Along the same lines, the HIV-positive lipodystrophy group had much higher metabolic risks than the HIV-positive group without lipodystrophy (35.2% versus 5.6% IGT; 26.5% versus 3.5% insulin level >18 μU/mL; 57.1% versus 16.7% cholesterol level; 57.1 versus 13.3% triglyceride level >200 mg/dL).

In 2014, Dragovic et al. [31] followed-up 840 HIV/AIDS patients who were commencing treatment between 2001 and 2010 for a mean period of 5.6 ± 2.8 years. During that time, they found the prevalence of lipodystrophy among the subjects to be 69.2%. Furthermore, they estimated the probability of developing lipodystrophy in the cohort increased with time, reaching 100% after 10 years of ART treatment [31].

During the pre-ART era, studies showed a high level of wasting syndrome, which was associated with shorter survival rates [32]. The incidence of wasting per 1,000 person-years increased from 7.5 between 1988 and 1990, to 22.1 between 1994 and 1995, and decreased again to 13.4 between 1996 and 1999, the initial years of ART [33]. In today's patient population, we can see less PLWH with wasting syndrome and many more PLWH struggling with HIV-associated overweight and obesity [34,35]. Although limited statistical data exist regarding the prevalence of wasting syndrome today, the dramatic decline is evident in a retrospective study conducted by Crum-Cianflone et al. [36] at two Navy HIV clinics between 2004 and 2005 to analyze the prevalence of overweight/obesity over approximately 10 years. On comparing the weight of participants at diagnoses versus the last clinic visit (mean time of 9.6 years), they found that 63% were overweight or obese compared with 54% at baseline. The authors also noted that 72% of participants gained weight (mean, 9.7 lb) over the course of 11 years (mean). Meanwhile, only 1% of the HIV-infected cohort was found to be underweight (BMI < 18.5). Three major physical problems accompany the increase in overweight/obesity, dyslipidemia, impaired glucose uptake, and insulin resistance, resulting in metabolic syndrome, which most likely leads to DM2.

17.2.1.1 Knowledge Gaps

Although more recent findings have shown that NNRTI-based therapy is less likely to result in lipodystrophy than NRTI or PI therapy [31], treatment toxicities continue to be a significant concern. Very few treatment options exist for treating lipodystrophy in PLWH due to a limited understanding of pathogenesis of adipose tissue function. Researchers are currently working to find novel therapies that are both potent and less toxic for individuals through the use of mouse models [37] and various drug combinations.

With obesity increasing among PLWH, lipohypertrophy, the accumulation of fat at the surface of the skin, is becoming a more common occurrence, creating a need for more research and therapeutic development in this area. Numerous studies cite the harmful effects of ARTs on body composition, but very few have looked at alternative methods of managing these metabolic abnormalities, such as diet and exercise.

17.2.2 Obesity

HIV-associated obesity is the abnormal redistribution of fat in the body, including increased trunk fat, and accumulation of fat in the dorsocervial region [38]. PLWH have significantly greater amounts of abdominal fat compared with age-matched HIV-uninfected individuals [39,40].

A study by Lakey et al. [35] found a 27% relative increase in overweight/obesity in the first 12 months of initial ART in HIV-infected participants, and they found no significant change in the HIV-seronegative control group. Another study conducted in Philadelphia looked at the intersection between obesity and HIV infection and concluded that although some HIV-infected patients are afflicted with wasting, obesity has become a more significant issue within the population, especially among women [34]. They found a positive correlation of BMI with elevated cholesterol, triglyceride, and glucose levels, which suggest an increased prevalence of metabolic syndrome in the overweight population. This evidence further suggests that obesity may also contribute to dyslipidemia and insulin resistance in PLWH.

Obesity is often linked to frailty and accelerated aging in the general population [41–43]. This makes obese OPLWH even more vulnerable for functional decline, as shown in a study of community-dwelling OPLWH [44]. This study found an association between greater fat mass and higher BMI with frailty and functional impairment in OPLWH. The authors concluded that central obesity and fat redistribution are important predictors of frailty in OPLWH, and that exercise and diet therapy may aid in decreasing frailty in this population.

17.2.2.1 Knowledge Gaps

Despite the evidence for an increase in obesity in the HIV population, many questions continue to be unanswered. Inconsistencies found in the current literature are common and must be addressed. For example, Lakey et al. [35] found that PI-based combination ART was associated with significantly higher weight gain than non PI-based treatment, a finding not consistent with the work of Amorosa et al. [34] and Crum-Cianflone et al. [32]. More research is necessary to elucidate the risk factors for weight gain and obesity associated with the type of ART used, as well as preventative steps that may be taken to reduce weight gain among PLWH.

In addition, women have been shown to have a higher prevalence of obesity than men, but more research is needed to study this gender gap and the variability in response to HIV infection and ART treatment in relation to risk factors. Little is known regarding how changes in body composition such as central obesity accelerate the incidence of frailty in OPLWH [44]. Further knowledge of what roles diet and exercise play in decreasing or preventing this occurrence would be very beneficial.

17.2.3 Dyslipidemia

Dyslipidemia is defined as having a high plasma triglyceride concentration, low high-density lipoprotein cholesterol (HDL-C) concentration, and decreased concentration of low-density lipoprotein cholesterol (LDL-C) [45]. Table 17.2 provides a range of optimal and nonoptimal lipid levels.

Changes in blood lipid levels have been described for more than a decade and are associated with PIs, which affect human adipose tissue and insulin resistance, and may contribute to the development of lipodystrophy and metabolic syndrome in PLWH [19,46–49]. The prevalence of dyslipidemia in PLWH using combination ART varies from 30% to 80% depending on the type of drug and definition criteria for diagnosis, with the most common being hypertriglyceridemia (40–80%) and hypercholesterolemia (10–50%) [47,50–52]. Many PIs lead to an increase in circulating triglyceride levels by impairing adipocyte differentiation and decreasing triglyceride accumulation in adipocytes [21,53,54]. An increase in triglycerides is often the most prominent lipid abnormality in PLWH and it appears to contribute independently to increased cardiovascular risk [21].

In the Multicenter AIDS Cohort Study (MACS), HIV-infected participants showed an increase in total cholesterol and LDL-C levels, and low HDL-C levels after initiation of ART [55]. Similarly, results from the Swiss HIV Cohort Study found PIs to be associated with an increase in total cholesterol and triglycerides [56]. In the Data Collection on Adverse Events of Anti-HIV Drugs (DAD) study, the authors found a 17% increase in the risk of myocardial infarction with each two-fold increase in triglyceride levels [57].

17.2.3.1 Knowledge Gaps

Dyslipidemia remains a challenging metabolic condition to treat and prevent in PLWH.

Although PIs have been linked with changing lipid profiles in PLWH, there is great variability in dyslipidemia outcomes within the different types of PIs. Lipid-lowering drugs such as statins are also useful in altering lipoprotein and triglyceride levels but may have negative interactions with many PIs, leading to high levels of statins in the body [58]. Combination therapies such as niacin and fish oils have been found to be effective in managing dyslipidemia [59,60], but more knowledge of the

TABLE 17.2 ATP III Classification of LDL, HDL-C, Total-C, Triglycerides (mg/dL)

LDL-C	
<100	Optimal
100–129	Near optimal/above optimal
130–159	Borderline high
160–189	High
≥190	Very high
HDL-C	
<40	Low
≥60	High
TOTAL CHOLESTEROL	
<200	Desirable
200–239	Borderline high
≥240	High
TRIGLYCERIDES	
<150	Normal
150–199	Borderline high
299–499	High
≥500	Very high

mechanisms involving dyslipidemia is necessary to provide the proper treatments targeted for each individual.

Additionally, we do not have sufficient information about how gender and ethnicity may alter lipid effects in different individuals. A 2002 study by Kumar and Thompson [61] found that black participants were more likely to have increased LDL-C levels compared with white or Hispanic patients, whereas Hispanic subjects had more significant levels of triglycerides. They also found that women were more likely than men to develop higher LDL-C levels. Very few studies within the past few years have measured similar gender and ethnicity outcomes, and more studies are warranted to provide better recommendations and care to all PLWH.

17.2.4 Glucose Uptake and Insulin Resistance

Abnormality in insulin–glucose function is common in PLWH, with estimates of diabetes mellitus (DM) prevalence in ART-naïve people being

3% and that in people with highly active ART being 10% [28]. Fasting glucose levels more than 126 mg/dL and 2-h plasma levels higher than 200 mg/dL generally indicate a diagnosis for diabetes [62]. There are numerous mechanisms by which ART may impair glucose function in PLWH, especially NRTIs and PIs [63,64]. NRTIs include drugs such as stavudine and zidovudine, which inhibit DNA polymerase-γ during mitochondrial replication, and may ultimately lead to mitochondrial dysfunction [65]. When this occurs, the inability of the muscle and liver to oxidize fat leads to lipotoxic insulin resistance [66].

Murata et al. [46] have shown that PIs selectively block the function of the glucose transporter 4 (Glut4), which impairs glucose signaling in muscle and adipose tissue. Glut4 activation by insulin is significant for glucose storage in muscle fat after a meal [67]. Therapeutic levels of PIs are also demonstrated to alter glucose sensing by beta-cells, causing impairment in insulin release [68].

Furthermore, a study by Brown et al. [69] found a link between inflammatory markers (including CRP and tumor necrosis factor receptors 1 and 2) and the development of diabetes in HIV infection, which suggests the role of chronic inflammation in impairing glucose metabolism [21]. Adipocytokines also play a significant role in glucose regulation. Adiponectin, an abundant protein secreted by adipocytes, is known to improve insulin sensitivity, increase cell survival through the regulation of glucose and lipid metabolism, and increase fatty acid oxidation [22,24]. In a study by Vigouroux et al. [70], low plasma adiponectin concentrations were linked with insulin resistance and metabolic alterations in HIV-infected males receiving PIs.

17.2.4.1 Knowledge Gaps

Treatment of glucose disorders in PLWH is a challenging feat. Knowledge of the intricate mechanisms involved in treating these disorders is limited. PIs have been shown to increase insulin resistance in PLWH, but more research is necessary to see if potential ART combinations could change this. We must also gain a better understanding of how mitochondrial dysfunction affects metabolism in PLWH, and how targeting this would impact metabolic function. Uncovering these current challenges will help find better treatment and preventative measures for PLWH in the future.

17.2.5 Metabolic Syndrome and Diabetes

The National Cholesterol Education Program (NCEP) Third Adult Treatment Panel (ATP III) guidelines define metabolic syndrome as having three of five risk factors that may lead to CD and DM. Table 17.3 lists these factors.

TABLE 17.3 NCEP ATP III panel Clinical Definition for Metabolic Syndrome

Risk factor	Defining level
Abdominal obesity	Waist circumference
Men	>102cm (>40in)
Women	>88cm (>35in)
HDL-C	
Men	<40mg/dL
Women	<50mg/dL
Triglycerides	≥150mg/dL
Blood pressure	≥130/85mmHG
Fasting glucose	100mg/dL

A study conducted by Alencastro et al. [71] demonstrated a high (24.7%) prevalence of metabolic syndrome in 1,240 HIV-infected individuals; this was attributed to the increasing number of ART agents, longer HAART use, and aging. Recent studies show a shift in the incidence of ART-related DM because of more contemporary drug therapies. In a 10-year study (1999–2009) conducted by Capeau et al. [72], the incidence of DM peaked in 1999–2000 and decreased during the following years. DM was attributed to ARTs (indinavir, stavudine, didanosine), adiposity, and aging in the cohort. Similarly, another study by Rasmussen et al. [73] followed-up a population of HIV-infected individuals and an HIV-seronegative cohort from 1996 to 2009; they found a 2.83-times higher risk of DM among the HIV-infected group compared with the control group between 1996 and 1999, but they found no difference between groups from 1999 to 2009. Like in the Capeau et al. study, Rasmussen et al. [73] also showed no difference in DM incidence in the years after 1999 between the HIV-infected versus HIV-seronegative control group. They concluded that ARTs including indinavir, saquinavir, stavudine, and didanosine increased the risk of DM, along with age, BMI, and lipoatrophy. The two studies suggest that the incidence of DM is decreasing in PLWH with the use of modern ARTs.

Despite this newly emerging data, many studies conducted in the 2000s found a high risk of DM related to ART. A 2008 study from the DAD group concluded that stavudine and zidovudine are significantly associated with diabetes, even after controlling for other risk factors [74]. Another study found that HIV-infected men receiving combination ART were 3.1-times more likely to develop DM than control subjects [75]. In an analysis of the MACS, Brown et al. [48] found a 14% prevalence of DM at baseline in HIV-infected men compared with only a 5% increase for HIV-seronegative men. Furthermore, they found a four-fold increase in the incidence of DM in HIV-infected men using ART compared with the control group.

17.2.5.1 *Knowledge Gaps*

More research is needed to test the long-term effects of ART and to develop drugs that are not only effective at minimizing metabolic symptoms in PLWH but also less toxic to the body. There is also inconsistency among studies reporting the cause of metabolic syndrome and diabetes in PLWH, and among which drugs lead to a higher incidence of these among individuals.

17.3 EXERCISE

Numerous studies have shown the positive effect of aerobic and resistance exercise training on metabolic indices in adults living with HIV. Thoni et al. [76] found significant decreases in total abdominal adipose tissue, total cholesterol, and triglycerides, and significant increases in HDL cholesterol. Another study found that exercise, coupled with the use of metformin (a diabetes medication) decreased muscle adiposity in PLWH [77]. Aerobic and resistance exercises are classified by the way in which they target certain muscle and organ groups. Aerobic involves lungs and cardiovascular system, whereas resistance more specifically targets bones and skeletal muscle.

17.3.1 Aerobic

Aerobic exercise interventions typically include jogging, cycling, swimming, stair stepping, and rowing. The American College of Sports Medicine (ACSM) recommends brisk walking, light jogging, and bicycling for 30–60 min, 3–4 days/week, at 40–60% Karvonen heart rate [78].

17.3.2 Resistance

Resistance exercise interventions include muscle-strengthening activities that involve the use of free weights and machines. The ACSM recommends resistance training of each major muscle group (chest, shoulders, back, hips, legs, trunk, and arms) 2–3 days/week, at 8–10 repetitions per exercise. Strength training plays a significant role in the body's glucose control by increasing lean muscle tissue, which is more metabolically active than adipose tissue [79].

Using the limited amount of current studies on the effects of exercise on OPLWH, Yahiaoui et al. [80] developed evidence-based exercise recommendations by analyzing three groups (frail older adults, elderly individuals with metabolic syndrome, and HIV-infected adults) whose clinical symptoms represent similar physiological effects of OPLWH. That exercise recommendation did not include any information on body weight management, metabolic indicators, and diet.

The purpose of this review was to critically analyze the existing literature on effects of aerobic and resistance exercise in OPLWH on body composition, obesity, dyslipidemia, glucose uptake, insulin resistance, metabolic syndrome, and diabetes, to identify gaps and make recommendations for additional research in the future.

17.4 METHODS

We searched the PubMed database for the key words "HIV, elderly and exercise," "exercise in older adults with HIV," and "metabolic function in elderly with HIV." We found 269, 27, and 694 publications, respectively. After close analysis of the abstracts, we included seven studies that matched our research criteria. Articles were selected for this review if:

1. Subjects included HIV-positive adults 18 years of age or older
2. Study included weekly aerobic and/or resistance exercise training
3. Study included metabolic measurements
4. Study included a control group.[1]

17.5 RESULTS

All seven of the studies included in this review measured the effect of exercise on metabolic function in PLWH (see Table 17.4 for demographic data). De Souza et al. [82] conducted the only trial that exclusively enrolled participants 60 years of age or older. Engelson et al. [81] and Terry et al. [83] were the only two teams to report a combined diet and exercise intervention. Of the exercise studies, four conducted both aerobic and resistance training [8,10,12,81], two conducted aerobic only [13,83], and one conducted resistance only [82].

17.5.1 Lipids

All seven of the studies included in this review measured lipid profiles before and after the exercise programs. However, Engelson et al. [81] did

[1] Engelson and colleagues [81] did not have a control group. They were included in this study because they conducted the only trial to test diet and exercise intervention on metabolic outcomes in an obese cohort. We found this data important to include.

not include lipid concentration data in the manuscript. Results for total cholesterol, LDL-C, HDL-C, and triglycerides are given in Table 17.5.

Mutimura et al. [10] found a slight decrease in total cholesterol in the exercise group compared with the control group at the end of the

TABLE 17.4 Demographic Data

Year and author	Population
De Souza et al. (2011)	N1 = 21 (Healthy > 60) N2 = 11 (HIV+ > 60)
Ogalha et al. (2011)	N1 = 28 N2(S) = 35 29 males/29 females Mean age: 44 ± 11(N1) 42 ± 7 (N2)
Lindegaard et al. (2008)	N1 (strength) = 10 N2 (endurance) = 8 Male only Mean age: 46 ± 8 (N1) 53 ± 8 (N2)
Mutimura et al. (2008)	N1 (BFR + noEXS) = 50 N2 (BFR + EX)(S, group) = 50 40 males/60 females Mean age: 37.5 ± 7 (N1) 38 ± 6 (N2)
Dolan et al. (2006)	N1 = 20 N2 (S, HB) = 20 All females Mean age: 40 ± 2 (N1) 43 ± 2 (N2)
Terry et al. (2006)	N1 = 15 N2 (S, group) = 15 20 males/10 females Mean age: 39 ± 7 (N1) 36 ± 5 (N2)
Engelson et al. (2006)	N = 18 All female Mean age: 41.8 ± 7.5

Note: N1, control group; N2, intervention group; HR, heart rate; UE, upper extremity; LE, lower extremity; S, supervised; HB, home-based.
Results charts.

TABLE 17.5 Lipids

	Total cholesterol	HDL-C	LDL-C	Triglycerides
De Souza et al.[a] (2011)	Baseline N1: 216 Final N1: 207.9 Baseline N2: 220.5 Final N2: 219.4	Baseline N1: 57.29 Final N1: 65.29 Baseline N2: 54.75 Final N2: 61.75	Baseline N1: 126.29 Final N1: 118.43 Baseline N2: 127.4 Final N2: 129.4	Baseline N1: 161.57 Final N1: 121.57 Baseline N2: 191.13 Final N2: 160
Ogalha et al. (2011)	Baseline N1: 189.8 mg/dL Final N1: 186.8 mg/dL Baseline N2: 222.7 mg/dL Final N2: 203.7 mg/dL	Baseline N1: 42.4 mg/dL Final N1: 44.8 mg/dL Baseline N2: 53.9 mg/dL Final N2: 53.7 mg/dL	Baseline N1:107.6 mg/dL Final N1:105.1 mg/dL Baseline N2: 126.1 mg/dL Final N2: 114.8 mg/dL	Baseline N1: 187.4 mg/dL Final N1: 204.3 mg/dL Baseline N2: 190.2 mg/dL Final N2: 172.1 mg/dL
Mutimura et al. (2008)	Baseline N1: 3.89 mmol/L Final N1§: 3.96 mmol/L Baseline N2: 3.78 mmol/L Final N2§: 3.75 mmol/L	Baseline N1: 1.27 mmol/L Final N1§: 1.34 mmol/L Baseline N2: 1.28 mmol/L Final N2§: 1.31 mmol/L	Baseline N1: 2.2 mmol/L Final N1§: 0.19 mmol/L Baseline N2: 2.1 mmol/L Final N2§: 2.24 mmol/L	Baseline N1: 1.34 mmol/L Final N1§: 1.41 mmol/L Baseline N2: 1.33 mmol/L Final N2§: 1.55 mmol/L
Lindegaard et al. (2008)	Baseline N1: 5.7 mmol/L Final N1: 5.9 mmol/L Baseline N2: 5.9 mmol/L Final N2: 5.8 mmol/L	Baseline N1: 1.18 mmol/L Final N1:1.2 mmol/L Baseline N2: 0.96 mmol/L Final N2:1.1 mmol/L	Baseline N1: 3.1 mmol/L Final N1: 3.3 mmol/L Baseline N2: 3.6 mmol/L Final N2: 3.5 mmol/L	Baseline N1: 2.1 mmol/L Final N1: 1.72 mmol/L Baseline N2: 2.04 mmol/L Final N2: 2.04 mmol/L
Dolan et al. (2006)	Baseline N1:162 mg/dL Final N1§:162 mg/dL Baseline N2: 191 mg/dL Final N2§: 189 mg/dL	Baseline N1: 47 mg/dL Final N1§: 44 mg/dL Baseline N2: 52 mg/dL Final N2§: 51 mg/dL	Baseline N1: 94 mg/dL Final N1§: 96 mg/dL Baseline N2: 112 mg/dL Final N2§: 109 mg/dL	Baseline N1: 107 mg/dL Final N1§: 107 mg/dL Baseline N2:141 mg/dL Final N2§: 147 mg/dL
Terry et al. (2006)	Baseline N1: 256 mg/dL Final N1: 251 mg/dL Baseline N2: 256 mg/dL Final N2: 243 mg/dL	Baseline N1: 38 mg/dL Final N1: 39 mg/dL Baseline N2: 42 mg/dL Final N2: 43 mg/dL	NA	Baseline N1: 338 mg/dL Final N1: 346 mg/dL Baseline N2: 325 mg/dL Final N2: 296 mg/dL

Note: N1, control group; N2, exercise group; HDL-C, high-density lipoprotein cholesterol; LDL-C, low-density lipoprotein cholesterol; §, final values calculated by adding baseline and change values.
[a]*For this study only: N1, HIV+ w/o protease inhibitors; N2, HIV+; and exercise before and after. Gray background denotes OPLWH study.*

study (3.96 versus 3.75; $P < 0.05$), but no significant change in HDL-C or LDL-C levels. For metabolic outcomes, De Souza et al. [82] divided participants into two groups: an HIV-positive group using PIs and an HIV-positive group not using PIs. The study did not find a significant change in lipid profile during the 1-year training program. Lindegaard et al. [12] measured outcomes for an aerobic exercise–only group versus a resistance-only group. The resistance group showed an improvement in triglycerides, whereas the aerobic training group demonstrated a decrease in total cholesterol, LDL-C, and free fatty acids, and an increase in HDL-C. Engelson et al. [81] reported no change in mean fasting lipid concentrations and no correlation between changes in weight and changes in lipids, with the exception of LDL-C, which correlated negatively with changes in weight and subcutaneous adipose tissue. There was also no correlation between changes in triglycerides and visceral adipose tissue.

Both Dolan et al. [8] and Terry et al. [83] reported no significant improvement in lipid levels between the exercise and control groups. Similarly, Ogalha et al. [12] showed no improvement in HDL-C or LDL-C levels.

17.5.2 Glucose

Mutimura et al. [10] found a significant decrease in fasting plasma glucose in the exercise group compared with the control group ($P < 0.0001$) (Table 17.6). De Souza et al. [82] also found a significant decrease in fasting glucose levels among PLWH after the 1-year program, and even more so in the participants not using PIs. Lindegaard et al. [12] showed an increase in insulin-mediated glucose uptake in both resistance and aerobic training groups. Engelson et al. [81], Dolan et al. [8], Terry et al. [83], and Ogalha et al. [13] did not show any significant change or improvement in glucose levels.

17.5.3 Strength

De Souza et al. [82] showed significant increases in strength for all exercises in the HIV-infected group (1.52- to 2.33-times baseline values), but they also found an increase in the control group, although to a lesser extent (1.21- to 1.48-times baseline values).

Lindegaard et al. [12] found a 30% increase in strength measures in the resistance group compared with the aerobic only group. Dolan et al. [8] found significant improvement in the upper and lower extremity muscle groups tested. The study showed an increase in total muscle area ($P = 0.02$) and total muscle attenuation ($P = 0.03$). Engelson et al. [81] reported a 30% increase in pectoral, latissiumus dorsi, and quadriceps strength from baseline ($P < 0.0001$).

TABLE 17.6 Glucose

Author	Glucose
De Souza et al.[a] (2011)	Baseline N1: 96 mg/dL Final N1: 89.5 mg/dL Baseline N2: 98.3 mg/dL Final N2: 92.4 mg/dL $P = 0.037$
Ogalha et al. (2011)	Baseline N1: 89.5 mg/dL Final N1: 86.7 mg/dL Baseline N2: 90.3 mg/dL Final N2: 87.6 mg/dL
Mutimura et al. (2008)	Baseline N1: 4.9 mmol/L Final N1[§]: 5.34 mmol/L Baseline N2: 4.8 mmol/L Final N2[§]: 5 mmol/L
Lindegaard et al. (2008)	Baseline N1: 5.5 mmol/L Final N1: 5.4 mmol/L Baseline N2: 5.4 mmol/L Final N2: 5.4 mmol/L
Dolan et al. (2006)	Baseline N1: 87 mg/dL Final N1[§]: 88 mg/dL Baseline N2: 85 mg/dL Final N2[§]: 84 mg/dL
Terry et al. (2006)	Baseline N1: 100 mg/dL Final N1: 106 mg/dL Baseline N2: 90 mg/dL Final N2: 97 mg/dL

[a]For this study only: N1, HIV+ w/o protease inhibitors; N2, HIV+; and exercise before and after. Gray background denotes OPLWH study.

17.5.4 Body Composition, Dietary Intervention, and Exercise

Engelson et al. [81] and Terry et al. [83] are among the few authors to have measured both the effects of exercise and a dietary component in PLWH.

Engelson et al. [81] included 18 obese HIV-infected women who received individual dietary counseling throughout the 12-week study. They followed a 5,024-kJ hypoenergetic diet that included 50% energy from carbohydrates, 30% from fat, and 20% from protein. After the study, subjects demonstrated an average weight loss of 7.3% of initial body weight, which resulted in a 2.6-kg/m^2 mean change in BMI. There was a 17% loss of visceral adipose tissue and a 15% loss in subcutaneous adipose tissue from baseline measure.

Study participants in the study by Terry et al. [83] were given dietary guidance by a registered dietitian to achieve a daily caloric intake of

30 kcal/kg of body weight for women and 40 kcal/kg of body weight for men, with a protein intake of 2.0 g/kg for women and 2.5 g/kg of body weight for men. Fifty-seven percent of calories were given as carbohydrates, 23% as unsaturated fat, 15% as saturated fat, and 5% as protein. The daily recommended cholesterol intake was 200 mg (approximately one large egg). During the 12-week study, they found a significant reduction in the percentage of saturated fatty acids, which the authors attributed to a low protein and carbohydrate intake. However, there was no significant overall change in plasma lipid levels, and both the exercise and diet group and the diet-only group showed similar changes in body composition. This suggests that body composition changes in this study were mostly attributed to dietary intervention and not to aerobic exercise.

Most studies did not include dietary recommendations but still reported body composition changes. Mutimura et al. [10] reported significant improvements in waist circumference, waist-to-hip ratio, sum of skin folds, and percentage of body fat. Ogalha et al. [13] found an improvement in muscle mass ($P = 0.001$) and hip circumference ($P = 0.001$) in the exercise group compared with the control group. Dolan et al. [8] showed no significant change in BMI, abdominal fat, or total fat between the exercise and control groups. Table 17.7 illustrates the exercise type and metabolic outcomes for each study.

TABLE 17.7 Metabolic Outcomes

Year and author	Study duration	Exercise program/duration		Metabolic outcomes
		Aerobic	Resistance	
De Souza et al. (2011)	3 × week for 1 year	NA	Free weight machines; 2 × week *Type*: Leg press; seated row; lumbar extension; *chest* press; seated abdominal 3 sets of 12, 10, and 8 repetitions at light, moderate, and heavy resistance	*Significant changes*: – *Fasting glucose* levels decreased (especially in non-PI participants) *Insignificant changes:* – Lipid profile – BMI – Weight
Ogalha et al. (2011)	3 × week for 24 weeks	treadmill at 75% of HRmax	NA	No significant improvements in this study *Insignificant Changes*: – BMI – Lipodystrophy – HDL-C or LDL-C

(continued)

TABLE 17.7 Continued

Year and author	Study duration	Exercise program/duration		Metabolic outcomes
		Aerobic	Resistance	
Lindegaard et al. (2008)	3 × week for 16 weeks	5 min warmup, 35 min interval training at 50–100% VO_2max	UE and LE exercises for 45–60 min	*Significant changes*: *Insulin-mediated glucose* uptake increased with aerobic ($P = 0.02$) and resistance training ($P = 0.05$) – Decrease in total cholesterol, LDL-C, and free fatty acids – Increase in HDL-C
Mutimura et al. (2008)	3 × week for 6 months	Progressive 30 min warmup/cooldown, 45–60 min (jogging, running, stair climbing)	Progressive UE exercises	*Significant changes*: – Fasting total cholesterol ($P < 0.05$) – Triglycerides ($P < 0.05$) – *Fasting glucose* levels ($P < 0.05$) *Insignificant changes*: – No change in HDL-C or LDL-C.
Dolan et al. (2006)	3 × week for 4 months	20 min run (first 2 weeks) at 60% of maximal HR, 30 min at 75% thereafter	UE and LE exercises	No significant change was seen in lipid levels, blood pressure, glucose level, or abdominal visceral fat between exercise and control groups.
Terry et al. (2006)	3 × week for 3 months	30 min warmup/cooldown, 30 min exercise at 70–85% of HRmax	NA	No significant change in triglyceride, cholesterol, or HDL-C levels between exercise and control groups.
Engelson et al. (2006)	3 × week for 12 weeks	5 min warmup; 30 min treadmill at 70–80% HRmax	7 major muscle groups: 3 sets of 8–10 repetitions; 10 exercises	↓ Daily food intake and body weight (95.5% fat) ↓ Resting energy expenditure ↑ Strength, fitness, and QOL ↔ CD4, viral load, fasting glucovse, insulin, insulin sensitivity, fasting lipids, TPA, PAI-1

17.6 DISCUSSION

Justice [84] developed a conceptual model that documents our current knowledge regarding the physical process of aging with HIV and the interactions between HIV, treatments, and other comorbidities. The diagram in Figure 17.1 depicts the interactions between the viral disease, chronic inflammation, treatment toxicity, and immunosenescence. With increased aging, these multiple disease manifestations lead to depletion in organ system reserves and eventually to functional decline, organ system failure, and ultimately to death. Regular exercise has been found to be beneficial for improving many physiologic indices in PLWH and may help counter the negative manifestations seen in HIV, aging, and the use of ART.

In this review, we found variable results in metabolic outcomes. Of the trials that tested glucose levels, three found significant changes after exercise and two found no change. De Souza et al. [82] (the only cohort to exclusively include EPLWH) found an increase in fasting glucose levels in the group. Similarly, there was no consistent result for lipid profile

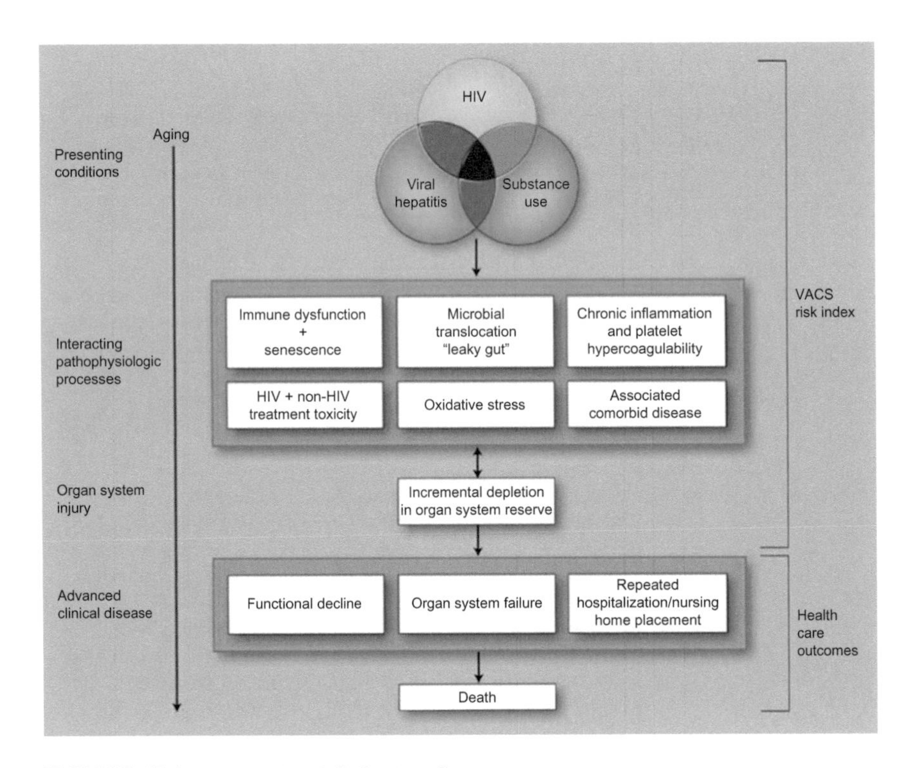

FIGURE 17.1 Justice (2010) [84] aging diagram.

through the seven studies. De Souza et al. [82], Ogalha et al. [13], Dolan et al. [8], Terry et al. [83], and Engelson et al. [81] found no significant change in cholesterol and triglycerides after exercise. Lindegaard et al. [12] reported a decrease in total cholesterol, LDL-C, and free fatty acids and an increase in HDL-C. Mutimura et al. [10] found significant changes in fasting total cholesterol and triglycerides, but no change in HDL-C and LDL-C. Exercise intervention showed an overall improvement in body composition in the studies included in this review. The only exception was the study by Terry et al. [83], whose positive outcomes were attributed primarily to diet.

As they age, PLWH experience many similar symptoms as the non-HIV-infected aging population. However, the toxicity of ARTs causes OPLWH to endure more severe and more rapid onset of functional decline. Malin and Kirwan [85] tested the efficacy of a 12-week exercise program on glucose metabolism in obese non-HIV-infected adults with impaired fasting glucose (IFG), IGT, and combined glucose intolerance (CGI) compared with normal glucose tolerant (NGT) and T2D groups. Exercise training lowered fasting and 2-h glucose levels in IFG, CGI, and T2D groups, but not to the same extent in the IGT group. Because PLWH tend to experience high levels of IGT due to the added toxicity of ARTs, they must face additional hurdles to overcome these metabolic abnormalities, setting them apart from non-HIV-infected individuals with similar symptoms.

This is not always the case, however. A study comparing the incidence of DM2 in a cohort of HIV-infected compared with non-HIV-infected persons found a significantly higher risk of diabetes among HIV-infected subjects using PIs (1.35 relative risk), but, interestingly, they found the incidence of diabetes to be higher in non-HIV participants compared with HIV-infected individuals using combination ARTs (13.60 versus 11.35 per 1,000 person-years) [86]. This suggests that although PIs must be avoided in the treatment of diabetes, combination ARTs are closing the gap in metabolic function between PLWH and the general population. Furthermore, Amorosa et al. [34] noted in their study that the rate of obesity or overweight status in an urban HIV population reflected the obesity epidemic in Philadelphia, further demonstrating how far PLWH have come since the days of wasting syndrome.

The review by Yahiaoui et al. [80] presents evidence-based exercise recommendations specifically geared toward OPLWH (Table 17.8). These correlate with exercise methods and intensities used by the authors in this review and should be used as guidelines for managing body weight in EPLWH. Although some of the studies in this review recommend an aerobic exercise intensity of 70–85% HRmax, it is important to adjust the intensity when developing exercise regimens for OPLWH by beginning with a lower intensity and gradually increasing it to reach the desired intensity level.

TABLE 17.8 Exercise Recommendations for OPLWH

	Mode	Frequency/duration	Intensity
Aerobic	Walking, cycling, swimming, stair climbing, rowing (may use machines such as treadmill, and stationary bicycle)	At least 6 weeks, 3 days per week for 20–40 min. 5–10 min of stretching before and after each session to prevent injury	50–90% of estimated maximum heart rate →Based on age and weight of individual →Begin at lower intensity and incrementally increase
Resistance	Knee extension, knee flexion, grip strength, shoulder flexion, chest press, seated bench press, seated row, leg press, leg curl, biceps curl, tricep pull, and extension	3 days per week for at least 6 weeks	1–2 sets of 6–8 repetitions at 60% 1-RM initially Increase to 3 sets of 8–10 repetitions at 80–90% of 1-RM - 20–30 seconds rest period between each set

Source: Yahiaoui et al. (2012).

However, exercise is not the only factor when it comes to maintaining an optimal body weight. The dietary intake of adequate amounts of fibers, saturated fats, and refined sugars plays an equally important role in a OPLWHs weight. Researchers in the United Kingdom found that the dietary habits of PLWH have a major impact on their overall health and HIV-associated metabolic comorbidities [87]. The authors reported that 43% of men and 36% of women did not consume enough energy [expressed as total kcal intake minus ((basal metabolic rate*1.3)/day)] to meet their basal metabolic requirements in terms of proteins, carbohydrates, and fats. The majority of the cohort consumed more than the recommended amount of saturated fats. A study in Brazil found similar results, with more than 20% of their PLWH cohort consuming higher than recommended amounts of saturated fat, cholesterol, and/or sodium and less than the recommended amounts of fiber in their diets [88].

A study conducted by Mason et al. [89] measured the effects of exercise and diet on weight loss and insulin resistance in obese, non-HIV-infected women aged 50–75 years old. With the exception of age and HIV status, this trial was similar to that of Engelson et al. [81], who tested diet and exercise intervention in an obese, HIV-infected group of women. Both studies documented weight loss in the diet and diet plus exercise groups. Whereas Engelson et al. [81] showed no differences in metabolic parameters, Mason et al. [89] found significant reductions in serum insulin and glucose in the diet (22.3%; 2.4%) and diet plus exercise (24%; 2.8%) groups compared with the control group (1.9%; 0.2%). They found that women in the diet group and the diet plus exercise group showed similar reductions in body weight, total body fat, and visceral fat. However, the diet plus exercise group showed a much greater improvement in insulin sensitivity compared with the other groups. Given the wide range of potential confounding factors, it is difficult to hypothesize what role HIV infection had in the metabolic outcomes between the two trials. However, it is important to note that the duration of the Mason et al. study was 12 months compared with 3 months in the Engelson et al. study. A longer trial of this type might show a greater improvement in metabolic indices in an HIV-infected cohort.

Engelson et al. [81] also reported significant changes in visceral and subcutaneous adipose tissue, which is important in managing body weight. Visceral adipose tissue was related to total fat loss, and it was greater in women who had more at baseline. Terry et al. [83] also conducted a diet and exercise intervention but did not find significant changes in adipose tissue. They noted that lipodystrophy presents as subcutaneous lipoatrophy and visceral adiposity, neither of which is adequately measured by the skinfold thickness test that they used in their study, suggesting that there may be a possible change that they did not measure. The study duration was also 12 weeks, which may not fully capture the benefit of a diet and exercise combination program. Future research is warranted to examine the impact of a longer combination trial on body composition and metabolic function. Stronger studies are also needed to compare which interventions (such as diet, diet and exercise, or potential drugs) may eliminate the risk factors involved in metabolic syndrome.

Poor dietary nutrient intake has also been associated with a higher level of depression symptoms in PLWH. Using the Center for Epidemiologic Studies Depression Scale to classify the risk of depression, Purnomo et al. [90] reported that depressed subjects had a significantly lower mean intake of fiber, vitamin A, magnesium, and folate compared with nondepressed subjects.

There are very few randomized controlled trials that analyze the effect of exercise and diet on body composition in PLWH, much less OPLWH. Some studies have begun to look at possible diet interventions that improve the lipid profiles of PLWH, as well as diet and exercise regiments to target risk factors such as lipoprotein-associated phospholipase A2 (Lp-PLA2), whose activity is associated with an increased risk for coronary heart disease [91]. However, there are currently only a few studies available to test the proper exercise and dietary rules and their effects on weight management and prevention of metabolic disorders for OPLWH.

There is no consensus in the current literature on the best type of interventions geared toward an aging HIV population. Future studies must develop long-term trials in OPLWH to understand the impact of exercise on physiological function, which will allow health care workers to develop specific diet and exercise recommendations for each individual.

The limitations of this review study include a small number of trials, small sample sizes, limited study durations, differing levels of adherence to exercise interventions, and variable results from study to study. The rapid development of trials to test these interventions will add critical knowledge regarding how OPLWH can maintain a stable weight, live healthier lives, and experience a better quality of life.

17.7 CONCLUSION

Over the past decade, the prevalence of obesity and metabolic changes has been increasing in PLWH as well as OPLWH. These changes in body composition and the decline in metabolic function lead to a higher rate of DM and CV, among other diseases. Aerobic and resistance exercise have shown to be safe and effective in improving body functions such as strength, cardiovascular capacity, and endurance. In addition to exercise, studies have shown that diet is an important factor in controlling body and fat mass. Currently, little is known about the intersection of diet and exercise in OPLWH. More work is needed in the development of comparative studies to test the impact of aerobic and resistance exercise with and without dietary restrictions in OPLWH. This will help us to better understand some of the underlying pathophysiological mechanisms and ultimately provide better preventative care and treatment in the future.

References

[1] Effros R. Aging and HIV disease: synergistic immunological effects? In: Fulop T, Franceschi C, Hirokawa K, Pawelec G, editors. Handbook on immunosenescence. The Netherlands: Springer; 2009. pp. 949–64.
[2] Farrant L, Gwyther L, Dinat N, Mmoledi K, Hatta N, Harding R. Maintaining wellbeing for South Africans receiving ART: the burden of pain and symptoms is greater with longer ART exposure. S Afr Med J 2014;104(2):119–23.
[3] Feeney ER, Mallon PWG. HIV and HAART-associated dyslipidemia. Open Cardiovasc Med J 2011;5:49–63.
[4] Nasi M, Pinti M, De Biasi S, et al. Aging with HIV infection: a journey to the center of inflammAIDS, immunosenescence and neuroHIV. Immunol Lett 2014.
[5] NIH. Guidelines for the Use of Antiretroviral Agents in HIV-1-Infected Adults and Adolescents. 2012. <http://aidsinfo.nih.gov/guidelines/html/1/adult-and-adolescent-arv-guidelines/277/hiv-and-the-older-patient>.
[6] Somarriba G, Neri D, Schaefer N, Miller TL. The effect of aging, nutrition, and exercise during HIV infection. HIV/AIDS 2010;2:191–201.
[7] Baigis J, Korniewicz DM, Chase G, Butz A, Jacobson D, Wu AW. Effectiveness of a home-based exercise intervention for HIV-infected adults: a randomized trial. J Assoc Nurses AIDS Care 2002;13(2):33–45.
[8] Dolan SE, Frontera W, Librizzi J, et al. Effects of a supervised home-based aerobic and progressive resistance training regimen in women infected with human immunodeficiency virus: a randomized trial. Arch Intern Med 2006;166(11):1225–31.

[9] Hand GA, Phillips KD, Dudgeon WD, William Lyerly G, Larry Durstine J, Burgess SE. Moderate intensity exercise training reverses functional aerobic impairment in HIV-infected individuals. AIDS Care 2008;20(9):1066–74.
[10] Mutimura E, Crowther NJ, Cade TW, Yarasheski KE, Stewart A. Exercise training reduces central adiposity and improves metabolic indices in HAART-treated HIV-positive subjects in Rwanda: a randomized controlled trial. AIDS Res Hum Retroviruses 2008;24(1):15–23.
[11] O'Brien K, Nixon S, Tynan AM, Glazier R. Aerobic exercise interventions for adults living with HIV/AIDS. Cochrane Database Syst Rev 2010(8):CD001796.
[12] Lindegaard B, Hansen T, Hvid T, et al. The effect of strength and endurance training on insulin sensitivity and fat distribution in human immunodeficiency virus-infected patients with lipodystrophy. J Clin Endocrinol Metab 2008;93(10):3860–9.
[13] Ogalha C, Luz E, Sampaio E, et al. A randomized, clinical trial to evaluate the impact of regular physical activity on the quality of life, body morphology and metabolic parameters of patients with AIDS in Salvador, Brazil. J Acquir Immune Defic Syndr 2011;57(Suppl. 3): S179–85. (1999).
[14] Jeon CY, Lokken RP, Hu FB, van Dam RM. Physical activity of moderate intensity and risk of type 2 diabetes: a systematic review. Diabetes Care 2007;30(3):744–52.
[15] Vogel T, Brechat PH, Lepretre PM, Kaltenbach G, Berthel M, Lonsdorfer J. Health benefits of physical activity in older patients: a review. Int J Clin Pract 2009;63(2): 303–20.
[16] Hahn V, Halle M, Schmidt-Trucksass A, Rathmann W, Meisinger C, Mielck A. Physical activity and the metabolic syndrome in elderly German men and women: results from the population-based KORA survey. Diabetes Care 2009;32(3):511–3.
[17] Stewart KJ, Bacher AC, Turner K, et al. Exercise and risk factors associated with metabolic syndrome in older adults. Am J Prev Med 2005;28(1):9–18.
[18] Han TS, Wu FC, Lean ME. Obesity and weight management in the elderly: a focus on men. Best Pract Res Clin Endocrinol Metab 2013;27(4):509–25.
[19] Grunfeld C, Saag M, Cofrancesco Jr. J, et al. Regional adipose tissue measured by MRI over 5 years in HIV-infected and control participants indicates persistence of HIV-associated lipoatrophy. AIDS (London, England) 2010;24(11):1717–26.
[20] Jacobson DL, Knox T, Spiegelman D, Skinner S, Gorbach S, Wanke C. Prevalence of, evolution of, and risk factors for fat atrophy and fat deposition in a cohort of HIV-infected men and women. Clin Infect Dis 2005;40(12):1837–45.
[21] Stanley TL, Grinspoon SK. Body composition and metabolic changes in HIV-infected patients. J Infect Dis 2012;205(Suppl. 3):S383–90.
[22] Palmer CS, Crowe SM. The role of glucose and lipid metabolism in the pathogenesis of HIV-1 infection. Curr Trends Immunol 2012;13:37–50.
[23] Unger RH. Minireview: weapons of lean body mass destruction: the role of ectopic lipids in the metabolic syndrome. Endocrinology 2003;144(12):5159–65.
[24] Flint OP, Noor MA, Hruz PW, et al. The role of protease inhibitors in the pathogenesis of HIV-associated lipodystrophy: cellular mechanisms and clinical implications. Toxicol Pathol 2009;37(1):65–77.
[25] Dube MP, Parker RA, Tebas P, et al. Glucose metabolism, lipid, and body fat changes in antiretroviral-naive subjects randomized to nelfinavir or efavirenz plus dual nucleosides. AIDS (London, England) 2005;19(16):1807–18.
[26] Mallon PW, Miller J, Cooper DA, Carr A. Prospective evaluation of the effects of antiretroviral therapy on body composition in HIV-1-infected men starting therapy. AIDS (London, England) 2003;17(7):971–9.
[27] Samaras K, Gan SK, Peake PW, Carr A, Campbell LV. Proinflammatory markers, insulin sensitivity, and cardiometabolic risk factors in treated HIV infection. Obesity (Silver Spring) 2009;17(1):53–9.

[28] Lake JE, Currier JS. Metabolic disease in HIV infection. Lancet Infect Dis 2013;13(11):964–75.
[29] Calvo M, Martinez E. Update on metabolic issues in HIV patients. Curr Opin HIV AIDS 2014;9(4):332–9.
[30] Hadigan C, Meigs JB, Corcoran C, et al. Metabolic abnormalities and cardiovascular disease risk factors in adults with human immunodeficiency virus infection and lipodystrophy. Clin Infect Dis 2001;32(1):130–9.
[31] Dragovic G, Danilovic D, Dimic A, Jevtovic D. Lipodystrophy induced by combination antiretroviral therapy in HIV/AIDS patients: a Belgrade cohort study. Vojnosanit Pregl 2014;71(8):746–50.
[32] Crum-Cianflone NF, Roediger M, Eberly LE, et al. Obesity among HIV-infected persons: impact of weight on CD4 cell count. AIDS 2010;24(7):1069–72.
[33] Smit E, Skolasky RL, Dobs AS, et al. Changes in the incidence and predictors of wasting syndrome related to human immunodeficiency virus infection, 1987–1999. Am J Epidemiol 2002;156(3):211–8.
[34] Amorosa V, Synnestvedt M, Gross R, et al. A tale of 2 epidemics: the intersection between obesity and HIV infection in Philadelphia. J Acquir Immune Defic Syndr 2005;39(5):557–61. (1999).
[35] Lakey W, Yang LY, Yancy W, Chow SC, Hicks C. Short communication: from wasting to obesity: initial antiretroviral therapy and weight gain in HIV-infected persons. AIDS Res Hum Retroviruses 2013;29(3):435–40.
[36] Crum-Cianflone N, Tejidor R, Medina S, Barahona I, Ganesan A. Obesity among patients with HIV: the latest epidemic. AIDS Patient Care STDS 2008;22(12):925–30.
[37] Mencarelli A, Francisci D, Renga B, et al. Ritonavir-induced lipoatrophy and dyslipidaemia is reversed by the anti-inflammatory drug leflunomide in a PPAR-gamma-dependent manner. Antivir Ther 2012;17(4):669–78.
[38] Anuurad E, Bremer A, Berglund L. HIV protease inhibitors and obesity. Curr Opin Endocrinol Diabetes Obes 2010;17(5):478–85.
[39] Shah K, Alio AP, Hall WJ, Luque AE. The physiological effects of obesity in HIV-infected patients. J AIDS Clin Res 2012;3:151.
[40] Kosmiski L, Kuritzkes D, Hamilton J, et al. Fat distribution is altered in HIV-infected men without clinical evidence of the HIV lipodystrophy syndrome. HIV Med 2003;4(3):235–40.
[41] Villareal DT, Banks M, Siener C, Sinacore DR, Klein S. Physical frailty and body composition in obese elderly men and women. Obes Res 2004;12(6):913–20.
[42] Fried LP, Tangen CM, Walston J, et al. Frailty in older adults: evidence for a phenotype. J Gerontol A Biol Sci Med Sci 2001;56(3):M146–56.
[43] Hubbard RE, Lang IA, Llewellyn DJ, Rockwood K. Frailty, body mass index, and abdominal obesity in older people. J Gerontol A Biol Sci Med Sci 2010;65A(4):377–81.
[44] Shah K, Hilton TN, Myers L, Pinto JF, Luque AE, Hall WJ. A new frailty syndrome: central obesity and frailty in older adults with the human immunodeficiency virus. J Am Geriatr Soc 2012;60(3):545–9.
[45] Mooradian AD. Dyslipidemia in type 2 diabetes mellitus. Nat Clin Pract End Met 2009;5(3):150–9.
[46] Murata H, Hruz PW, Mueckler M. The mechanism of insulin resistance caused by HIV protease inhibitor therapy. J Biol Chem 2000;275(27):20251–20254.
[47] Sprinz E, Lazzaretti RK, Kuhmmer R, Ribeiro JP. Dyslipidemia in HIV-infected individuals. Braz J Infect Dis 2010;14:575–88.
[48] Brown TT, Cole SR, Li X, et al. Antiretroviral therapy and the prevalence and incidence of diabetes mellitus in the Multicenter AIDS Cohort Study. Arch Intern Med 2005;165(10):1179–84.
[49] Grinspoon S. Diabetes mellitus, cardiovascular risk, and HIV disease. Circulation 2009;119(6):770–2.

[50] Dubé MP, Stein JH, Aberg JA, et al. Guidelines for the evaluation and management of dyslipidemia in human immunodeficiency virus (HIV)-infected adults receiving antiretroviral therapy: recommendations of the HIV medicine association of the infectious disease society of America and the adult AIDS clinical trials group. Clin Infect Dis 2003;37(5):613–27.
[51] Saves M, Raffi F, Capeau J, et al. Factors related to lipodystrophy and metabolic alterations in patients with human immunodeficiency virus infection receiving highly active antiretroviral therapy. Clin Infect Dis 2002;34(10):1396–405.
[52] Carr A, Samaras K, Thorisdottir A, Kaufmann GR, Chisholm DJ, Cooper DA. Diagnosis, prediction, and natural course of HIV-1 protease-inhibitor-associated lipodystrophy, hyperlipidaemia, and diabetes mellitus: a cohort study. Lancet 1999;353(9170):2093–9.
[53] Kim RJ, Wilson CG, Wabitsch M, Lazar MA, Steppan CM. HIV protease inhibitor-specific alterations in human adipocyte differentiation and metabolism. Obesity (Silver Spring) 2006;14(6):994–1002.
[54] Jones SP, Waitt C, Sutton R, Back DJ, Pirmohamed M. Effect of atazanavir and ritonavir on the differentiation and adipokine secretion of human subcutaneous and omental preadipocytes. AIDS 2008;22(11):1293–8.
[55] Riddler SA, Smit E, Cole SR, et al. Impact of HIV infection and HAART on serum lipids in men. JAMA 2003;289(22):2978–82.
[56] Young J, Weber R, Rickenbach M, et al. Lipid profiles for antiretroviral-naive patients starting PI- and NNRTI-based therapy in the Swiss HIV cohort study. Antivir Ther 2005;10(5):585–91.
[57] Worm SW, Kamara DA, Reiss P, et al. Elevated triglycerides and risk of myocardial infarction in HIV-positive persons. AIDS 2011;25(12):1497–504.
[58] Tungsiripat M, Aberg JA. Dyslipidemia in HIV patients. Cleve Clin J Med 2005;72(12): 1113–20.
[59] Wohl DA, Tien HC, Busby M, et al. Randomized study of the safety and efficacy of fish oil (omega-3 fatty acid) supplementation with dietary and exercise counseling for the treatment of antiretroviral therapy-associated hypertriglyceridemia. Clin Infect Dis 2005;41(10):1498–504.
[60] Balasubramanyam A, Coraza I, Smith EO, et al. Combination of niacin and fenofibrate with lifestyle changes improves dyslipidemia and hypoadiponectinemia in HIV patients on antiretroviral therapy: results of "heart positive," a randomized, controlled trial. J Clin Endocrinol Metab 2011;96(7):2236–47.
[61] Kumar P, Rodriguez-French A, Thompson M. Prospective study of hyperlipidemia in ART-naive subjects taking combivir/abacavir (COM/ABC), COM/nelfinavir (NFV), or stavudine (d4t)/lamivudine (3TC)/NFV (ESS40002) [abstract 7.3/7]. 9th Conference on Retroviruses and Opportunistic Infections, Seattle, WA; 2002.
[62] Executive summary: Standards of medical care in diabetes—2013. Diabetes care 2013; 36 Suppl. 1: S4–10.
[63] Hruz PW. Molecular mechanisms for insulin resistance in treated HIV-infection. Best Pract Res Clin Endocrinol Metab 2011;25(3):459–68.
[64] Paik IJ, Kotler DP. The prevalence and pathogenesis of diabetes mellitus in treated HIV-infection. Best Pract Res Clin Endocrinol Metab 2011;25(3):469–78.
[65] Lewis W, Day BJ, Copeland WC. Mitochondrial toxicity of NRTI antiviral drugs: an integrated cellular perspective. Nat Rev Drug Discov 2003;2(10):812–22.
[66] Shikuma CM, Day LJ, Gerschenson M. Insulin resistance in the HIV-infected population: the potential role of mitochondrial dysfunction. Curr Drug Targets Infect Disord 2005;5(3):255–62.
[67] Grunfeld C. HIV protease inhibitors and glucose metabolism. AIDS 2002;16(6):925–6.
[68] Koster JC, Remedi MS, Qiu H, Nichols CG, Hruz PW. HIV protease inhibitors acutely impair glucose-stimulated insulin release. Diabetes 2003;52(7):1695–700.

[69] Brown TT, Tassiopoulos K, Bosch RJ, Shikuma C, McComsey GA. Association between systemic inflammation and incident diabetes in HIV-infected patients after initiation of antiretroviral therapy. Diabetes Care 2010;33(10):2244–9.
[70] Vigouroux C, Maachi M, Nguyen TH, et al. Serum adipocytokines are related to lipodystrophy and metabolic disorders in HIV-infected men under antiretroviral therapy. AIDS 2003;17(10):1503–11.
[71] Alencastro P, Wolff F, Oliveira R, et al. Metabolic syndrome and population attributable risk among HIV/AIDS patients: comparison between NCEP-ATPIII, IDF and AHA/NHLBI definitions. AIDS Res Ther 2012;9(1):29.
[72] Capeau J, Bouteloup V, Katlama C, et al. Ten-year diabetes incidence in 1046 HIV-infected patients started on a combination antiretroviral treatment. AIDS 2012;26(3):303–14.
[73] Rasmussen LD, Mathiesen ER, Kronborg G, Pedersen C, Gerstoft J, Obel N. Risk of diabetes mellitus in persons with and without HIV: a Danish nationwide population-based cohort study. PLoS One 2012;7(9):e44575.
[74] De Wit S, Sabin CA, Weber R, et al. Incidence and risk factors for new-onset diabetes in HIV-infected patients: the Data Collection on Adverse Events of Anti-HIV Drugs (D:A:D) study. Diabetes Care 2008;31(6):1224–9.
[75] Grinspoon S, Carr A. Cardiovascular risk and body-fat abnormalities in HIV-infected adults. N Engl J Med 2005;352(1):48–62.
[76] Thoni GJ, Fedou C, Brun JF, et al. Reduction of fat accumulation and lipid disorders by individualized light aerobic training in human immunodeficiency virus infected patients with lipodystrophy and/or dyslipidemia. Diabetes Metab 2002;28(5):397–404.
[77] Driscoll SD, Meininger GE, Ljungquist K, et al. Differential effects of metformin and exercise on muscle adiposity and metabolic indices in human immunodeficiency virus-infected patients. J Clin Endocrinol Metab 2004;89(5):2171–8.
[78] Perry AC, LaPerriere A, Klimas N. Acquired immune deficiency syndrome (AIDS). In: Durstine JL, Moore GE, Painter PL, Roberts SO, editors. ACSM's exercise management for persons with chronic diseases and disabilities (3rd ed.). Champagne, IL: Human Kinetics; 2009.
[79] Westcott WL. Resistance training is medicine: effects of strength training on health. Curr Sports Med Rep 2012;11(4):209–16.
[80] Yahiaoui A, McGough EL, Voss JG. Development of evidence-based exercise recommendations for older HIV-infected patients. J Assoc Nurses AIDS Care 2012;23(3):204–19.
[81] Engelson ES, Agin D, Kenya S, et al. Body composition and metabolic effects of a diet and exercise weight loss regimen on obese, HIV-infected women. Metabolism 2006;55(10):1327–36.
[82] De Souza PM, Jacob-Filho W, Santarem JM, Zomignan AA, Burattini MN. Effect of progressive resistance exercise on strength evolution of elderly patients living with HIV compared to healthy controls. Clinics (Sao Paulo, Brazil) 2011;66(2):261–6.
[83] Terry L, Sprinz E, Stein R, Medeiros NB, Oliveira J, Ribeiro JP. Exercise training in HIV-1-infected individuals with dyslipidemia and lipodystrophy. Med Sci Sports Exerc 2006;38(3):411–7.
[84] Justice AC. HIV and aging: time for a new paradigm. Curr HIV/AIDS Rep 2010;7(2):69–76.
[85] Malin SK, Kirwan JP. Fasting hyperglycaemia blunts the reversal of impaired glucose tolerance after exercise training in obese older adults. Diabetes Obes Metab 2012;14(9):835–41.
[86] Tripathi A, Liese AD, Jerrell JM, et al. Incidence of diabetes mellitus in a population-based cohort of HIV-infected and non-HIV-infected persons: the impact of clinical and therapeutic factors over time. Diabet Med 2014.
[87] Klassen K, Goff LM. Dietary intakes of HIV-infected adults in urban UK. Eur J Clin Nutr 2013;67(8):890–3.

[88] Giudici KV, Duran AC, Jaime PC. Inadequate food intake among adults living with HIV. Sao Paulo Med J 2013;131(3):145–52.
[89] Mason C, Foster-Schubert KE, Imayama I, et al. Dietary weight loss and exercise effects on insulin resistance in postmenopausal women. Am J Prev Med 2011;41(4):366–75.
[90] Purnomo J, Jeganathan S, Begley K, Houtzager L. Depression and dietary intake in a cohort of HIV-positive clients in Sydney. Int J STD AIDS 2012;23(12):882–6.
[91] Wooten JS, Nambi P, Gillard BK, et al. Intensive lifestyle modification reduces Lp-PLA2 in dyslipidemic HIV/HAART patients. Med Sci Sports Exerc 2013;45(6):1043–50.

CHAPTER

18

Exercise Treadmill Test for the Assessment of Cardiac Risk Markers in HIV

Andrea De Lorenzo[1,2,3]
and Filipe Penna de Carvalho[3]

[1]Instituto Nacional de Cardiologia, Rio de Janeiro, RJ, Brazil,
[2]Universidade Federal do Rio de Janeiro, Rio de Janeiro, RJ, Brazil,
[3]Clinica de Diagnostico por Imagem, Rio de Janeiro, RJ, Brazil

18.1 INTRODUCTION

The survival of persons living with HIV has increased considerably after the advent of antiretroviral therapy; currently, HIV-infected patients are as prone to common chronic diseases as their noninfected counterparts, more likely dying from those diseases and their complications than from opportunistic infections [1]. Cardiovascular illness is one of the most important conditions in this scenario [2–6], because antiretroviral therapy frequently results in metabolic abnormalities such as dyslipidemia and glucose intolerance, which increase the risk of coronary artery disease [7,8]. Furthermore, when compared with age-matched controls, HIV-infected patients have higher rates of other conventional cardiovascular risk factors such as hypertension and smoking [9,10]. Finally, the virus itself is associated with increased atherosclerotic risk [11].

The exercise treadmill test has been extensively used both in general populations and in specific patient groups (e.g., diabetics, postmyocardial infarction patients) for the stratification of cardiovascular risk or as a guide for the institution of therapies and exercise programs [12,13]. For HIV-infected persons, the evaluation with the exercise treadmill test

Health of HIV Infected People, Volume 2.
DOI: http://dx.doi.org/10.1016/B978-0-12-800767-9.00018-2

may be useful for screening for underlying cardiac disease or as a means of assessing cardiovascular fitness, with the latter as a preparation for exercise programs or simply as a guide for patients and care providers regarding patient management.

18.2 EXERCISE TESTING

Exercise testing is most frequently performed for the diagnosis of coronary artery disease or evaluation of its prognosis, two pieces of information that are in parallel. In any case, exercise testing also serves as a guide for the prescription of exercise training or for the adjustment of patients' activities to their diseases (according to their ischemic threshold).

Although exercise testing may be performed on a treadmill, bicycle, or even an arm ergometer, the first is more widely available. There are several exercise treadmill protocols, with the Bruce protocol being one of the most popular [14,15]. For the purposes of diagnosing underlying coronary artery disease, drugs with negative chronotropic properties such as ß-blockers and some calcium-channel blockers, which are often prescribed for hypertensive patients, should be withdrawn 48h before the test. In the usual protocols used in exercise stress testing, the test begins with the treadmill set to a low speed and incline, which increase periodically. The test may be stopped due to exhaustion, exercise-limiting leg discomfort or chest pain, severe blood pressure increase (systolic blood pressure ≥240mmHg or diastolic blood pressure ≥140 in previously hypertensive patients, or diastolic blood pressure ≥120mmHg in individuals without baseline hypertension), or if life-threatening arrhythmias occur [16].

During exercise several variables are evaluated, with the most common being exercise duration, the occurrence of chest pain or angina equivalents, electrocardiographic changes, heart rate response to exercise and after exercise cessation, blood pressure response to exercise, and oxygen consumption. The most well-known markers of ischemia used for diagnosis are ST segment depression and angina. Nonetheless, other variables such as chronotropic incompetence and heart rate recovery, among others, are also markers of underlying coronary artery disease and powerful predictors of outcome [17]. Along with exercise duration, these variables likewise assess general fitness and function of the autonomic nervous system. The most relevant of them are discussed later.

18.2.1 Ischemic Electrocardiographic Response to Exercise

The electrocardiographic response to exercise may be considered ischemic if patients develop ≥1.5mm ascending ST segment depression or ≥1mm horizontal ST segment depression, 80ms after the J point in 3

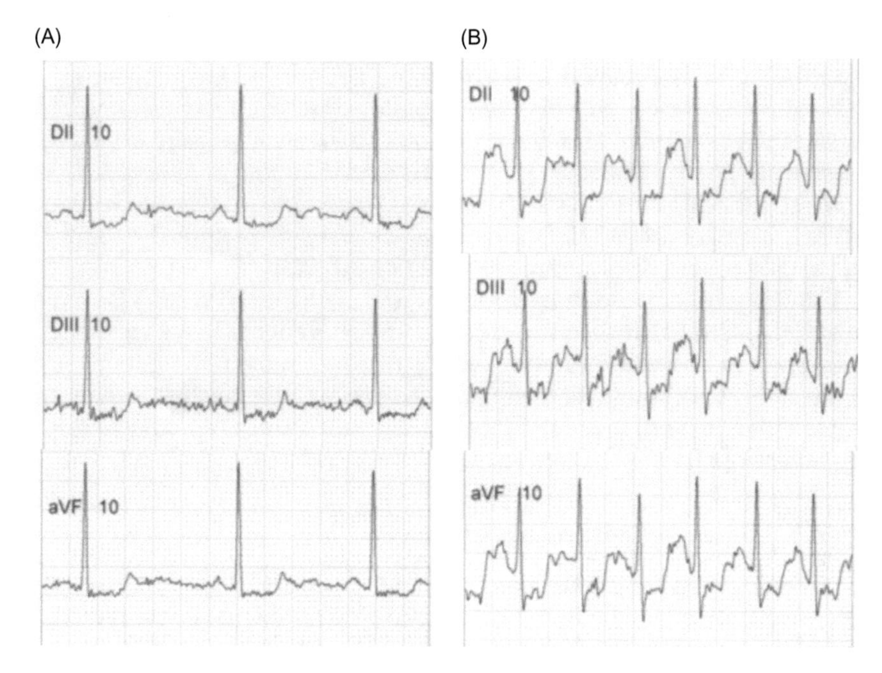

FIGURE 18.1 ECG recordings during a treadmill graded exercise test of a 58-year-old man with minor repolarization abnormalities at rest (A). During peak exercise (B), there is a marked downsloping ST segment depression.

consecutive beats [18] (Figure 18.1). Although exercise-induced ST depression does not localize the site of ischemia, ST segment elevation localizes ischemia and indicates the coronary artery is most likely involved. ST elevation is a sign of transmural ischemia if Q waves are absent; in the presence of Q waves, ST elevation usually does not indicate myocardial ischemia, but that it is a marker of myocardial viability [19].

18.2.2 Abnormal Exercise Duration, Functional Capacity, Peak Oxygen Consumption, Metabolic Equivalent

Average exercise time for a middle-aged adult is 8–10 min. Exercise duration (the time in minutes a patient can perform the exercise test) is a good measure of *functional capacity*, analogous to *peak oxygen consumption* or *metabolic equivalents* (MET).

Peak oxygen consumption (VO_2 peak, displayed as mL/kg/min) may be either measured in cardiopulmonary testing (exercise testing with respiratory gas analysis) or estimated, as occurs in the overall majority of exercise tests. When estimated, it is automatically calculated by exercise test software using the Foster equation [20]. Whereas directly measured

VO_2 is more precise, it is less often available because it requires additional expertise and costs related to the required equipment. On the contrary, VO_2 estimates based on validated equations are routinely obtained in most clinical facilities and have demonstrated an important role as a functional capacity indicator [21]. In this situation, functional capacity is expressed in MET, with 1 MET = 3.5 mL O_2/kg/min. Categories of poor (<5 MET) or good (>8 MET) functional capacity, as previously defined, are usually reported for prognostic assessment [22].

The prognostic value of exercise duration, METs, and peak VO_2 have been demonstrated in healthy subjects and in patients being evaluated for suspected or known coronary artery disease, in men, in women, and in the elderly. Although all decrease with age and are generally lower in women than in men, they retain their prognostic value after adjusting for age and sex [23].

18.2.3 Chronotropic Incompetence

Physiologically, heart rate increases with exercise. Chronotropic incompetence is defined as the inability to reach 85% of the maximal predicted heart rate, according to age and gender [24]. The latter may be generally calculated as 220 minus age in years. Different criteria for defining chronotropic incompetence have been used based on resting heart rate, exercise protocol, patient age, and medications (especially ß-blockers). Chronotropic incompetence is predictive of all-cause and cardiovascular death [24–26].

18.2.4 Abnormal Heart Rate Recovery

Also, physiologically, after exercise heart rate decreases and gradually returns to baseline levels. Abnormal heart rate recovery after exercise is defined as a heart rate decrease of less than 12 bpm in the first minute after exercise compared with peak heart rate [27] when recovery from exercise is active. Abnormal heart rate recovery is also a marker of cardiovascular risk, either for coronary artery disease or for all-cause death, and independently of coronary artery disease severity [24,28].

18.2.5 Abnormal Blood Pressure Response to Exercise

Blood pressure response during exercise is considered abnormal either when systolic blood pressure decreases ≥10 mmHg [29] or when systolic BP reaches ≥220–240 mmHg [30]. Exercise hypotension reflects a failure of cardiac output to increase during exercise and may be associated with severe coronary artery disease, left ventricular systolic dysfunction, or both [31,32], and it is a predictor of increased risk of cardiac events [29].

For exercise hypertension, whereas thresholds vary according to different studies, in general it is considered predictive of future systemic hypertension in people who are normotensive [33,34].

18.3 EXERCISE TESTING AND HIV

Whereas there are numerous studies and clinical indications for the use of the exercise treadmill test for cardiovascular risk evaluation either in healthy populations or in patients with known cardiovascular disease [35], few have focused on the (increasingly large) population of HIV-infected patients. Table 18.1 displays a summary of these data.

18.3.1 Exercise Responses in HIV

18.3.1.1 Electrocardiographic

In line with the higher risk of coronary artery disease in HIV-infected individuals [36–39], Duong et al. [40] found 11% of ischemic electrocardiographic responses in the exercise treadmill test of HIV-infected patients. However, their population had a higher proportion of males and some met AIDS-defining criteria; therefore, they were in a more advanced stage of infection, which might have increased the probability of coronary artery disease. In the study by De Lorenzo et al. [41], among patients undergoing long-term antiretroviral therapy and low viral load, none had electrocardiographic evidence of ischemia. However, these studies have in common the evidence of a link between central fat accumulation or increased weight and cardiovascular abnormalities elicited at the exercise test (either at the level of ST segment changes, in the case of Duong et al., or at heart rate variability, as in the study by De Lorenzo et al.).

18.3.1.2 Exercise Capacity

Lower functional capacity in HIV patients, whether receiving antiretroviral therapy, has been frequently reported [42–44]. Aerobic exercise intolerance in HIV has been attributed to chronic disease–related deconditioning, anemia, smoking, or even nucleoside reverse-transcriptase inhibitor–related peripheral oxidative dysfunction [45].

Although muscle wasting and severe loss of functional capacity were very frequent before antiretroviral therapy was available, both have become less common [46–48]. In the study by De Lorenzo et al. [41], among HIV-infected patients receiving antiretroviral therapy, 90% reached more than 8 METs. Also, age and body mass index were inversely correlated with estimated peak VO_2, indicating that effective antiretroviral therapy, although increasing risk because of several metabolic effects [7,8], may also "match" HIV-infected patients to noninfected individuals of the same

TABLE 18.1 Results of exercise testing in individuals living with HIV

				Stress test variables					Other findings
Author (ref#)	Subjects	Age (years)[a]	ARVT	Fx Capacity (peak VO_2)	Abnormal HRR	CI	Ischemic ECG	Abnormal BP response	
Duong et al. ([40])	99 HIV	42.0 ± 9.0	100%				11%		
De Lorenzo et al. ([41])	49 HIV	46.4 ± 8.4	100%	31.4 ± 4.8 (estimated)	10.2%	24.9%	None	15.0%	
Cade et al. ([42])	15 HIV 15 controls	18.3 ± 0.3	100%	24.9 ± 1.3 32.9 ± 1.1					Lower peak HR in HIV vs. controls (175.7 ± 2.5 vs. 193.7 ± 2.2)
Cade et al. ([43])	15 HIV 15 controls	41.9 ± 1.7 36.1 ± 1.8	100%	24.6 ± 1.2 32.0 ± 1.2					Lower peak HR in HIV vs. controls (167.8 ± 3.5 vs. 180.1 ± 3.5)
Keyser et al. ([44])	17 HIV	18.0 ± 2.0		22.9 ± 8.3					Peak VO_2 42 ± 19% less than expected values
Hand et al. ([49])	40 HIV 44 controls	41.2 ± 2.3 42.4 ± 1.4	72.5%	31.6 ± 2.1 29.4 ± 0.3					
Raso et al. ([50])	39 HIV (males) 25 controls	40.6 ± 1.4 44.4 ± 2.1		34.2 ± 0.9 32.2 ± 0.9					
Cade et al. ([51])	38 HIV 15 controls	41.0 ± 9.0 (with PI) 43.0 ± 6.0 (without PI) 40.0 ± 10.0	100%	26.0 ± 5.0 28.8 ± 8.6 33.1 ± 9.7					Impaired HRR in HIV Lower peak HR In HIV (with PI: 161 ± 15; without PI: 162 ± 15) vs. controls (175 ± 10) Higher peak SBP in HIV(with PI: 129 ± 15; without PI: 122 ± 13) vs. controls (111 ± 7)

ARVT, antiretroviral therapy; BP, blood pressure; CI, chronotropic incompetence; HRR, heart rate recovery; PI, protease inhibitor; SBP, systolic blood pressure.
[a] *Mean ± SD.*

age—including the effects of aging and obesity on functional capacity. Exercise training, among other beneficial effects, may reverse functional aerobic impairment in HIV-infected persons [49,50].

18.3.1.3 Chronotropic Incompetence and Abnormal Heart Rate Recovery

Chronotropic incompetence and abnormal heart rate recovery have been reported in HIV-infected patients. Cade et al. [51] observed impaired postexercise heart rate recovery in HIV-infected patients using antiretroviral therapy and suggested a link with autonomic neuropathy. In the study by De Lorenzo et al. [41], 25% of the patients had chronotropic incompetence and 10% had abnormal heart rate recovery. Chronotropic incompetence and abnormal heart rate recovery may be linked in HIV-infected patients either to coronary artery disease [52,53] or to autonomic dysfunction due to several reports of autonomic neuropathy in these patients [54–57]. Abnormal heart rate recovery, a sign of reduced vagal tone, matches findings of ineffective vagal response to cold-face test and abnormal sympathovagal balance, described by Correia et al. [58]. Any of these findings, even in the absence of electrocardiographic signs of ischemia, may allocate patients to a higher risk category [23–28].

18.3.1.4 Blood Pressure Response

Scarce data are available regarding blood pressure responses to exercise in HIV-infected patients. In our study, exercise hypertension was found in 15% of the patients and none had exercise-induced hypotension [41]. The paucity of data regarding blood pressure response to exercise may be partly due to the frequently found low accuracy of blood pressure measurements during exercise, secondary to noise from the treadmill or the lack of standards for the definition of abnormal responses.

18.4 THE ETT AS A SCREENING TOOL IN HIV-INFECTED INDIVIDUALS

The evaluation of cardiovascular risk in HIV-infected patients is relevant for a number of reasons. First, because of the interaction between antiretroviral therapy and coronary artery disease, there are advocates of cardiovascular risk stratification before starting treatment and also during treatment [59].

The stratification of cardiovascular risk with the Framingham risk score—the most disseminated [60]—may not be the best way to assess cardiovascular risk in persons living with HIV. This score was developed in middle-aged, mostly Caucasian Americans free of coronary artery disease at baseline and therefore is mostly unsuitable for the HIV-infected population. Also, the latter are, on average, younger, thus resulting in a low score because age is strongly associated with cardiovascular risk and one of the main drivers of the Framingham score. Even in general populations, it has been pointed out that the 10-year risk model may underestimate lifetime risk [61].

Plenty of data regarding subclinical cardiovascular abnormalities may be found with exercise testing, allowing early appropriate management and/or rehabilitation [62]. Interventions to decrease cardiovascular risk have well-recognized importance and include exercise programs, smoking cessation, and pharmacologic measures such as aspirin and lipid-lowering medications; the level of aggressiveness for initiating these measures may be tailored by exercise test results [59,63–67].

In this sense comes another important practical application of exercise testing: to plan interventions aimed at improving cardiovascular prognosis. Recommendations for rehabilitation of older adults living with HIV have been released [59,68]. A combination of aerobic and resistive exercise was recommended for older adults living with HIV who are medically stable and living with comorbidities, including bone and joint disorders, cancer, stroke, cardiovascular disease, mental health, cognitive impairment, chronic obstructive pulmonary disease, and diabetes. The recommendations stated that "frequency, intensity, time, and type of exercise should be individually tailored to the specific goals and capacity of the individual and the specific comorbidity." In that sense, the exercise treadmill test has unique value to define each patient's limits and adequately plan exercise training. The exercise program should be modified according to the individual's physical function, health status, exercise response, and programmed goals.

Several initiatives regarding exercise training in the HIV-infected population [64–67] have been reported. In the study by Garcia et al. [64], the number of $CD4^+$ cells, lean body mass, muscle strength, HDL cholesterol levels, as well as VO_2max increased after exercise training. Studies have found favorable effects of exercise on metabolic indices and autonomic function, as well as a decrease of body mass index and an increase in oxygen consumption in HIV-infected patients [65–67].

Currently, there are neither well-established nor disseminated strategies of searching for cardiovascular disease in persons living with HIV. Yet, pooled results indicate a subgroup of patients with HIV receiving antiretroviral therapy—the older, overweight/obese HIV-infected patients—who may deserve periodic cardiovascular screening with exercise treadmill test [69–71]. Recent evidence showed that older adults living with HIV frequently experience frailty at a much younger age than the general older population, with central obesity and fat redistribution appearing as important predictors of frailty [72]. Notwithstanding, physical frailty in HIV-infected patients may be amenable to lifestyle interventions, especially exercise and diet therapy. Accordingly, awareness of the need of risk assessment strategies is growing [73,74], and further studies are still necessary.

18.5 CONCLUSIONS

The burden of cardiovascular disease in persons living with HIV is a reality. Therefore, even though the global management of HIV-infected individuals is quite challenging, the importance of prevention or early diagnosis of cardiovascular disease should not be overlooked. Risk stratification strategies including the exercise test may prove useful in detecting subclinical abnormalities and/or in tailoring exercise programs as a part of a global risk-reduction management effort that may result in improved cardiovascular prognosis.

References

[1] The Joint United Nations Programme on HIV/AIDS. AIDS epidemic update. Available from: <http://www.unaids.org/en/media/unaids/contentassets/documents/epidemiology/2013/gr2013/unaids_global_report_2013_en.pdf>[accessed on July 2014].
[2] Henry K, Melroe H, Huebsch J, et al. Severe premature coronary artery disease with protease inhibitors. Lancet 1998;351:1328.
[3] Currier JS, Taylor A, Boyd F, et al. Coronary heart diseases in HIV- infected individuals. J Acquir Immune Defic Syndr 2003;33:506–12.
[4] Palella FJ, Baker RK, Moorman AC, et al. Mortality in the highly active antiretroviral therapy era: changing causes of death and disease in the HIV outpatient study. J Acquir Immune Defic Syndr 2006;43:27–34.
[5] Lau B, Gange SJ, Moore RD. Risk of non-AIDS-related mortality may exceed risk of AIDS-related mortality among individuals enrolling into care with CD4+ counts greater than 200 cells/mm3. J Acquir Immune Defic Syndr 2007;44:179–87.
[6] Triant VA, Lee H, Hadigan C, Grinspoon SK. Increased acute myocardial infarction rates and cardiovascular risk factors among patients with human immunodeficiency virus disease. J Clin Endocrinol Metab 2007;92:2506–12.
[7] Carr A, Samaras K, Burton S, et al. A syndrome of peripheral lipodystrophy, hyperlipidaemia and insulin resistance in patients receiving HIV protease inhibitors. AIDS 1998;12:F51–8.
[8] Calza L, Manfredi R, Chiodo F. Dyslipidaemia associated with antiretroviral therapy in HIV-infected patients. J Antimicrob Chemother 2004;53:10–14.
[9] Kaplan RC, Kingsley LA, Sharrett AR, et al. Ten-year predicted coronary heart disease risk in HIV-infected men and women. Clin Infect Dis 2007;45:1074–81.
[10] Gazzaruso C, Rruno R, Garzaniti A, et al. Hypertension among HIV patients: prevalence and relationships to insulin resistance and metabolic syndrome. J Hypertens 2003;21:1377–82.
[11] Lang S, Mary-Krause M, Simon A, et al. HIV replication and immune status are independent predictors of the risk of myocardial infarction in HIV-infected individuals. Clin Infect Dis 2012;55:600–7.
[12] Villella A, Maggioni AP, Villella M, et al. Prognostic significance of maximal exercise testing after myocardial infarction treated with thrombolytic agents: the GISSI-2 data-base: gruppo italiano per lo studio della sopravvivenza nell'infarto. Lancet 1995;346:523–9.

[13] Heller GV. Evaluation of the patient with diabetes mellitus and suspected coronary artery disease. Am J Med 2005;118(Suppl. 2):9S–14S.
[14] Bruce RA, Lovejoy Jr. FW, Yu PN, Mc Dowell ME. Observations of cardiorespiratory performance in normal subjects under unusual stress during exercise. AMA Arch Ind Hyg Occup Med 1952;6:105–12.
[15] Myers J, Buchanan N, Walsh D, et al. Comparison of the ramp versus standard exercise protocols. J Am Coll Cardiol 1991;17:1334–42.
[16] Gibbons RJ, Balady GJ, Bricker JT, et al. ACC/AHA 2002 guideline update for exercise testing: summary article: a report of the American college of Cardiology/American heart association task force on practice guidelines (committee to update the 1997 exercise testing). Circulation 2002;106:1883–92.
[17] Ellestad MH. Stress testing: principles and practice, 5th ed. New York, NY: Oxford University Press; 2003.
[18] Okin PM, Prineas RJ, Grandits G, et al. Heart rate adjustment of exercise-induced ST segment depression identifies men who benefit from a risk factor reduction program. Circulation 1997;96:2899.
[19] Li RA, Leppo M, Miki T, et al. Molecular basis of electrocardiographic ST segment elevation. Circ Res 2000;87:837.
[20] Foster C, Crowe AJ, Daines E, et al. Predicting functional capacity during treadmill testing independent of exercise protocol. Med Sci Sports Exerc 1996;28:752–6.
[21] Snader CE, Marwick TH, Pashkow FJ, et al. Importance of estimated functional capacity as a predictor of all-cause mortality among patients referred for exercise thallium single photon emission computed tomography: report of 3,400 patients from a single center. J Am Coll Cardiol 1997;30:641–8.
[22] Myers J, Prakash M, Froelicher V, et al. Exercise capacity and mortality among men referred for exercise testing. N Engl J Med 2002;346:793–801.
[23] Chang JA, Froelicher VF. Clinical and exercise test markers of prognosis in patients with stable coronary artery disease. Curr Probl Cardiol 1994;19:533–87.
[24] Lauer MS, Okin PM, Larson MG, et al. Impaired heart rate response to graded exercise. Prognostic implications of chronotropic incompetence in the Framingham heart study. Circulation 1996;93:1520–6.
[25] Lauer MS, Francis GS, Okin RM, et al. Impaired chronotropic response to exercise stress testing as a predictor of mortality. JAMA 1999;281:524–9.
[26] Elhendy A, Mahoney DW, Khanderia BK, et al. Prognostic significance of impairment of heart rate response to exercise: impact of left ventricular function and myocardial ischemia. J Am Coll Cardiol 2003;42:823–30.
[27] Cole CR, Blackstone EH, Pashkow FJ, et al. Heart rate recovery immediately after exercise as a predictor of mortality. N Engl J Med 1999;341:1351–7.
[28] Vivekananthan DP, Blackstone EH, Pothier CE, Lauer MS. Heart rate recovery after exercise is a predictor of mortality, independent of the angiographic severity of coronary disease. J Am Coll Cardiol 2003;42:831–8.
[29] Dubach P, Froelicher VF, Klein J, et al. Exercise-induced hypotension in a male population. Criteria, causes, and prognosis. Circulation 1988;78:1380–7.
[30] Tzemos N, Lim PO, MacDonald TM. Is exercise blood pressure a marker of vascular endothelial function? QJM 2002;95:423–9.
[31] Hammermeister KE, DeRouen TA, Dodge HT, Zia M. Prognostic and predictive value of exertional hypotension in suspected coronary artery disease. Am J Cardiol 1983;51:1261–6.
[32] Hakki AH, Munley BM, Hadjimiltiades S, et al. Determinants of abnormal blood pressure response to exercise in coronary artery disease. Am J Cardiol 1986;57:71–5.
[33] Wilson NV, Meyer BM. Early prediction of hypertension using exercise blood pressure. Prev Med 1981;10:62–8.
[34] Dlin RA, Hanne N, Silverberg DS, Bar-Or O. Follow-up of normotensive men with exaggerated blood pressure response to exercise. Am Heart J 1983;106:316–20.

[35] Lauer M, Froelicher ES, Williams M, Kligfield P. Exercise testing in asymptomatic adults: a statement for professionals from the American heart association council on clinical cardiology, subcommittee on exercise, cardiac rehabilitation, and prevention. Circulation 2005;112:771–6.
[36] Fris-Møller N, Sabin CA, Weber R, et al. Data collection on adverse events of anti-HIV drugs (DAD) study group. Combination antiretroviral therapy and the risk of myocardial infarction. N Engl J Med 2003;349:1993–2003.
[37] Kamin DS, Grinspoon SK. Cardiovascular disease in HIV-positive patients. AIDS 2005;19:641–52.
[38] Currier JS, Lundgran JD, Carr A, et al. Epidemiological evidence for cardiovascular disease in HIV-infected patients and relationship to highly active antiretroviral therapy. Circulation 2008;118:e29–35.
[39] Escarcega RO, Franco JJ, Mani BC. Cardiovascular disease in patients with chronic human immunodeficiency virus infection. Int J Cardiol 2014;175:1–7.
[40] Duong M, Cottin Y, Piroth L, et al. Exercise stress testing for detection of silent myocardial ischemia in human immunodeficiency virus–infected patients receiving antiretroviral therapy. Clin Infect Dis 2002;34:523–8.
[41] De Lorenzo A, Meirelles V, Vilela F, Souza FC. Use of the exercise treadmill test for the assessment of cardiac risk markers in adults infected with HIV. J Int Assoc Provid AIDS Care 2013;12:110–6.
[42] Cade WT, Peralta L, Keyser RE. Aerobic capacity in late adolescents infected with HIV and controls. Pediatr Rehabil 2002;5:161–9.
[43] Cade WT, Fantry LE, Nabar SR, Keyser RE. Decreased peak arteriovenous oxygen difference during treadmill exercise testing in individuals infected with the human immunodeficiency virus. Arch Phys Med Rehabil 2003;84:1595–603.
[44] Keyser RE, Peralta L, Cade WT, et al. Functional aerobic impairment in adolescents seropositive for HIV: a quasiexperimental analysis. Arch Phys Med Rehabil 2000;81:1479–84.
[45] Stringer WW. Mechanisms of exercise limitation in HIV+ individuals. Med Sci Sports Exerc 2000;32:S412–21.
[46] Stanton DL, Wu AW, Moore RD, et al. Functional status of persons with HIV infection in an ambulatory setting. J Acquir Immune Defic Syndr 1994;7:1050–6.
[47] Wilson IB, Cleary PD. Clinical predictors of decline in physical functioning in persons with AIDS: results of a longitudinal study. J Acquir Immune Defic Syndr Hum Retrovirol 1997;16:343–9.
[48] Crystal S, Fleishman JA, Hays RD, et al. Physical and role functioning among persons with HIV: results from a nationally representative survey. Med Care 2000;38:1210–23.
[49] Hand GA, Phillips KD, Dudgeon WD, et al. Moderate intensity exercise training reverses functional aerobic impairment in HIV-infected individuals. AIDS Care 2008;20:1066–74.
[50] Raso V, Shephard RJ, Casseb J, et al. Association between muscle strength and the cardiopulmonary status of individuals living with HIV/AIDS. Clinics (Sao Paulo) 2013;68:359–64.
[51] Cade WT, Reeds DN, Lassa-Claxton S, et al. Post-exercise heart rate recovery in HIV-positive individuals on highly active antiretroviral therapy. Early indicator of cardiovascular disease? HIV Med 2008;9:96–100.
[52] Vittecoq D, Escaut L, Monsuez JJ. Vascular complications associated with use of HIV protease inhibitors. Lancet 1998;351:1959.
[53] Boccara F, Lang S, Meuleman C, et al. HIV and coronary artery disease. J Am Coll Cardiol 2013;61:511–23.
[54] Ruttimann S, Hilti P, Spinas GA, Dubach UC. High frequency of human immunodeficiency virus-associated autonomic neuropathy and more severe involvement in advanced stages of human immunodeficiency virus disease. Arch Intern Med 1991;151:2441–3.

[55] Lin-Greenberg A, Taneja-Upal N. Dysautonomia and infection with the human immunodeficiency virus. Ann Intern Med 1987;106:167.
[56] Freeman R, Roberts MS, Friedman LS, Broadbridge C. Autonomic function and HIV. Neurology 1990;40:575–80.
[57] Rogstad KE, Shah R, Tesfaladet G, et al. Cardiovascular autonomic neuropathy in HIV infected patients. Sex Transm Infect 1999;75:264–7.
[58] Correia D, Rodrigues de Resende LA, Molina RJ, et al. Power spectral analysis of heart rate variability in HIV-infected and AIDS patients. Pacing Clin Electrophysiol 2006;29:53–8.
[59] Grinspoon SK, Grunfeld C, Kotler DP, et al. State of the science conference: initiative to decrease cardiovascular risk and increase quality of care for patients living with HIV/AIDS: executive summary. Circulation 2008;118:198–210.
[60] D'Agostino Sr RBD, Vasan RS, Pencina MJ, et al. General cardiovascular risk profile for use in primary care: the Framingham heart study. Circulation 2008;117:743–53.
[61] Schlendorf KH, Nasir K, Blumenthal RS. Limitations of the Framingham risk score are now much clearer. Prev Med 2009;48:115–6.
[62] Schuster I, Thöni GJ, Edérhy S, et al. Subclinical cardiac abnormalities in human immunodeficiency virus-infected men receiving antiretroviral therapy. Am J Cardiol 2008;101:1213–7.
[63] O'Brien KK, Solomon P, Trentham B, et al. Evidence-informed recommendations for rehabilitation with older adults living with HIV: a knowledge synthesis. BMJ Open 2014;4:e004692. doi: http://dx.doi.org/10.1136/bmjopen.
[64] Garcia A, Fraga GA, Vieira Jr RC, et al. Effects of combined exercise training on immunological, physical and biochemical parameters in individuals with HIV/AIDS. J Sports Sci 2014;32:785–92.
[65] Engelson ES, Agin D, Kenya S, et al. Body composition and metabolic effects of a diet and exercise weight loss regimen on obese, HIV-infected women. Metabolism 2006;55:1327–36.
[66] Multimura E, Crowther NJ, Cade TW, et al. Exercise training reduced central adiposity and improves metabolic indices in HAART-treated HIV-positive subjects in Rwanda: a randomized controlled trial. AIDS Res Hum Retroviruses 2008;24:15–23.
[67] O'Brien K, Nixon S, Tynan AM, Glazier R. Aerobic exercise interventions for adults living with HIV/AIDS. Cochrane Database Syst Rev 2010;4:CD001796.
[68] Steinn JH, Hadigan CM, Brown TT, et al. Prevention strategies for cardiovascular disease in HIV-infected patients. Circulation 2008;118:e54–60.
[69] Rusch M, Nixon S, Schilder A, et al. Impairments, activity limitations and participation restrictions: prevalence and associations among persons living with HIV/AIDS in British Columbia. Health Qual Life Outcomes 2004;2:46.
[70] Oursler KK, Sorkin JD, Smith BA, Katzel LI. Reduced aerobic capacity and physical functioning in older HIV-infected men. AIDS Res Hum Retroviruses 2006;22:1113–21.
[71] Oursler KK, Goulet JL, Leaf DA, et al. Association of comorbidity with physical disability in older HIV-infected adults. AIDS Patient Care STDS 2006;20:782–91.
[72] Shah K, Hilton TN, Myers L, et al. A new frailty syndrome: central obesity and frailty in older adults with the human immunodeficiency virus. J Am Geriatr Soc 2012;60:545–9.
[73] High KP, Bradley S, Loeb M, et al. A new paradigm for clinical investigation of infectious syndromes in older adults: assessment of functional status as a risk factor and outcome measure. Clin Infect Dis 2005;40:114–22.
[74] Oursler KK, Katzel LI, Smith BA, et al. Prediction of cardiorespiratory fitness in older men infected with the human immunodeficiency virus: clinical factors and value of the six-minute walk distance. J Am Geriatr Soc 2009;57:2055–61.

CHAPTER

19

Measures of Physical Function in the Management of Individuals Living with HIV/AIDS

Vagner Raso[1] *and Roy Jesse Shephard*[2]

[1]School of Medicine of the University of Western Sao Paulo, UNOESTE, Brazil, Masters Program on Body Balance Rehabilitation of the Anhanguera University, UNIAN, Brazil [2]Faculty of Kinesiology and Physical Education of the University of Toronto, Toronto, ON, Canada

19.1 INTRODUCTION

Measures that include the promotion of condom use, needle exchanges for drug users, more careful control of blood transfusions, and early antiretroviral/protease inhibitor treatment for those individuals who do become infected with the human immunodeficiency virus (HIV) have reduced the incidence of infection and its progression to the acquired immunodeficiency syndrome (AIDS) in developed countries [1]. Many of those who receive the latest treatment modalities show little disturbances in physical function. In contrast, HIV/AIDS remains a pandemic in Africa; in 2012, 35.3 million people were living with HIV/AIDS, with at least 1.6 million dying in 2012 alone [2]. Moreover, in many African countries where a large percentage of the population is infected, treatment is inadequate by modern standards [3–5]. Such individuals are liable to develop many measurable physical manifestations [6], including decreases in lean tissue mass and muscle strength, vital capacity, arterial oxygen saturation, and maximal aerobic power and bone density, together with lipodystrophy that increases the risks of cardiovascular disease in longer-term survivors.

The objectives of this chapter are to explore the overall physiopathology of impaired functional capacity, to evaluate the specific physiopathology of functional changes in muscle strength and maximal aerobic power,

Health of HIV Infected People, Volume 2.
DOI: http://dx.doi.org/10.1016/B978-0-12-800767-9.00019-4

to consider how far such changes can be assessed by the simple tests likely to be available in third world countries, and to determine the extent to which such information plays a useful role in the assessment of disease severity, evaluation of prognosis, and the management of nutrition and exercise rehabilitation.

19.2 OVERALL BASIS OF POOR FUNCTIONAL CAPACITY IN HIV/AIDS

Many factors contribute to the poor muscular and cardiovascular fitness of patients with HIV/AIDS [7]. In general, habitual physical activity is limited and insufficient to maintain physical condition [8,9]. Many patients are unemployed and/or unable to cultivate the small-holding that normally provides much of their daily diet [8,10–12], so the balanced food intake needed for optimal muscle and cardiovascular function is lacking. The ingestion of nutritious food may be reduced because of financial problems, but also because of depression, fatigue, and social isolation. The problem of an inadequate diet is often exacerbated by a tumor necrosis factor alpha (TNF-α)-mediated suppression of appetite [13], dysphagia resulting from ulceration of the mouth or inflammation of the esophagus [14,15], malabsorption of food due to HIV enteropathy, decreased gut transit time, and diarrhea due to opportunistic infections such as salmonella [15]. Other metabolic factors limiting functional capacity include general mitochondrial dysfunction and cellular toxicity, with a blunting of lipolysis and fatty acid oxidation during submaximal effort [16] and impaired muscle oxidative phophorylation, including a rapid build-up of lactate and early fatigue when exercising [17].

19.3 LEAN TISSUE MASS AND MUSCULAR STRENGTH

19.3.1 Specific Physiopathology

The loss of muscle tissue and the decrease in muscle strength and endurance have multiple causes. Tissue loss may reflect a combination of impaired absorption of food and increased catabolism, although, unfortunately, the provision of nutritional supplements sometimes exacerbates a deleterious accumulation of fat rather than correcting the loss of lean tissue [18]. Adverse humoral factors militating against the maintenance and synthesis of muscle protein include elevated levels of cortisol and cytokines such as TNF-α, a breakdown of binding proteins and, thus, insulin-like growth factor-1 (IGF-1) activity, and decreased testosterone levels [10].

Other metabolic issues include a "futile" mobilization of peripheral fat by inflammatory cytokines, with subsequent hepatic resynthesis of triglycerides, increased muscle catabolism [10,19], and a reduced antioxidant activity, and thus greater oxidant stress [20]. The strength developed for any given lean tissue mass may also be low because of restricted habitual physical activity [8] and poorly understood impairment of central, coordinated motor unit activation, possibly reflecting a direct effect of the virus on the motor areas of the cerebral cortex [21].

19.3.2 Determinations of Lean Tissue Mass

The modern laboratory uses a wide variety of techniques for the determination of lean tissue mass [22], but most of these methodologies are unlikely to be available to third world patients. Perhaps the simplest approach in a clinic with limited resources is simply to determine the individual's body mass, either as an absolute value relative to the person's standing height or as a change relative to when the patient was in good health. If the absolute value is to be considered, then it will be necessary to use local body mass/height tables; prior malnutrition and/or regional differences of limb length will make North American or European norms inappropriate as baseline data [23]. If a change in body mass is considered, then it is likely that the "healthy" weight will have been exaggerated by 1–2 kg, because the person was wearing shoes and some clothing when the measurement was taken. Despite these problems, several investigators have concluded that ratios of mass to height provide not only the simplest but also one of the best epidemiological indices of body composition [24–26]. The loss of lean tissue in a severe case of HIV/AIDS can be as large as 10–15 kg [27–29], and a portable scale will indicate current weight with a precision of perhaps 0.5 kg. Simple weight measurements thus should give some indication of immediate disease severity, although a part of the loss of lean tissue may be masked by an accumulation of fat. Equally, during rehabilitation, weight gain should provide a measure of clinical progress, although much will depend on concomitant changes in fat stores; progressive exercise may reduce excess body fat, but the use of nutritional supplements may increase unwanted fat deposits [18].

An alternative approach is to estimate lean tissue mass more directly from total body mass and skinfold determinations of the percentage of body fat [22]. Precision skinfold calipers may be outside the budget of some third world clinics, but reasonably accurate skinfold determinations can be made with simple plastic skinfold calipers that retail for $15 to $30. Estimates of lean tissue mass are likely to give a more precise indication of clinical condition than simple weighing and, in particular, should circumvent the issue of increased fat storage in HIV/AIDS. Nevertheless, there are several important caveats when assessing HIV/AIDS patients in the third world. In particular, the conversion of skinfold readings into estimates of body fat is compromised because equations for the prediction of body fat are based on either European or North American populations, and they assume a normal bone density. Unfortunately, many patients with HIV/AIDS show a decrease in bone density [30]; this has multiple causes, but a 2–6% deficit of bone mineral content has been reported over the first 2 years of antiviral treatment.

19.3.3 Determinations of Muscular Strength

Direct determinations of muscle strength have the attraction of face validity in the assessment of a patient's functional ability, and if there is a decrease in central motor unit activation, then this would be reflected in the score obtained. However, the strength that is recorded depends not simply on the patient's muscle function but also on technical factors such as subject motivation and the learning of test techniques (both of which can change over successive evaluations).

In modern laboratories, strength is commonly evaluated using expensive devices such as isokinetic dynamometers and force plates, but in the third world the only likely options are various jump tests to assess explosive force and simple mechanical dynamometers to measure handgrip and leg isometric extension force and endurance.

The scores obtained on jump tests depend substantially on the learning of an optimal technique and are likely to show a decrease as the individual gains lean body mass during recovery. They are not well-suited to either the immediate or the longitudinal evaluation of patients with HIV/AIDS. Dynamometer measurements evaluate only one muscle group, and the question of how far the data obtained are representative of the body muscles as a whole arises. The most commonly used field device is the handgrip dynamometer, and a recent analysis concluded that the handgrip force was well-correlated with overall muscular strength [31]. Certainly, widespread practical experience has shown this measure to be effective in evaluating many other types of clinical population, including the elderly, with substantial losses of muscle strength [32–35]. Even after a healthy person has practiced the test sufficiently to reach a stable maximal value, the standard deviation of handgrip measurements over an interval of a few weeks is likely to be at least 5% and may be somewhat greater in patients with HIV/AIDS. Thus, if this test is applied to the assessment of an individual patient, then it can only detect change in muscle strength with a confidence of 10%. Nevertheless, this may be sufficient precision to indicate current status and response to therapy. It can also provide information about prognosis because approximately three-quarters of the variance in performance of the activities of daily living (e.g., gait speed and the tying of shoe laces) in individuals living with HIV/AIDS is explained by handgrip strength [31]. Current levels of handgrip force can indicate patients who are at risk for losing their physical independence [31], offering not only an immediate assessment of functional status but also a prediction of longer-term prognosis [36–39].

19.4 CARDIORESPIRATORY FUNCTION

19.4.1 Specific Physiopathology

Patients with HIV/AIDS often show substantial impairment in maximal oxygen transport. Treadmill $\dot{V}O_{2peak}$ were from 24% to 44% below anticipated age-related normal values [40] and that 6-min walk predictions of maximal aerobic power averaged only 18.4 mL/[kg·min] in HIV-infected men with a median age of 57 years [41]. Others have commented on slow recovery of exercise heart rates relative to uninfected controls [42]. The deterioration of aerobic function is commonly marked by poor cardiac stroke volume, slowed oxygen kinetics [11,12], widening of the A–V oxygen difference, and impaired muscle oxygenation [43–45]. These abnormalities may reflect either a primary effect of the disease or a side effect of treatment. Several studies have linked such changes to the administration of HAART and/or protease inhibitor, with these agents either acting directly on the mitochondria in skeletal and cardiac muscle [11,12,42,46,47] or causing longer-term pathologies associated with lipodystrophy and the promotion of atherosclerosis [48,49]. A further issue limiting sustained aerobic activity is that because of muscle weakness, patients reach their anaerobic threshold at an unusually low fraction of peak aerobic power. This leads to an early accumulation of lactate, with an increase in fatigue that limits peak oxygen uptake, sustained aerobic activity, and performance of the activities of daily living [50,51].

19.4.2 Determinations of Cardiorespiratory Performance

Measurements of oxygen on-transients and arteriovenous oxygen differences are limited mainly to the experimental laboratory. In the developed world, the cardiorespiratory performance of a patient with HIV/AIDS is usually assessed by a graded treadmill stress test, although because of muscle weakness, early fatigue, and sometimes poor motivation, the data obtained are peak rather than centrally limited maximal oxygen intakes [52]. In a healthy person able to reach an oxygen consumption plateau, the test–retest variation over an interval of several weeks is likely to be approximately 4–5% [53], but in patients who only attain peak readings the variance is likely to be larger.

In the third world, treadmill testing is unlikely to be available; weaker options will include measures of maximal or habitual walking speed and simple submaximal step tests. The self-paced distance walked in 6 min has commonly been used as a simple measure of aerobic function in the elderly and in a variety of clinical patients [54,55]. It is attractive in terms of face validity, although in terms of objective laboratory data it has a relatively low coefficient of correlation with the directly measured maximal oxygen intake (0.3–0.4). Exercise physiologists have also developed a large number of submaximal step tests; the Canadian Aerobic Fitness Test is perhaps the most widely used [56]. If an electrocardiograph is available to provide an accurate determination of the exercise heart rate, then the directly measured maximal oxygen intake can be predicted with a standard deviation of approximately ±10%. However, if the heart rate is obtained by wrist or carotid palpation, then errors are much greater, to the point that it is recommended to simply make a five-level categorization of fitness from test scores [56].

Because patients with HIV/AIDS are likely to show variations in body fat content during treatment, it seems desirable to express oxygen transport in units of L/min as well as the more customary mL/[kg·min]. In patients who are able to attain a plateau of maximal oxygen intake during treadmill testing, the laboratory data can plainly detect a 10% deficit of cardiorespiratory function relative to expected norms, and it should also be competent to detect a 10–20% gain of function in response to a training regimen. Observations are particularly relevant to the prognosis for independent living because a maximal oxygen transport of approximately 15 mL/[kg·min] is needed to allow a patient to live independently [57,58].

The ability to make parallel inferences from walking speeds and step tests has yet to be clearly established; both types of data should probably be interpreted directly, rather than attempting to predict maximal oxygen intake, as is commonly done. The preferred walking speed varies with age, sex, and body size, but it may be possible to establish norms based on these variables, and thus to make an assessment of a patient's current status; for instance, there have been claims that walking speed offers a measure of life expectancy [59]. However, such tests seem likely to have a large test/retest standard deviation, and thus only limited ability to detect changes in cardiorespiratory function.

Step tests have much smaller face validity in a third world environment—many dwellings do not contain stairs, and rapid stair climbing has limited relevance to most daily activities. Interpretation is further limited by the categoric rather than numeric classification of patient status.

19.5 PERSPECTIVE ON THE LIMITATIONS OF FUNCTIONAL TESTING

There are important limitations to the interpretation of most laboratory tests, and it is important for these limitations to be acknowledged before any attempt is made to use the numerical data in an assessment of current status, prognosis, or the response to treatment. Even assuming that the measure is appropriate relative to the function under evaluation (content validity), there are many sources of error that cause instability in the reported numbers. In terms of the patient, the test commonly requires learning a technique and maximal motivation, with further variations in personal response introduced by environmental factors and circadian and circaseptan rhythms, independently of any effects of illness. Further, these largely unavoidable sources of variance are boosted by changes in calibration of the apparatus and random errors of measurement. Even when healthy, well-motivated subjects are using the latest types of laboratory equipment, most test results differ by at least 5% when repeated after an interval of several weeks. With anxious and/or poorly motivated subjects, and when using simple field equipment, errors are likely to be much larger. In some situations, useful information can still be obtained by functional testing, but the test data must always be regarded with skepticism and analyzed in tandem with careful clinical examination.

19.6 CONCLUSION

HIV/AIDS can lead to a substantial loss of lean tissue, with decreases in the strength and maximal aerobic power of the patient. In parts of the world where the disease is most prevalent, practical considerations limit measures of such changes to body mass, skinfold thicknesses, dynamometer assessments of handgrip force, and walking speed or step estimates of aerobic function. The data may still provide some indication of current status, prognosis, and response to dietary and exercise treatments, but interpretation is severely limited by an inherent large month-to-month variance in test score.

References

[1] Palella FJ, Delaney KM, Moorman AC, Loveless MO, Fuhrer J, Satten GA, et al. Declining morbidity and mortality among patients with advanced human immunodeficiency virus infection. N Engl J Med 1998;338:853–60.

[2] World Health Organization Global health observatory. Geneva, Switzerland: World Health; 2014.

[3] UNAIDS. Global report fact sheet, <http://www.unaids.org/documents/20101123_FS_Global_em_en.pdf>[accessed 07.08.14].

[4] UNAIDS. 2011 World AIDS day report, <www.unaids.org/.../unaids/.../unaidspublication/2011/jc2216_worldaidsday_report_2011_en.pdf>[accessed 07.08.14].

[5] Kallings LO. The first postmodern pandemic: 25 years of HIV/AIDS. J Intern Med 2008;263:218–43.

[6] Shephard RJ. Physical impairment in HIV infections and AIDS: responses to resistance and aerobic training. J Sports Med Phys Fitness 2014 June 20 [E-pub ahead of print].

[7] Arey BD, Beal MW. The role of exercise in the prevention and treatment of wasting in acquired immune deficiency syndrome. J Assoc Nurses AIDS Care 2002;13:29–49.
[8] Smit E, Crespo CJ, Semba RD, Jaworowicz D, Vlahov D, Ricketts EP, et al. Physical activity in a cohort of HIV-positive and HIV-negative injection drug users. AIDS Care 2006; 18:1040–5.
[9] Clingerman EM. Participation in physical activity by persons living with HIV disease. J Assoc Nurses AIDS Care 2003;14:59–70.
[10] Dudgeon WD, Phillips KD, Carson JA, Brewer RB, Durstine JL, Hand GA. Counteracting muscle wasting in HIV-infected individuals. HIV Med 2006;7:299–310.
[11] Cade WT, Fantry LE, Nabar SR, Shaw DK, Keyser RE. Impaired oxygen on kinetics in persons with human immunodeficiency virus are not due to highly active antiretroviral therapy. Arch Phys Med Rehabil 2003;84:1831–8.
[12] Cade WT, Fantry LE, Nabar SR, Shaw DK, Keyser RE. A comparison of Qt and a-vO2 in individuals with HIV taking and not taking HAART. Med Sci Sports Exerc 2003;35:1108–17.
[13] Van Rossum AMC, Gaakeer MI, Verweel G, Hartwig NG, Wolfs TF, Geelen SP, et al. Endocrinologic and immunologic factors associated with recovery of growth in children with human immunodeficiency virus type 1 infection treated with protease inhibitors. Pediatr Infect Dis J 2003;22:70–6.
[14] de Pee S, Semba RD. Role of nutrition in HIV infection: review of evidence for more effective programming in resource-limited settings. Food Nutr Bull 2010;31:S313–44.
[15] Duggal S, Chugh TD, Duggal AK. HIV and malnutrition: effects on immune system. Clin Dev Immunol 2012;784740. http://dx.doi.org/10.1155/2012/784740.
[16] Cade WT, Reeds DN, Mittendorfer B, Patterson BW, Powderly WG, Klein S, et al. Blunted lipolysis and fatty acid oxidation during moderate exercise in HIV-infected subjects taking HAART. Am J Physiol 2007;292:E812–9.
[17] Duong M, Dumas JP, Buisson M, Martha B, Piroth L, Grappin M, et al. Limitation of exercise capacity in nucleoside-treated HIV-infected patients with hyperlactataemia. HIV Med 2007;8:105–11.
[18] Sharpstone DR, Murray C, Ross H, Phelan M, Crane R, Lepri AC, et al. The influence of nutritional and metabolic status on progression from asymptomatic HIV infection to AIDS-defining diagnosis. AIDS 1999;13:1221–6.
[19] Dudgeon WD, Phillips KD, Durstine JL, Burgess SE, Lyerly GW, Davis JM, et al. Individual exercise sessions alter circulating hormones and cytokines in HIV-infected men. Appl Physiol Nutr Metab 2010;35:560–8.
[20] Deresz LF, Sprinz E, Kramer AS, Cunha G, de Oliveira AR, Sporleder H, et al. Regulation of oxidative stress in response to acute aerobic and resistance exercise in HIV-infected subjects: a case-control study. AIDS Care 2010;22:1410–7.
[21] Scott WB, Oursler KK, Katzei LI, Ryan AS, Russ DW. Central activation, muscle performance, and physical function in men with human immunodeficiency virus. Muscle Nerve 2007;36:374–83.
[22] Shephard RJ. Body composition in biological anthropology. Cambridge, UK: Cambridge University Press; 1991.
[23] Shephard RJ, Rode A. Cardiorespiratory status of the Canadian Eskimo. In: Edholm OG, Gunderson EKE, editors. Polar human biology. London, UK: Heinemann Medical Books; 1973. p. 216–39.
[24] Billewicz WZ, Kemsley WF, Thomson AM. Indices of obesity. Br J Prev Soc Med 1962;16:183–8.
[25] Roche AF, Siervogel RM, Chumlea WC, Webb F. Grading body fatness from limited anthropometric data. Am J Clin Nutr 1981;34:2831–8.
[26] Murray S, Shephard RJ. Possible anthropometric alternatives to skinfold measurements. Hum Biol 1988;60:73–282.

[27] Suttman U, Ockenga J, Selberg O, Hoogestraat L, Helmuth D, Muller MJ. Incidence and prognostic value of malnutrition and wasting in human immunodeficiency virus-infected outpatients. J Acquir Immune Defic Syndr Hum Retrovirol 1995;8:239–46.
[28] Semba RD, Caiaffa WT, Graham NM, Cohn S, Vlahov D. Vitamin A deficiency and wasting as predictors of mortality in human immunodeficiency virus-infected injection drug users. J Infect Dis 1995;171:1196–202.
[29] Kotler DP, Tierney AR, Wang J, Pierson Jr RN. Magnitude of body-cell mass depletion and the timing of death from wasting in AIDS. Am J Clin Nutr 1989;50:444–7.
[30] McComsey GA, Tebas P, Shane E, Yin MT, Overton ET, Huang JS, et al. Bone disease in HIV infection: a practical review and recommendations for HIV care providers. Clin Infect Dis 2010;8:937–46.
[31] Raso V, Shephard RJ, Casseb JSR, Duarte AJS, Greve JMD'A. Handgrip force offers a measure of physical function in individuals living with HIV/AIDs. J Acquir Immune Defic Syndr 2013;63:e60–2.
[32] Franke MF, Murray MB, Muñoz M, Hernández-Díaz S, Sebastián JL, Atwood S, et al. Food insufficiency is a risk factor for suboptimal antiretroviral therapy adherence among HIV-infected adults in urban Peru. AIDS Behav 2011;15:1483–9.
[33] Ling CH, Taekema D, de Craen AJ, Gussekloo J, Westendorp RG, Maier AB. Handgrip strength and mortality in the oldest old population: the Leiden 85-plus study. CMAJ 2010;182:429–35.
[34] Sydall H, Cooper C, Martin F, Briggs R, Aihie Sayer A. Is grip strength a useful single marker of frailty? Age Ageing 2003;32:650–6.
[35] Fried LP, Tangen CM, Walston J, Newman AB, Hirsch C, Gottdiener J, et al. Cardiovascular health study collaborative research group. Frailty in older adults: evidence for a phenotype. J Gerontol A Biol Sci Med Sci 2001;56:M146–56.
[36] Roubenoff R. Acquired immunodeficiency syndrome wasting, functional performance, and quality of life. Am J Manag Care 2000;6:1003–16.
[37] Fleishman J, Crystal S. Functional status transitions and survival in HIV disease: evidence from the AIDS cost and service utilization survey. Med Care 1998;36:533–43.
[38] Justice AC, Aiken LH, Smith HL, Turner BJ. The role of functional status in predicting inpatient mortality with AIDS: a comparison with current predictors. J Clin Epidemiol 1996;49:193–201.
[39] Stanton DL, Wu AW, Moore RD, Rucker SC, Piazza MP, Abrams JE, et al. Functional status of persons with HIV infection in an ambulatory setting. J Acquir Immune Defic Syndr 1994;7:1050–6.
[40] Keyser RE, Peralta L, Cade WT, Miller S, Anixt J. Functional aerobic impairment in adolescents seropositive for HIV: a quasi-experimental analysis. Arch Phys Med Rehabil 2000;81:S1479–S1484.
[41] Oursler KK, Katzel LI, Smith BA, Scott WB, Russ DW, Sorkin JD. Prediction of cardiorespiratory fitness in older men infected with the human immunodeficiency virus: clinical factors and value of the six-minute walk distance. J Am Geriatr Soc 2009;57:2055–61.
[42] Cade WT, Reeds DN, Lassa-Claxton S, Davila-Roman VG, Waggoner AD, Powderly WG, et al. Post-exercise heart rate recovery in HIV-positive individuals on highly active antiretroviral therapy. Early indicator of cardiovascular disease? HIV Med 2008;9:96–100.
[43] Thöni GJ, Schuster I, Walther G, Nottin S, Vinet A, Boccara F, et al. Silent cardiac dysfunction and exercise intolerance in HIV+ men receiving combined antiretroviral therapies. AIDS 2008;22:2537–40.
[44] Pothoff G, Wassermann K, Ostmann H. Impairment of exercise capacity in various groups of HIV-infected patients. Respiration 1994;61:80–5.
[45] Johnson JE, Anders GT, Blanton HM, Hawkes CE, Bush BA, McAllister CK, et al. Exercise dysfunction in patients seropositive for the human immunodeficiency virus. Am Rev Respir Dis 1990;141:618–22.

[46] Schuster I, Thoni GJ, Ederhy S, Walther G, Nottin S, Vinet A, et al. Subclinical cardiac abnormalities in human immunodeficiency virus-infected men receiving antiretroviral therapy. Am J Cardiol 2008;101:1213–7.
[47] Zareba KM, Miller TL, Lipshultz SE. Cardiovascular disease and toxicities related to HIV infection and its therapies. Expert Opin Drug Saf 2005;4:1017–25.
[48] Giannarelli C, Klein RS, Badsimon JJ. Cardiovascular implications of HIV-induced dyslipidemia. Atherosclerosis 2011;219:384–9.
[49] Manuel O, Thiebaut R, Darioli R, Tarr PE. Treatment of dyslipidaemia in HIV-infected persons. Expert Opin Pharmacother 2005;6:1619–45.
[50] Raso V, Casseb JSR, Duarte AJS, Greve A, Shephard RJ. Aerobic power and muscle strength of individuals living with HIV/AIDS. J Sports Med Phys Fitness 2014;54:100–7.
[51] Raso V, Shephard RJ, Casseb JSR, Duarte AJS, Silva PRS, Greve JMD. Association between muscle strength and the cardiopulmonary status of individuals living with HIV/AIDS. Clinics 2013;68:359–64.
[52] Shephard RJ. Awrobic fitness and health. Champaign, IL: Human Kinetics; 1994.
[53] Wright GR, Sidney KH, Shephard RJ. Variance of direct and indirect measurements of aerobic power. J Sports Med Phys Fitness 1978;18:33–42.
[54] Cunningham DA, Rechnitzer PA, Donner A. Exercise training and the speed of self-selected walking pace in retrirement. Can J Aging 1986;5:19–26.
[55] Bassey EJ, Fentem PH, MacDonald IC, Sccriven PM. Self-paced walking as a method for exercise testing in elderly and young men. Clin Sci 1976;51:609–12.
[56] Shephard RJ. A brief history of exercise and phytsical activity participatiin clearance and prescription. 2. Canadian contributions to the development of objective, evidence-based procedures. Health Fit J Can 2014;7:101–5.
[57] Paterson DH, Stathokostas L. Physical activity, fitness and gender in relation to morbidity, survival, quality of life, and independence in old age. In: Shephard RJ, editor. Gender, physical activity and aging. Boca Raton, FL: CRC Press; 2001.
[58] Shephard RJ. Aging, physical activity and health. Champaign, IL: Human Kinetics; 1997.
[59] Harmon K. Walking speed predicts life expectancy of older adults. Scientific Am. 2011, <http://www.scientificamerican.com/article/walking-speed-survival/>[accessed 08.08.14].

SECTION IV

MODELS OF HIV: LESSONS TO BE LEARNED FROM ANIMAL VIRUSES

CHAPTER

20

Animal Lentiviruses: Models for Human Immunodeficiency Viruses and Nutrition

Mitchel Graham Stover[1] *and Ronald Ross Watson*[2]

[1]Department of Veterinary Science and Microbiology, University of Arizona, Tucson, AZ, USA, [2]Mel and Enid Zuckerman College of Public Health, School of Medicine, University of Arizona, Tucson, AZ, USA

20.1 INTRODUCTION

Lentiviruses are a genus of retroviruses (family *Retroviridae*) that infect several mammalian species, including humans. Although most commonly known for the human immunodeficiency virus (HIV), this genus includes several other lentiviruses that trigger serious persistent and chronic infections in their hosts [1,2]. Since the discovery of HIV-induced acquired immunodeficiency syndrome (AIDS) in the 1980s, there has been a substantial increase in the amount of research focused on HIV infections in humans, along with related viral infections in nonhuman animals [2]. In-depth characterizations of lentiviruses and host interactions across a range of biological scales have been established in a number of mammalian species [2]. Such lentiviruses include HIV, simian immunodeficiency virus (SIV), feline immunodeficiency virus (FIV), bovine immunodeficiency virus (BIV), maedivisna virus (MVV), equine infectious anemia virus (EIAV), Jembrana disease virus (JDV), and caprine arthritis–encephalitis virus (CAEV). Currently, there are no known animal model systems that reproduce the entire infectious process of HIV from viral entrance to manifestations of the disease. However, there are a number of lentiviral infections in nonhuman species that do reproduce one or more

Health of HIV Infected People, Volume 2.
DOI: http://dx.doi.org/10.1016/B978-0-12-800767-9.00020-0

of the characteristic events of HIV infections [3]. These animal models are essential for exploring problems that cannot be addressed in human subjects, such as initial testing of potential therapeutic and preventative strategies for HIV. Therefore, studying these infections in a comparative manner could provide beneficial insights into the treatment and research of HIVs.

This review analyzes several aspects of the different HIV-related lentiviral infections in various mammalian hosts. Focus will be placed on SIV and FIV because they possess many of the pathogenic characteristics of HIV, as well as BIV, a lentiviral infection in cattle that, despite a close phylogenic relationship, does not share many pathogenic similarities with HIV. Areas of emphasis include the historical background, morphology, genomic organization and expression, transmission events, viral infectious cycles, clinical and pathological characteristics, and nutritional effects of these lentiviruses.

20.2 SIMIAN IMMUNODEFICIENCY VIRUSES

20.2.1 SIV Background Information

The first primate species determined to be natural hosts of SIV were the sooty mangabey, African green monkey, chimpanzee, and mandrill [4]. Serological studies have now shown that 40 of the 69 African nonhuman primates (NHPs) are natural hosts of SIV [1,4]. In various populations of both captive and wild African primates, prevalence of SIV infections can exceed 80% [5]. Although SIV has not yet been found in wild Asian and New World primate populations, Asian macaques in captivity have been infected with SIV as a result of cross-species transmission from African species [1,6]. Complete genomic sequences and in-depth characterizations of six lineages of primate lentiviruses are available, including: SIVcpz/SIVgor/HIV-1 infecting chimpanzees, gorillas, and humans; SIVsmm/HIV-2 infecting sooty mangabey and humans; SIVagm infecting African green monkeys; SIVsyk infecting Sykes' monkeys; SIVlhoest infecting mandrills, l'Hoest's monkeys, and sun-tailed monkeys; and SIVcol infecting Colobus monkeys [1,7].

20.2.2 SIV Morphology, Genomic Organization, and Expression

As a result of the highly divergent nature of primate lentiviruses, some of the SIV strains' viral proteins share less than 30% amino acid identity [1]. Regardless, most of the molecular, structural, and biological features are conserved among the different strains [1]. All of the primate lentiviral particles are surrounded by a host cell–derived lipid membrane with viral glycoproteins and have an overall diameter of approximately 100–150 nm [1,8,9]. These envelope glycoproteins have evolved structural features that help provide resistance to neutralizing antibodies in the natural hosts [8]. On the inside of the SIV particle, a cone-shaped capsid surrounds the highly ordered and complex viral genome, which consists of two copies of positive ssRNA [1]. The viral ssRNA are associated with a tRNA primer, the nucleocapsid protein, and enzymes involved in reverse transcription and viral integration into the host cell [1].

The primate lentivirus genomes are complex and consist of approximately 10,000 nucleotides containing eight or nine genes encoding for approximately 15 different protein products [1]. SIV contains the *gag*, *pol*, and *env* genes, like all other lentiviruses [10]. The *gag* (group-specific antigen) gene encodes for the Gag polyprotein, whose cleavage products are important in the assembly of the viral core and structural products [10]. The *pol* gene encodes for viral enzymes, such as protease (PR), integrase (IN), and reverse transcriptase (RT) [10]. The *env* gene encodes for viral envelope surface glycoproteins and transmembrane proteins involved in cellular binding and fusion with host cell membranes [10]. SIV genomes contain several additional small open reading frames (ORFs) that encode for regulatory proteins [10]. Of all the lentiviruses, SIV and HIV both have the largest number of these ORFs, which are involved in viral genome transcription, counteracting host cell restriction factors, and the processing of RNA [1,10,11]. These ORFs, found in both HIV and SIV, include *tat* (trans-activator factor of transcription), *rev* (regulator of virus expression), *vif* (viral infectivity factor), *nef* (negative factor), *vpu*, *vpr*, and *vpx* [10–12]. Although all of these ORFs are not found in every SIV strain, most of the strains have at least three and all of them contain the *tat* and *rev* genes, which encode essential regulatory proteins [1].

20.2.3 SIV Transmission and Cross-Species Transmission

The most common mode of SIV transmission in wild African NHPs is horizontal, usually via sexual contact and bite wounds [4]. Although possible, vertical transmission of SIV is less common and seropositivity is rare in young animals [4,5]. Studies involving experimentally infected mandrill dams show that breastfeeding does not result in SIV transmission, most likely as a result of low levels of CCR5 co-receptors in infants, which play an important role in the binding of SIV virions to host cells [5]. Successful experimental infections with SIV have been accomplished through oral, vaginal, rectal, transplacental, intravenous, and mucosal administration of the virus [13]. Additionally, the route of transmission usually does not appear to effect the progression of SIV, unless intravenous infection occurs, in which case rapid transport of the virus to lymphatic tissues results [4].

Closely related primate species normally transmit closely related lentiviruses among one another [5,14]. This is seen through phylogenetic tree analyses that suggest several SIVs may have co-evolved with their African NHP hosts over long periods of time [1]. A relevant example is the high prevalence of very similar SIVagm strains infecting all four species of African green monkeys [1]. An explanation for this is that ancient SIV infections of the common ancestor of the African green monkey species was followed by co-divergence and virus–host adaptation, resulting in the similar viruses infecting closely related species [1]. However, several occasional cases of cross-species transmission of SIV between different primate species have been reported, showing that not all strains of primate lentiviruses are the result of long-term co-evolution of the viruses with their hosts [1,5]. For example, numerous cases of SIVsmm transmission from captive sooty mangabey to Asian macaques have been documented, resulting in the SIV strain, SIVmac [1,5]. Other examples of more recent cross-species transmissions are those between African green monkeys to patas monkeys, white-crowned mangabeys, and baboons [1]. Additionally, two SIV strains infecting chimpanzees and gorillas have been transmitted to the human population on several different occasions, resulting in HIV-1 and HIV-2 strains, as discussed in more depth later in this chapter [1].

20.2.4 Clinical and Pathological Aspects of SIV Infections

Although the majority of lentiviruses are primarily macrophage-tropic, SIVs, like HIVs and FIVs, are primarily lymphotropic, although they do also target macrophages [5,13]. This affinity for lymphocytes is an explanation for the associated immunodeficiency of certain strains of these virus groups [5]. Once in the host species, the viral membrane glycoproteins mediate virus entry by binding with certain chemokine receptors on the surface of the host cell [8,10]. SIV glycoproteins usually bind primarily to the T-cell CD4 receptors and the co-receptor CCR5 of the host [5,10]. The virus particles use these receptors located on host lymphocytes primarily in the lymphoid compartments (i.e., blood, intestines, and lymph nodes) to begin the cellular infection process [5].

Most SIV infections in their natural host species are often subclinical, rarely resulting in disease or notable histological lesions [6]. However, introduction of SIV into populations of captive rhesus macaques and other atypical hosts have resulted in epidemics of severe immunodeficiency disease often characterized by a substantial reduction in $CD4^+$ T lymphocytes, hematologic irregularities, infections by opportunistic organisms, and lymphoma, all of which are also seen in human AIDS patients [5,6]. SIV-infected macaques usually have significantly altered cytokine expression involving an increase in production of interferons and interleukins (e.g., IL-12 and IL-18) [6]. Also, SIV infections in macaques have been associated with changes in cell surface markers, including alterations in expression of CCR5, CD38, CD69, Ki-67, and HLA-DR, which are involved in signaling and immune system activation [5,6]. Similarities between SIV infections in rhesus macaques and HIV infections in humans have resulted in experimental infections in macaques serving as the primary NHP model for AIDS-related research [6].

20.2.5 SIV and HIV

The discovery that HIV initially emerged as a result of cross-species transmission events from SIV-infected NHP species to humans has resulted in an increased interest in the relationships between these viruses [5]. The major form of the AIDS virus in humans, HIV-1 group M, has been traced to the strain of SIV, SIVcpz/SIVgor, which infects central subspecies of chimpanzees and gorillas [1]. Studies suggest that SIVcpz/SIVgor was initially transmitted from NHPs to humans during the early 20th century in southeastern regions of Cameroon [1,14]. A similar cross-species transmission event of SIVsmm from the sooty mangabey to humans may have resulted in the emergence of HIV-2 [5]. It is likely that, in addition to cross-species transmission, several other factors exist that play a role in the emergence of new primate lentivirus strains, such as HIV [5,15,16]. For example, serial passages leading to viral adaptations that allow lentiviral strains to bypass the intrinsic restriction factors of new hosts most likely contributed to the development and success of new strains [5,15,16]. Although current research strongly suggests that cross-species transmission leads to the emergence of novel primate lentiviral diseases, factors leading to the success and pathogenicity of these diseases have not been entirely described [5].

As previously mentioned, although genetically similar to HIV, most SIV strains in their natural NHP hosts do not result in AIDS [5]. As a result, studying the lack of disease progression in SIV-infected African NHP hosts could provide therapeutic approaches aimed at controlling HIV disease progression in humans [5]. Through the comparison of natural SIV infections that do not result in pathogenesis (e.g., SIVagm in African green monkeys) with AIDS-causing SIV infections (e.g., SIVmac in rhesus macaques), correlations might be identified to manipulate different aspects of the pathogenic HIV infections toward nonpathogenic situations [5]. In other words, comparing natural and pathogenic SIV infections to delineate significant differences might allow for identification of aspects of lentiviral infections that are critical for lentiviral disease progression and prevention.

20.2.6 SIV Effects on Gastrointestinal Tract and Nutrition

Approximately 90% of HIV-induced AIDS patients have some form of gastrointestinal dysfunction and wasting syndrome characterized by weight loss and malnutrition [17,18]. Specifically, decreased digestive enzymes, severe protein energy malnutrition, micronutrient deficiencies, and nutrient malabsorption are seen in HIV-infected individuals [17,18]. Some of these nutrient deficiencies include decreased absorption of vitamin B_{12}, fats, D-xylose, and lactose [18]. Decreased absorption of D-xylose is often used as a tool to test for and characterize the small intestinal malabsorptive defects in HIV patients that also lead to other more important nutrient deficiencies such as vitamin B_{12} deficiency [19,20]. Vitamin B_{12} deficiencies can cause serious and sometimes irreversible problems such as dementia, anemia, and neuropathy [20,21]. Studies have shown that SIV infections in macaques result in similar malabsorption complications, also associated with diarrhea and weight loss, making them an ideal model to study HIV-associated intestinal dysfunction [13,17,18]. HIV infections in humans and SIV infections in macaques cause mucosal immunodeficiency, resulting in associated opportunistic infections of the gastrointestinal tract, along with opportunistic infections of other mucosal regions [22]. In addition to these opportunistic infections, there is evidence that both HIV and SIVmac cause direct damage to the small intestine, even without the presence of opportunistic pathogens [13,18,22]. Because a substantial amount of enzymatic digestion and nutrient absorption occurs in the small intestine, this damage is most likely one of the major causes of nutrient deficiencies in SIV- and HIV-infected individuals.

Mucosal linings of the gastrointestinal tract possess highly specialized immune systems involving T and B cells that differ from lymphocytes in their function and differentiation in other regions of the body [22]. Both HIV and SIVmac infections cause significant changes in the gut-associated immune system, most likely adding to the pathogenesis of these infections [22]. Significant losses of $CD4^+$ T cells in intestinal mucosa occur in HIV/SIVmac cases [22]. This decrease in important regulatory T lymphocytes is a probable explanation for mucosal immunodeficiency and associated opportunistic infections of the gastrointestinal tract [22]. A study found that SIV infections specifically influence the functioning of the stomach, duodenum, jejunum, ileum, cecum, and colon [17]. Also, it is believed that functional interrelationships exist between the mucosal immune system and the gut epithelial cells [22]. In the later stages of HIV in infected humans, villous atrophy and hyporegeneration of intestinal epithelial cells occur [22]. Although SIV infections in rhesus macaques have similar enteropathy, villus atrophy is an earlier event and is accompanied by crypt cell hyperproliferation and inflammatory infiltrates [17,18,22]. Thus, these infections alter the development and function of absorptive epithelial cells in the intestinal mucosa [17,18,22]. These alterations in mucosal and epithelial anatomy and physiology accompanied by changes in gut-associated immunity lead to the opportunistic infections that cause gastrointestinal dysfunctions and nutrient malabsorption [18]. Studies suggest that the overall failure to thrive and wasting observed in SIV-infected rhesus macaques is the result of multiple factors, including, but not limited to, altered food intake, opportunistic infections, malabsorption, energy expenditure, and cytokine production [17,18,22,23]. Taking these factors into consideration, nutrition becomes a critical aspect of the overall health of humans and NHPs infected with pathogenic lentiviruses.

20.2.7 Alcohol Consumption and SIV

HIV-infected individuals are more likely to consume alcohol and be categorized as alcohol abusers than the general population [24–26]. Alone, alcohol consumption has been reported to significantly compromise the efficiency of the immune system response, alter nutritional state by producing malabsorption and decreasing food intake, and cause incidences of skeletal muscle myopathy, possibly from accelerated muscle proteolysis and a decrease in muscle protein synthesis [24–26]. Additionally, these alcohol-induced disorders impact circulating and tissue growth factors, as well as micronutrient availability [25]. It is suspected that the sum of these negative effects of chronic alcohol consumption is the cause of alcohol-induced muscle wasting and that, when coexisting with HIV and SIV infections, produces an accelerated muscle wasting syndrome and exacerbates these diseases [25,26].

As previously discussed, SIV-infected rhesus macaques are an ideal model for HIV infections because they replicate many aspects of the infection, produce similar symptoms, and result in AIDS as in infected individuals [5,6,26]. Therefore, multiple studies have been performed using the SIVmac model to better elucidate the effects of alcohol consumption on HIV progression [24–26]. Studies utilizing SIVmac-infected rhesus macaques suggest that excessive alcohol consumption influences the progression of and accelerates HIV/SIV disease as a result of immune cell alterations that produce a disease-susceptible environment [24–26]. A study found that although alcohol consumption does not have a substantial effect on the acute plasma viral load, it does result in a reduction of circulating memory $CD4^+$ T cells and an increase in the levels of monocytes that express the viral co-receptor CCR5 [26]. Also, alcohol consumption by SIV-infected macaques impacted immune cells in organs such as the liver and other lymphatic and nonlymphatic tissues in which $CD4^+$ T cells were primarily affected [26]. Another study suggests that chronic alcohol consumption by SIV-infected rhesus macaques accelerates nutritional and metabolic dysregulation and produces a skeletal muscle proinflammatory state, most likely explaining the observed muscle wasting of both SIV-infected and HIV-infected individuals [25]. In conclusion, animal models suggest it is likely that alcohol consumption accelerates HIV/SIV infections and should be avoided by individuals with the disease.

20.3 FELINE IMMUNODEFICIENCY VIRUSES

20.3.1 FIV Background Information

The first cases of FIV (initially referred to as feline T-lymphotropic lentivirus [FTLV]) were isolated from the peripheral blood leukocytes of a group of domestic cats in a rescue facility in Petaluma, California, in 1986 [27–29]. Although these cats were not infected with the common immunosuppressive feline leukemia virus, they were still showing signs typical of immunodeficiency-causing diseases [27]. Since the initial discovery of this lymphotropic virus in California, many cases of FIV have been found in domestic cat populations worldwide, as well as in several wild and captive large cat species [27]. Some countries, such as Japan, have substantially higher rates of FIV infections and studies have shown up to 12% of healthy cat populations as carriers of the virus in these regions [27]. Although it is known that FIV causes AIDS in the domestic cat, it has not been explicitly determined if FIV results in AIDS in any of the free-ranging species of Felidae that are endemic with FIV strains [30]. The following FIV strains have been identified in their respective hosts: FIVfca (infecting domestic cats, pumas, and Asian leopard cats); FIVlpa (infecting ocelots); FIVpco (infecting pumas and bobcats); FIVpya (infecting jaguarundis); FIVoma (infecting Pallas cats); FIVaju (infecting cheetah); FIVppa (infecting leopards); FIVple (infecting lions and snow leopards); and FIVccr (infecting spotted hyena) [31].

FIV is biochemically and morphologically similar to HIVs, SIVs, and BIVs, but it does have distinct antigenic properties [27]. Regardless, the infectious process of FIV in domestic cats also closely resembles HIV infections humans [3,27]. FIV-infected domestic cats are said to be one of the most desirable and extensively studied models for HIV as a result of the similarities between these viruses and the small size and ability to breed cats easily and quickly [3,27]. This model appears to be particularly valuable for exploring new therapeutic strategies, antiviral drug evaluation, novel vaccinations, and preventative strategies, and for further exploration of viral-associated immunodeficiency pathogenesis [3,27].

20.3.2 FIV Morphology, Genomic Organization, and Expression

As previously mentioned, FIV is morphologically similar to other lentiviruses that result in AIDS in human and NHPs [28]. The overall size of an FIV virion is approximately 105–125 nm in diameter and is spherical to ellipsoid in shape [28]. The FIV virion's membrane is derived from infected host cells in a manner similar to that of other lentiviruses and contains short envelope projections [28]. An electron-lucent space separates the FIV viral core from this overlying plasma membrane [28]. The FIV viral core consists of a conical shell, which is surrounded by an electron-dense nucleoid [28].

At least three complete nucleotide sequences of different proviral clones of FIV (including the first discovered Petaluma strain) have been sequenced, and several other strains have been partially sequenced [27]. The overall genomic structure of FIV also parallels that of HIV, with a few important distinctions, although it is said to be more similar to the lentiviruses of the ungulate species (visna virus) in its genetic organization and regulation [28,32,33]. Several studies suggest that the common genomic features between the two viruses may serve as common targets for the production of broad-based intervention strategies [3,32]. Important enzymes that are encoded for in both FIV and HIV include RT, PR, IN, endonuclease, and RNAse H [28,32]. FIV has a slightly smaller genome than that of HIV and is approximately 9,400 nucleotides long [32]. The integrated FIV provirus includes the *gag*, *pol*, and *env* genes bordered by long terminal repeats (LTRs), which are found in all other retroviruses [27,28,32]. The LTRs of lentiviruses are important for gene expression and regulation of viral replication; they contain the promoter, enhancer, and terminator regions that are critical for transcription [34]. However, the LTRs of FIV are significantly shorter than HIV and SIV strains and are approximately 355 base pairs long [27]. The LTRs of FIV also have several transcriptional signal elements that vary among isolates [27]. Certain promoter–enhancer elements that have been found among all FIV isolates and are thought to be necessary for FIV replication include the AP-1, ATF, and second AP-4 sites [27]. Other promoters that are not conserved among all FIV isolates, such as NF-κB, LBP-1, and the first AP-4 site, could be used to determine certain biological characteristics of the different FIC isolates [27].

The variation within and among subtypes of FIV and HIV strains are strikingly similar, although there are several important distinctions [35]. Although both HIV and FIV possess *vif* and *rev* genes, which are essential for virus replication, the accessory genes *vpr*, *vpu*, and *nef*, which are found in HIV, are lacking in FIV [32]. Another distinction in the FIV genome is the presence of an apparent transactivator, called orf2, which increases the net translation of gene products whose transcription is driven by a LTR [32]. However, FIV orf2 does not utilize a TAR element, as seen with HIV-1 Tat, and enhances transcription and translation by mechanisms that are distinct from those of other lentiviruses [32]. Some studies suggest that orf2 might be similar to HIV Vpr in that it could also be involved in virus release from host cells during replication [32]. Therefore, current research suggests that FIV orf2 could have multiple functions, which is in line with the need for genes of a relatively small genome encoding for versatile products [32].

20.3.3 FIV Transmission and Cross-Species Transmission

FIV transmission is similar to HIV in that it can be transmitted horizontally via blood transfer and mucosal exposure and vertically through prenatal and postnatal routes [32]. However, the main mechanism in which FIV is spread is through bites, because FIV is also shed in the saliva [31,35]. Therefore, the majority of FIV-infected cats are adults (older than 5 years of age), males are twice as likely to be infected, and free-roaming and feral cats are more frequently infected [35]. Although transmission from queens to kittens via breastfeeding does occur, it does not seem to be the major contributor of field infections [35]. Experimentally, cats have been infected with both cell-associated and cell-free FIV via most mucosal routes, including vaginal, rectal, and oral, and subcutaneous, intramuscular, intraperitoneal, and intravenous injections [35].

Fortunately, because FIV is usually transmitted via direct contact, a behavioral and ecological barrier to cross-species transmission in the wild exists [31]. Additionally, the presence of host intracellular antiviral proteins contributes to the species-specific nature of FIVs and further limits the spread of these viruses between species [31]. Also, phylogenetic analyses support the prediction that FIV is rarely transmitted between cat species, although it has been observed in captive settings [31]. A recent study has documented that wild puma and bobcat populations in Southern California do share an FIV strain, which provides for an opportunity to determine evolutionary aspects of both viral strains and the activity and presence of intracellular restriction proteins [31]. Further investigation of cross-species transmissions of wild free-range cat populations can provide an invaluable model system to evaluate the evolutionary history of FIV along with aspects of transmission and host cell tropism [31].

20.3.4 Clinical and Pathological Aspects of FIV Infections

FIV causes an AIDS-like pathology accompanied by immune suppression, $CD4^+$ depletion, and death [31]. Cells that are most susceptible to FIV infection include $CD4^+$ T cells, $CD8^+$ T cells, macrophages, B lymphocytes, and astrocytes [35]. Some studies suggest that the CD4 antigen is not necessary for infection and that an alternate receptor could be the feline CD9 antigen [35]. FIV disease progression parallels a pattern similar to that observed in HIV infections, possibly even more so than SIV [27,32,35]. Pathologies involving the skin, oral cavity, respiratory tract, intestinal tract, liver, kidneys, and central nervous system have all been observed in FIV-infected cats [33]. The infection cycle includes an acute, asymptomatic, and terminal phase.

The infection begins with an acute phase denoted by an increase in viral loads ($CD8^+$ lymphocytes, macrophages, B cells), which is relatively short, beginning 4–6 weeks after inoculation and lasting for several months [27,29,32,35]. The acute FIV phase is often accompanied by febrile episodes, lymphadenopathy, leukopenia (neutropenia), and weight loss [27,29,32]. The pyrexia is usually mild and intermittent, developing approximately 5 weeks after the initial infection and able to last for several days [27]. The acute phase lymphadenopathy is normally more generalized and develops with pyrexia, but it typically persists for several months [27]. Although the cats do not usually die during the acute phase, some cases have been reported in which cats developed fatal bacterial infections, usually as a result of the associated leukopenia [27].

After the acute phase is an asymptomatic phase that can last for several years, during which the cats can appear healthy [32,35]. The period of time that FIV-infected cats can remain in this asymptomatic phase can differ substantially, most likely because of differences in exposures to secondary pathogens [27]. This asymptomatic phase in FIV infections is often associated with lower viral titers, significant antiviral immune responses, minimal clinical symptoms, and a gradual decline in $CD4^+$ cell numbers [32]. The final, terminal stage is denoted by exacerbation of plasma viral load, immunologic deterioration, and numerous clinical symptoms typical of immunodeficiency and secondary infections [32,35]. Some of the more frequently reported clinical signs reported in cats in the terminal stage of FIV include chronic respiratory disease, stomatitis, weight loss, and pyrexia [35].

FIV infections, like SIV and HIV, result in alterations in lymphoid tissues [32]. Such alterations include lymphoid hyperplasia, thymic depletion, plasmacytosis, and terminal lymphoid depletion [32]. FIV manifestations can also be associated with the nervous system [32]. Neurological problems caused by FIV infections include alterations in sleep patterns and delayed auditory and visual responses [32]. Although these clinical symptoms are usually most notable in the acute phases and resolve as the cats proceed into the latent stages, neurological abnormalities usually persist throughout the course of the infection [32]. Cats that are not euthanized in the early stages of the disease usually die of opportunistic infections rather than the associated neurological disorders [32].

20.3.5 Nutrition and FIV

FIV produces pathological changes of the intestinal tract and oral cavity [33,35]. In some accounts, FIV-infected cats with intestinal dysfunction have been observed with chronic diarrhea and wasting, as seen in both HIV and SIV infections [17,33]. This could suggest that FIV has effects on nutritional and dietary intakes that are similar to HIV and SIV. Additionally, intestinal abnormalities such as small intestinal villous blunting, crypt dilatation, and loss of villi are frequently associated with FIV [33]. Other intestinal disorders that have been observed in FIV-infected cats include ulceration, necrotizing pyogranulomatous inflammation of the large intestine, and submucosal infiltration of macrophages, neutrophils, and histiocytes [33]. Several cases of FIV infections accompanied by necrotizing typhlitis and colitis that are associated with acute diarrhea and resulting in death have been documented [33]. Although attempts have been made to discover opportunistic infections that might be responsible for the effects that FIV has on the intestinal tracts, no studies have been successful in describing these pathogens [33]. Thus, it has been speculated that FIV infection in the intestinal epithelium could be directly responsible for the intestinal dysfunction, even without the presence of opportunistic infections. It is possible that these intestinal maladies could prevent proper functioning of the digestive tract in acquiring proper nutrition, explaining the frequently associated weight loss and chronic diarrhea observed in FIV-infected cats. As a result, nutrition and dietary intake become critical aspects of FIV-infected cat health.

20.4 BOVINE IMMUNODEFICIENCY VIRUS

20.4.1 BIV Background Information

The first documented isolation of BIV occurred in 1969 in a progressively deteriorating 8-year-old pregnant Holstein dairy cow named R-29 [34]. This cow displayed signs of wasting syndrome, initially suggesting bovine leucosis [12,34]. R-29 also showed clinical signs of lymphadenopathy, elevated white blood cell counts, mild persistent lymphocytosis, fatigue, lesions of the central nervous system, and emaciation [12,34]. Histological tissue examination from the infected cow determined the presence of perivascular cuffing of the brain and generalized follicular hyperplasia of lymph nodes [12]. Initially, the disease was designated as bovine visna-like virus due to the virus being structurally similar to MVV and inducing formation of syncytia in cell cultures [12].

The virus remained unstudied until the discovery of HIV-1 in 1983 [34]. The bovine R-29 isolate was demonstrated to be a lentivirus, similar to HIV, 20 years later [12]. BIV was named as a result of its genetic, morphologic, and serologic features that possess similarities to SIV and HIV-1 [12]. Since the discovery of the BIV R-29 isolate, several other BIV strains (including BIV-106, BIV-127, FL-491, and FL-112) have also been documented worldwide and extensively studied for their development of leukocytosis [12,34,36]. Infections with these different strains can vary in prevalence, from rare occurrences in the northern regions of the United States to up to 40% of beef and 64% of dairy herd cows being infected in southern regions [36]. Regardless of the availability of different isolates, the majority of molecular, pathological, and serological information on BIV has been obtained from the original BIV R-29 isolate [12,34].

20.4.2 BIV Morphology, Genomic Organization, and Expression

Several aspects of BIV morphology are comparable with HIV. Regarding size, both HIV and BIV are approximately 120–130 nm. Additionally, the viral bilayer envelope contains the transmembrane gp45 and surface gp100 proteins, which encompass a conical capsid and nucleocapsid structures that protect the BIV genome [34]. The virions contain two copies of capped and polyadenylated single-stranded RNA, which are protected by the bilayer envelope, transmembrane, and surface proteins [12,34]. The BIV linear proviral DNA genome consists of 8,960 base pairs [12,36].

A complete genetic map of BIV has been developed from the molecular cloning and sequencing of proviruses obtained from BIV-infected cells [12,36]. Various analytical techniques such as Northern blotting and cDNA cloning experiments have been used to characterize many aspects of the genetic complexity of BIV viral transcripts [36]. These experiments have determined that among the lentiviruses, the genomic organization of BIV is the most complex, containing numerous regulatory genes [12,36]. The proviral BIV genome contains the obligatory *gag*, *pol*, and *env* retroviral structural genes with viral LTR segments on the 5′ and 3′ ends and additional nonstructural and regulatory genes [36,37]. BIV LTRs are organized in a similar manner as other retroviruses in that they contain typical U3, R, and U5 regions and are created during the reverse transcription of genomic RNA [34]. BIV nonstructural accessory genes are found in the central region between and overlapping the *pol* and *env* genes, which consist of short ORFs, similar to those found in other lentiviruses [36,37].

The central region is a common characteristic of lentiviruses (although certain deviations have been noted) and is thought to have importance in the role of their pathogenesis [37]. The coding exons found in this region of BIV include *vif*, *tat*, *rev*, *vpw*, *vpy*, and *tmx* [12,34,36]. A few of these nonstructural accessory genes in BIV have been thought to be nonessential because the inactivation or deletion of these genes *in vitro* has insignificant effects on viral replication [36]. However, substantial effects have been noted when these genes are deleted *in vivo* [36]. Despite the lack of sequence similarities, the genome locations, conserved traits in translated products, and functional studies suggest that the majority of BIV nonstructural accessory genes (*tat*, *rev*, *vif*, *vpr*, and *vpw*) are analogous to those found in primate lentiviruses (*tat*, *rev*, *vif*, *vpr*, *vpu*, and *vpx*) [36]. Although BIV does not have an equivalent *nef* ORF, which is found in primate lentiviruses, cDNA analysis of BIV transcripts suggest that a unique gene found in BIV, called *tmx*, could be analogous to *nef* [36]. Further analysis of these genes could provide beneficial insight into the similarities between BIV and its lentiviral counterparts.

20.4.3 BIV Transmission and Cellular Infection

In vivo BIV usually infects cells of the immune system, such as monocytes, macrophages, and lymphocytes [36]. BIV is introduced into its host via vertical (*in utero*) or horizontal transmission (from body fluids such as blood and colostrum) [34]. After transmission, exogenous BIV particles attach to specific cell surface proteins via viral envelope glycoproteins, initiating the cellular infection process [36]. The virus then enters the cell by directly fusing the viral envelope with the cell's plasma membrane [36]. After the virus fuses with the cell membrane, it releases the BIV genomic RNA along with mature *pol* gene products from within the viral core into the cell's cytoplasm [12]. At this time, viral RNA is converted into double-stranded DNA by viral RT and ribonuclease [36]. This viral double-stranded DNA, also known as the BIV provirus, is then transported into the nucleus and incorporated into the host genome by the viral protein IN [12,36]. After integration into the host genome, the BIV provirus can remain transcriptionally inactive until appropriate cellular signals activate gene expression from the LTR portions of the provirus [12,36]. The expression of these LTRs is substantially increased by the action of the encoded viral Tat protein [36]. The cellular splicing machinery and the virally encoded protein, Rev, splice the primary genome-length BIV mRNA into sub-genomic messages and transport them into the host cell's cytoplasm [12,36]. Once in the cytoplasm, sub-genomic BIV mRNA is translated by ribosomes into viral precursors [12]. These viral precursors are for *gag* and *gag-pol* genes and are assembled beneath the plasma membrane and package viral genomic RNA during the budding process of immature virions [12,34]. During the budding process, the viral envelope is also covered with transmembrane and surface glycoproteins [12]. After the immature virion is released from the host cell, *gag*-related precursors are cleaved by the viral PR into function subunits as the virus undergoes morphogenesis, allowing the viral particle to finish maturation [34]. The mature BIV particle can then begin the infectious cycle again when it comes in contact with another host cell displaying the appropriate surface proteins for binding [12].

20.4.4 Clinical and Pathological Aspects of BIV Infections

BIV is more pathologically similar to the lentiviruses that are associated with chronic inflammatory diseases, such as CAEV and EIAV, as compared with those associated with severe immunodeficiency, such as HIV, SIV, and FIV [34]. However, most infections of BIV in cattle occur with no evidence of disease, resulting in an absence of clearly established clinical signs [34]. This is a result of cattle being production animals and having a high turnover rate, as well as common dual infections with bovine leukemia virus (BLV), which further complicates determining what effects BIV infections have on cattle health [36]. As a result, the effects of natural BIV infections on the overall health of herds have not yet been distinctly explained [36]. However, because BIV infects monocyte and macrophage cells, it is believed that the virus does produce slight dysfunction of the immune system [34]. The fact that numerous secondary conditions (pododermatis, mastitis, and other bacterial diseases) are associated with BIV infections further suggests that this virus can impair the immune system [34]. Increased occurrences of similar secondary diseases are also seen in HIV infections, and finding ways to prevent and treat them could be beneficial to hosts infected with either HIV or BIV.

Several studies have been conducted to better characterize the pathological manifestations of BIV in cattle. A long-term study of a dairy herd with significant BIV infection was accompanied with high cull rates and prevalence of skin infections that were unresponsive to treatment [36]. Other studies used the BIV R-29 isolate to experimentally infect calves demonstrated a transient lymphocytosis and lymphadenopathy without any other noticeable clinical signs [36]. Several studies have found enlarged lymph nodes, substantial follicular hyperplasia of germinal centers, and nonsuppurative perivascular cuffing in the cerebrum through necropsies and histopathological examination [36]. *In vitro*, mononuclear cells isolated from sheep and cattle that were experimentally infected with BIV showed a reduction in lymphoproliferative responses to certain antigens [34]. Further studies focusing on pathological manifestation could provide further insights into BIV infections and their clinical and pathological effects, as well as any potential effects on nutrition and correlations with HIV.

20.5 CONCLUSION

Extensive amounts of research have been performed on HIV-related animal lentiviruses since the 1980s. These viruses have the potential to serve as models for investigating new means of therapeutic and preventative strategies for HIV. Although there are no animal lentiviral models that perfectly replicate the HIV/AIDS infectious cycle in humans, SIV and FIV infections are two promising models that share many characteristics with HIV infections. These viruses display potentially valuable similarities regarding morphology, genomic organization and expression, transmission, clinical and pathological manifestations, and effects on nutrition. Further investigation of these viruses could provide promising insights into areas that cannot be addressed directly in human subjects.

References

[1] Munch J, Kirchhoff F. Natural SIV infection: virological aspects. Pancino G, Silvestri G, Fowke K, editors. Models of protection against HIV/SIV: avoiding AIDS in humans and monkeys. London: Elsevier Inc; 2012. pp. 3–45.
[2] Gifford RJ. Viral evolution in deep time: lentiviruses and mammals. Trends Genet 2012;28:89–100.
[3] Miller RJ, Cairns JS, Bridges S, Sarver N. Human immunodeficiency virus and AIDS: insights from animal lentiviruses. J Virol 2000;74:7187–95.
[4] Jacquelin B, Zahn RC, Barré-Sinoussi F, Schmitz JE, Kaur A, Müller-Trutwin MC. Natural SIV infection: immunological aspects. Pancino G, Silvestri G, Fowke K, editors. Models of protection against HIV/SIV: avoiding AIDS in humans and monkeys. London: Elsevier Inc; 2012. pp. 47–79.
[5] Pandrea I, Landay A. Implications for therapy. Pancino G, Silvestri G, Fowke K, editors. Models of protection against HIV/SIV: avoiding AIDS in humans and monkeys. London: Elsevier Inc; 2012. pp. 81–131.
[6] Lerche NW, Osborn KG. Simian retrovirus infections: potential confounding variables in primate toxicology studies. Toxicol Pathol 2003;31:103–10.
[7] Hirsch VM, et al. A distinct African lentivirus from Sykes' monkeys. J Virol 1993;67:1517–28.
[8] Evans DT, Desrosiers RC. Immune evasion strategies of the primate lentiviruses. Immunol Rev 2001;183:141–58.
[9] Etemad-Moghadam B, Rhone D, Steenbeke T, et al. Understanding the basis of CD4+ T-cell depletion in macaques infected by a simian–human immunodeficiency virus. Vaccine 2002;20:1934–7.
[10] Affranchino JL, González SA. Understanding the process of envelope glycoprotein incorporation into virions in simian and feline immunodeficiency viruses. Viruses 2014;6:264–83.
[11] Fultz PN, Anderson DC. The biology and immunopathology of simian immunodeficiency virus infection. Curr Opin Immunol 1990;2:403–8.
[12] Bhatia S, Patil SS, Sood R. Bovine immunodeficiency virus: a lentiviral infection. Indian J Virol 2013;24:332–41.
[13] Whetter LE, et al. Pathogenesis of simian immunodeficiency virus infection. J Gen Virol 1999;80:1557–68.
[14] Castro-Nallar E, Pérez-Losada M, Burton GF, Crandall KA. The evolution of HIV: inferences using phylogenetics. Mol Phylogenet Evol 2012;62:777–92.
[15] Marx PA, Apetrei C, Drucker E. AIDS as a zoonosis? Confusion over the origin of the virus and the origin of the epidemics. J Med Primatol 2004;33:220–6.
[16] Drucker E, Alcabes PG, Marx PA. The injection century: massive unsterile injections and the emergence of human pathogens. Lancet 2001;358:1989–92.
[17] Heise C, Vogel P, Miller CJ, Halsted CH, Dandekar S. Simian immunodeficiency virus infection of the gastrointestinal tract of rhesus macaques: functional, pathological, and morphological changes. Am J Pathol 1993;142:1759–71.

[18] Stone JD, Heise CC, Miller CJ, Halsted CH, Dandekar S. Development of malabsorption and nutritional complications in simian immunodeficiency virus-infected rhesus macaques. AIDS 1994;8:1245–56.
[19] Craig RM. D-xylose testing. J Clin Gastroeneterol 1999;29:143–50.
[20] Ehrenpreis ED, Carlson SJ, Boorstein HL, Craig RM. Malabsorption and deficiency of vitamin B12 in HIV-infected patients with chronic diarrhea. Dig Dis Sci 1994;39:2159–62.
[21] Truswell AS. Vitamin B12. Nutr Diet 2007;64:S120–5.
[22] Zeitz M, Ullrich R, Schneider T, Kewenig S, Hohloch K, Riecken EO. HIV/SIV enteropathy. Ann NY Acad Sci 1998;859:139–48.
[23] Freeman LM, et al. Body-composition changes in the simian immunodeficiency virus-infected juvenile rhesus macaque. J Infect Dis 2004;189:2010–5.
[24] Bagby GJ, Stoltz DA, Zhang P, Bohm RP, Nelson S. Simian immunodeficiency virus, infection, alcohol, and host defense. Alcohol Clin Exp Res 1998;22:193S–95S.
[25] Molina PE, et al. Chronic alcohol accentuates nutritional, metabolic, and immune alteration during asymptomatic simian immunodeficiency virus infection. Alcohol Clin Exp Res 2006;30:2065–78.
[26] Marcondes MG, et al. Chronic alcohol consumption generates a vulnerable immune environment during early SIV infection in rhesus macaques. Alcohol Clin Exp Res 2008;32:1583–92.
[27] Harbour DA. Feline immunodeficiency virus infection as a model for HIV infection in man. Rev Med Virol 1992;2:43–9.
[28] Pederson NC, Yamamoto JK, Ishida T, Hansen H. Feline immunodeficiency virus infection. Vet Immunol Immunopathol 1989;21:111–29.
[29] Friend SCE, Birch CJ, Lording PM, Marshall JA, Studdert MJ. Feline immunodeficiency virus: prevalence, disease associations and isolation. Aust Vet J 1990;67:237–43.
[30] Roelke ME, et al. Pathological manifestations of feline immunodeficiency virus (FIV) infection in wild African lions. Virology 2009;290:1–12.
[31] Troyer JL, et al. FIV cross-species transmission: an evolutionary prospective. Vet Immunol Immunopathol 2008;123:159–66.
[32] Elder JH, et al. Molecular mechanisms of FIV infection. Vet Immunol Immunopathol 2008;123:3–13.
[33] Sparger EE. Current thoughts on feline immunodeficiency virus infection. Hoskins JD, Loar AS, editors. The veterinary clinics of North America: small animal practice, feline infectious diseases. Philadelphia, PA: W.B. Saunders Company; 1993. pp. 173–91.
[34] Corredor AG, St-Lous MC, Archambault D. Molecular and biological aspects of the bovine immunodeficiency virus. Curr HIV Res 2010;8:2–13.
[35] Bennet M, Hart CA. Feline immunodeficiency virus infection—a model for HIV and AIDS? J Med Microbiol 1995;42:233–6.
[36] Gonda MA, Luther DG, Fong SE, Tobin GJ. Bovine immunodeficiency virus: molecular biology and virus–host interactions. Virus Res 1994;32:155–81.
[37] Garvey KJ, Oberste MS, Elser JE, Braun MJ, Gonda MA. Nucleotide sequence and genome organization of biologically active proviruses of bovine immunodeficiency-like virus. Virology 1990;175:391–409.

CHAPTER

21

T-Cell Number, Nutritional Status, and HIV: The Cuban Experience in the Provision of Food and Nutrition Care to People with HIV/AIDS

Elisa Maritza Linares Guerra[1] *and Sergio Santana Porbén*[2]

[1]Universidad de Ciencias Médicas de Pinar del Río, Pinar del Río. Cuba, [2]Hermanos Ameijeiras Hospital, Havana, Cuba

21.1 T-CELL NUMBER, NUTRITIONAL STATUS, AND HIV

Malnutrition poses a real threat to those patients living with HIV/AIDS from the very onset of the infection, and it becomes the gravity center of a vicious circle linking nutritional disorders and immune deficiencies [1]. Incidence and severity of malnutrition associated with HIV/AIDS are directly related to stage of viral infection and are more frequent and overt in the advanced stages of the disease [2,3].

Several causes might unleash malnutrition in HIV/AIDS. However, cell immune depression with a decline in $CD4^+$ T lymphocytes represents the main determinant [2,4]. Hence, nutritional status is a key factor for survival and life quality of subjects infected with HIV, and should become a fundamental pillar in the comprehensive treatment of them.

Health of HIV Infected People, Volume 2.
DOI: http://dx.doi.org/10.1016/B978-0-12-800767-9.00021-2

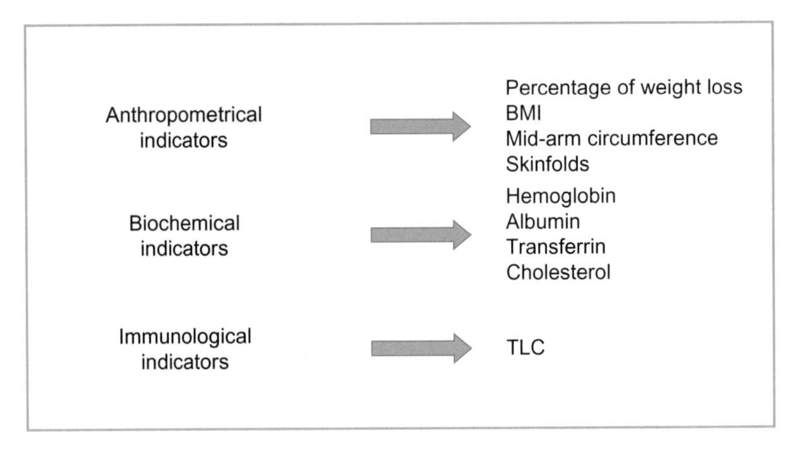

FIGURE 21.1 Nutritional indicators with predictive value in the progression of HIV/AIDS disease.

In the same manner as for individuals not infected with HIV, assessment of nutritional status of patients with HIV/AIDS is performed by means of anthropometric, biochemical, and immunological indicators, many of them within the reach of any medical outpatient practice, even in low-incomes countries. Simple tools initially designed for use in hospitalized patients, such as the Subjective Global Assessment (SGA) and Chang's algorithm, have also been applied in the nutritional assessment of those infected with HIV/AIDS [3,5,6].

Keeping in mind that risk of malnutrition increases considerably as infection progresses [3], and also that nutritional status is related to $CD4^{+}$ T-lymphocyte-mediated immunity, several studies have evaluated the role of different nutritional indicators as markers of progression of HIV/AIDS disease. Only a few of them have been found with demonstrable predictive value for HIV/AIDS, and they are summarized in Figure 21.1.

21.1.1 Percentage of Weight Loss

Percentage of weight loss is a simple anthropometric indicator recognized as a significant prognostic factor for progression of HIV/AIDS disease since the epidemic's outbreak [7]. Its relationship with survival is important, with wasting syndrome (usually defined as a nonintentional weight loss of 10% or more of normal body weight) being considered as definitive for AIDS diagnosis, in keeping with the disease scaling advanced by the United States Centers for Diseases Control (CDC) in 1993 [8]; it represents one of the main causes of death in these patients. As a matter of fact, mortality is so closely associated with loss of metabolically active tissues that it is possible to reasonably predict occurrence of death as a function of weight loss, whereas restoration of weight improves survival [4,9,10]. Curtailing weight loss could lead to improvement in the patient's response to antiretroviral therapy (ART) and result in lower morbidity and mortality rates.

21.1.2 Body Mass Index

Body mass index (BMI) is a simple indicator commonly used to assess nutritional status of adult patients [11]. Several studies have shown that BMI represents a powerful indicator to be used as evolution criterion of HIV/AIDS infection, and for determining initiation of antiretroviral therapy in low-income countries [12].

Earlier in the present century, the results of a cohort study were reported in which the role of BMI was assessed as a predictor of survival of 630 HIV/AIDS subjects. After adjusting for other usual prognostic factors, it was shown that BMI less than 18.5 kg/m^2 increased the risk of death [9]. In 2001, this same team of researchers replicated the study with a larger sample and found that relative risk of clinical AIDS increased as BMI cutoff decreased (4.7 for a BMI <16 kg/m^2) [10].

Others studies have shown a rapid decline in BMI values over the course of the 6 months preceding AIDS onset [13]. Predictive value of BMI might vary with sex. In this regard, these same researchers showed that a BMI cutoff less than 20.3 kg/m^2 for men and less than 18.5 kg/m^2 for women predicted an increase in the risk of death [13]. In addition, several ethnically mixed cohort studies have shown that declining BMI values from 17–18 kg/m^2 to less than 16 kg/m^2 were associated with a two-fold to five-fold increase in the risk of developing AIDS, respectively [14].

Before antiretroviral drugs were made available, studies showed a protective effect of obesity on both progression toward clinical AIDS and risk of mortality. In this regard, Koethe and Heimburger [15] referred to the results of a cohort of drug-consuming people infected with HIV-1. In this study, obesity was associated with a slower progression of the disease and a higher survival rate, regardless of the CD4$^+$ T-lymphocyte count.

After the introduction of antiretroviral drugs, results of research stating a convergence between ART and obesity can be found [16,17]. However, there are others studies pointing to an association between ART and lower values of BMI. In African patients, a decreased BMI at the start of ART represented an independent predictor of early mortality [15,18]. The increase in early mortality among HIV/AIDS African patients with low BMI started on ART might be multifactorial in its etiology, but several causes have been proposed. ART is started when the person with HIV/AIDS has reached the advanced stages of the disease, and low BMI reflects cachexia, as described in clinical AIDS [19]. Early mortality can also be the result of effects aggregated to malnutrition induced by dysfunction of the immune system, as is the case for a higher burden of opportunistic infections, metabolic derangement, and insufficient food ingestion in adults living in areas characterized by food scarcity [15].

Resembling AIDS in many ways, energy–nutrient malnutrition is associated with suppression of specific antigen immune response, reactivation of viral infections, diminishment of the primary response by T-cell-dependent antibodies as well as the memory response, inversion of CD4/CD8 ratio, atrophy of lymphoid tissues, and reduction of the number of peripheral lymphocytes and eosinophiles, along with a decrease in the activity of natural killer cells [4]. All these (along with other more) events make those with HIV/AIDS who are also malnourished more prone to suffer from opportunistic infections and higher mortality. The aforementioned explains why HIV-related opportunistic infections in individuals with low values of BMI further compromise the immune response and result in increased early mortality when they are placed on ART.

Another possible explanation for the association between low BMI and ART could be the lipodystrophia phenomenon caused by prolonged use of specified antiretroviral drugs such as stavudine (D4T) and zidovudine (AZT) [19].

Given the existing relationship between low BMI and early mortality at the start of ART, it is only natural to ask if weight gain should be a priority when treating these patients. A study conducted in Zambia with 27,915 patients who survived after 6 months on ART showed an inverse relationship between initial weight gain and 6-month mortality risk [20]. In this study, patients with BMI less than 16 kg/m^2 who initiated ART and did not gain weight during the 6-month observation period had a 10-fold increase in mortality risk when compared with those who gained more than 10 kg. A similar study with a cohort combining patients from Kenya (n = 2,681) and Cambodia (n = 2,451) reported an association between weight gain at 3 and 6 months and a subsequently increased survival [21].

We recently concluded a follow-up study with 118 persons living with HIV/AIDS who were nutritionally evaluated at two different times by means of anthropometric and biochemical indicators. Changes between the two observations were calculated. A binary logistic regression tool was used to predict CD4$^+$ T-cell counts after 1 year of follow-up using changes in nutritional indicators. The stepwise predictor selection method only found BMI gradient as a useful independent variable. When incorporating logistic equation baseline immune status with CD4$^+$ T-cell count (<350 versus ≥350) and ART use (yes/no), a significant increase in the sensitivity of BMI gradient [i.e., $gBMI = (BMI_{final\ value} - BMI_{initial\ value})/BMI_{initial\ value}$] was observed reaching values close to those obtained independently for CD4 gradient [22]. This result is of extraordinary importance for the follow-up of HIV/AIDS patients exposed to ART, and those unexposed, in low-income countries where CD4$^+$ T-cell counts can be performed at the onset of infection and at the start of ART, but costs and existing technologies might prevent additional tests as part of the follow-up protocol. In this regard, changes experienced in BMI values within 1 year of follow-up might represent a simple, easy-to-perform alternative within the reach of health care units in these low-income countries [22]. Combined with other simple markers such as hemoglobin (Hb), clinical status, and total lymphocyte count (TLC), BMI less than 18.5 kg/m^2 has been proven as useful as $CD4^+$ T-cell counts and plasma viral load for predicting patient response to ART [12].

21.1.3 Mid-Arm Circumference

Mid-arm circumference (MAC) is an easy-to-obtain anthropometric measure as well as a good predictor of risk of imminent death; it has been used for monitoring the nutritional status of patients in emergency situations and recommended for the assessment of acute malnutrition in adults [23].

In a study conducted in Guinea Bissau between May 1996 and April 2001, which aimed to assess easy-to-monitor predictors for tuberculosis (TB) mortality, 440 males and 260 females diagnosed with pulmonary TB were followed-up for 8 months. Highly significant differences in average MAC values were found between deceased and surviving patients, even after adjusting for sex, age, presence of HIV/AIDS, and stage of infection [24]. For every 10-mm reduction in MAC value, a 13% increase in risk of death from TB was observed for HIV-positive patients compared with a 22% increase in HIV-negative patients [24]. It was concluded that reduced MAC value can be considered an easy-to-monitor predictor of mortality in TB patients, independently of HIV/AIDS condition.

21.1.4 Skinfolds

After adjusting for sex-dependent differences, body fat is responsible for 20–30% of body weight. Skinfolds comprise as much as two-thirds of body fat. Consequently, skinfold measurement could be an important anthropometric indicator in the assessment of nutritional status of HIV/AIDS patients.

Depletion/loss of skinfolds is identified with wasting. Wasting could be the result of the patient's incapability to naturally sustain his/her nutritional status with foods taken by mouth and/or an increase in nutritional demands/requirements. Thus, wasting could be a marker of disease progression in non-ART-treated HIV/AIDS patients.

Body fat size and distribution could be dramatically altered by ART. Lypodystrophy is a localized disorder of body fat distribution that can be recognized after inspection of a patient's face, particularly Bichat's fat deposits giving form to patient's cheeks.

ART can also promote fat deposition at waist level [25], increasing the patient's risk for metabolic syndrome and cardiovascular disease. Use of protease inhibitors might partly explain this phenomenon [26].

21.1.5 Hemoglobin

Hb values reflect how rapid HIV disease progresses [27,28]. However, it has been suggested that increase in Hb value is of predictive value for therapeutic success when it is combined with TLC. In this regard, Anastos et al. [29] assessed the predictive value of TLC, and of Hb, for patient response to ART. The authors found that an Hb value less than 10.6 g/dL before the start of ART was independently associated with death as well as AIDS-defining diseases [29]. Hence, monitoring of Hb values is useful for predicting progression of HIV disease before as well as after starting ART.

The aforementioned can be explained with the studies of Obirikorang and Yeboah, who found a positive, significant correlation between Hb values and $CD4^+$ T-cell counts in a sample of 228 individuals with HIV/AIDS [30]. These authors suggested that, given the strong relationship between Hb values and AIDS-defining diseases and death, this biochemical marker should be used when more sophisticated laboratory resources are not available.

21.1.6 Albumin

Normal values of serum total protein have been described in HIV infection, accompanied by a significant decrease of serum albumin and a concomitant increase in globulins [31]. A study performed by us found that serum albumin was significantly diminished in the asymptomatic phase of HIV infection when compared with HIV-negative subjects serving as controls [32]. Thus, serum albumin could be considered as a possible marker of HIV presence in the earlier stages of infection, as well as a possible marker of disease progression, given the fact that albumin values decreased significantly as clinical stage of HIV infection progressed [32].

In the ART era, diminishing of serum albumin in HIV patients could also be related to microalbuminuria that these patients might suffer, particularly as a consequence of tubular dysfunction caused by use of certain antiretroviral drugs such as tenofovir [33].

Other researchers have proposed serum albumin as an adequate indicator of survival in HIV/AIDS patients; there was an average survival of 3 years for those patients with serum albumin more than 3.5 g/dL when compared with those with values less than 2.5 g/dL, who exhibited survival less than 3 weeks [34]. In a study conducted in Iran with 111 individuals coinfected with HIV and TB who were observed between 2004 and 2007, an association was found between low serum albumin values and increased mortality [35].

21.1.7 Transferrin

Transferrin (TFN) is a β-globulin responsible for transportation and deposition of serum iron. This protein has a half-life of 8–10 days, and the liver is the main (although not the exclusive) site of its synthesis [36]. TFN can be used as a negative acute reactant protein for its value decreases in chronic diseases, inflammatory status, infections, and cancer [37]. TFN value might also reflect nutritional status of the patient [37].

It is believed that TFN values reflect changes in the pool of visceral proteins more accurately than serum albumin, given its lower body content and a shorter half-life [37]. Hence, TFN, in the same manner as serum albumin, has been integrated into morbidity–mortality prognostic indexes [38]. It has been shown that serum TFN exhibits different phenotypes, and these phenotypes might be differentially expressed in HIV/AIDS patients [39]. Accordingly, it is important not only to measure serum TFN but also to determine the prevailing protein phenotype. TFN phenotype might be dependent on serum protein values, and it is associated with prevalence of opportunistic infections in these patients [39].

We completed a study in 2011 aimed at assessing changes brought about by ART on selected biochemical indicators of nutritional status of 142 persons living with HIV/AIDS in the province of Pinar del Río (250 km westward from Havana City, Cuba). There were no differences in average albumin and TFN values between ART-treated and non-ART-treated subjects [40].

21.1.8 Total Lymphocytes Count

TLC represents a marker that is readily available in low-incomes countries. In view of this, TLC has been investigated as an alternative for $CD4^+$ T-cell counts [12]. TLC less than 1,200 cells/mm^3 has been recommended as a surrogate cutoff value for starting ART in symptomatic HIV patients. A significant association between TLC less than 1,200 cells/mm^3 and subsequent progression of the disease (ending in mortality) has been confirmed [29,41]. Other authors have proposed that rate of decline in TLC should be used for monitoring progression of the disease: a 33% year reduction of TLC precedes onset of AIDS in 1–2 years [42].

Although TLC has been validated for predicting progression of disease in non-ART-treated HIV patients, its use for monitoring the response to pharmacological therapy has been questioned and abandoned [43]. Anastos et al. [29] examined if TLC (among others markers) could predict clinical response to ART in a cohort study with 873 women followed-up during 1 year preceding the start of ART. They produced three different multivariate analysis models (two of them excluded CD4 counts) with cutoff values of TLC less than 850 and less than 1,250 cells/μL, respectively. All models were similar in their power when predicting death as well as incidence of AIDS-defining diseases. The authors concluded that pre-ART TLC is an independent predictor of morbidity and mortality after starting ART [29].

21.1.9 Cholesterol

The term "cholesterol" denotes several complex aggregations of proteins and lipids circulating in the blood differing in not only nature and quantities of lipids but also nature, quantities, and amino acidic composition of proteins. Thus, total cholesterol comprises high-density lipoprotein (HDL) cholesterol, low-density lipoprotein (LDL) cholesterol, and very-low-density lipoprotein (VLDL) cholesterol; these names were assigned after studying the behavior of fractions during density centrifugation analysis.

Total cholesterol is not a classical nutritional marker, but it has gained attention in recent years after research reporting its relationship with nutritional demands, presence of inflammation, and changes in body weight and tissue compartments. Cholesterol can behave as a negative reactant molecule in cases of active inflammation, and this circumstance might obscure this marker's prognostic value [44].

Low cholesterol values can signal those patients at risk for complications after surgery [45]. Low cholesterol values can be found in non-ART-treated HIV/AIDS patients [32], but the total cholesterol can increase significantly in people with HIV who use ART [40].

ART might affect blood lipid values in the same manner as that previously described for skinfolds. ART drugs can cause a decrease in HDL, with a concomitant increase in LDL and triglycerides values, increasing the risk of atherosclerosis and cardiovascular damage [46,47].

We assessed the risk of lipid and lipoprotein disorders in HIV/AIDS patients on ART and how this risk is related to time of exposure to drugs. A significant increase in total cholesterol and VLDL was found in the ART group, and it was much more severe in those with 24 months (or more) of exposure to drugs. The study showed no differences between treated and untreated patients regarding serum LDL and HDL levels [48].

21.2 TOOLS FOR NUTRITIONAL ASSESSMENT OF PERSONS WITH HIV/AIDS

It is important in clinical settings to have the required tools for assessing the nutritional status of a particular patient because of the intimate relationship between nutrition and health [37,49]. Tools combining markers of different types (clinical, anthropometric, biochemical, immunological) have been proposed for assessment of the nutritional status of HIV/AIDS patients. We limit our discussion in this section to Chang's algorithm [50] and the SGA designed by Detsky et al. [51] and modified by Polo et al. [52] for use in those infected with HIV.

Chang's algorithm manipulates several anthropometric, biochemical, and immunological markers by organizing them within a scale according to the "crude" value observed in the patient. Information from ranked values is integrated into a numerical result expressing presence (yes/no), severity (mild/moderate/severe), and type (Marasmus/Kwashiorkor/mixed) of malnutrition.

We reported in 2005 the results found after using Chang's algorithm as a tool for assessing the nutrition status of non-ART-treated HIV patients living in Pinar del Río and going through different clinical stages of the disease [3]. Malnutrition was present in 40.0% of the patients. Malnutrition rates increased with disease stage: *asymptomatic*, 21.7%; *stage IVC2*, 42.7%; and *stage IVC1*, 87.5%. Two-thirds of the malnourished patients were marasmatic [3].

SGA was a nutritional assessment tool originally designed for use in patients undergoing elective gastrointestinal surgery, but it has been applied in other different populations of patients because of its ease of administration and reliability. As part of nutritional profiling of 22 HIV/AIDS patients assisted in a Buenos Aires hospital, BMI was calculated from current height and weight values. SGA was applied independently [1]. Although the small sample size prevented the investigators from extrapolating obtained results to a bigger population, it was nevertheless interesting to find discrepant malnutrition rates with the tools used. According with BMI values, only 36% of the sample was malnourished. On the contrary, SGA identified 85% of the people as showing malnutrition. The observed discrepancy in malnutrition estimates by these two tools are in line with other studies [5].

We recently determined nutritional status of HIV/AIDS patients by indistinctly using BMI calculation, Chang's algorithm, and SGA and assessing the association between the resulting nutritional diagnosis and $CD4^+$ T lymphocyte count [53]. The malnutrition rate (albeit small) was dependent on nutritional assessment method, as shown in Figure 21.2. However, the three methods converged when reporting the highest frequency of malnourished patients among those non-ART-treated individuals presenting with $CD4^+$ T lymphocyte counts less than 350 cells/mm^3 [53]. In any case, the association between nutritional status and $CD4^+$ T lymphocyte counts was weak, even after adjusting for the effect of ART [53]. Overweight and obesity were more prevalent in the studied patients.

21.3 THE IMPORTANCE OF HEALTHY FEEDING FOR HIV/AIDS PATIENTS

Even though the symptoms of viral infection are not always visible, HIV virus noticeably affects nutritional status. Consequently, satisfaction of nutritional needs is essential from the very moment the diagnosis is made to prevent future malnutrition.

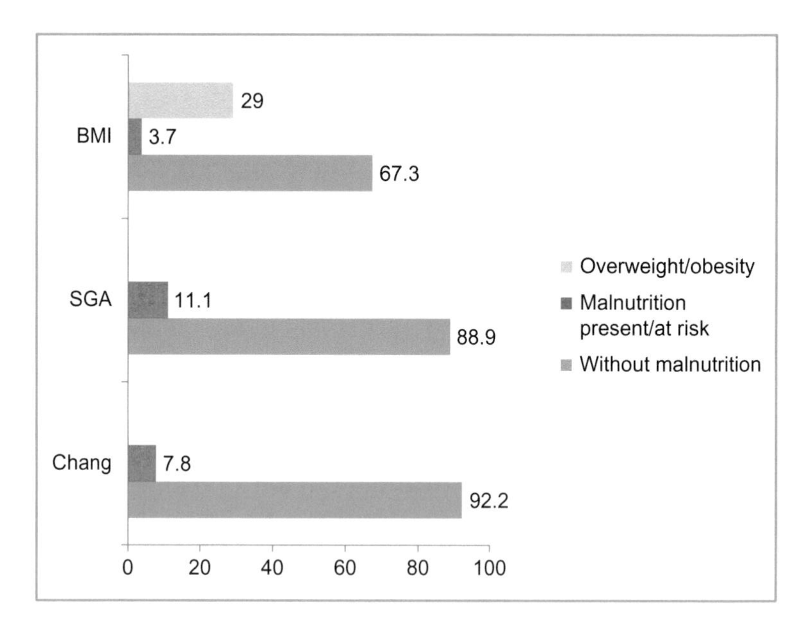

FIGURE 21.2 Nutritional status of patients as assessed by means of different methodologies. Data from Linares (2013) [53].

The role of feeding in HIV/AIDS patients is still a subject of study and debate, although from the initial moments of the disease it was perceived that adequate feeding could be relevant given the fact that HIV directly strikes the immune system. Good feeding is not a cure for the disease or protection from contagion. However, good feeding might help to preserve and improve a patient's nutritional status and to slow progression of HIV infection toward clinical AIDS.

HIV individuals are vulnerable to malnutrition because of impaired nutrient absorption due to intestinal damage manifesting as diarrhea and reduced food intake as a result of vomiting and painful swallowing. Malnutrition associated with HIV/AIDS might also be related to food insecurity as well as medication side effects such as loss of appetite, depression, or abdominal pain [54]. HIV/AIDS and malnutrition may compound (or cause) severe immune deficiencies that ultimately increase susceptibility to opportunistic infections [54]. Opportunistic infections can affect food intake, absorption, and metabolism, thus causing further weight loss and wasting.

Much of the attention has always been directed to examining quantity and quality of protein, fat, and carbohydrate intake without discussing the needs and current intakes of micronutrients such as minerals, vitamins, and trace elements. Micronutrients are involved in virtually every aspect of tissue metabolism and immunocompetence. Several reports have stated micronutrient deficiencies in HIV/AIDS patients. Lack of essential

TABLE 21.1 Several Studies Showing the Role of Micronutrients Deficiencies in Progression of HIV/AIDS Disease

Study	Results
Giraldo (2003) [56]	Low serum vitamin A is a risk factor in the progression of HIV infection toward clinical AIDS
	Low serum vitamin A is a predictor of mortality among HIV/AIDS patients
	Low values of vitamins A and B12 are directly associated with reduced T $CD4^+$ cells count
Anish et al. (2011) [57]	Frequent intakes of legumes and eggs might serve as nutritional protection factors against disease progression
Allavena et al. (1995) [58]	Serum selenium is a major determinant of rapid disease progression
Delmas-Beauvieux et al. (1996) [59]	Supplementation with selenium significantly increases glutathione-peroxidase enzyme activity in HIV/AIDS patients, hence slowing disease progression
Lake and Adams (2011) [60]	There is a risk for vitamin D deficiency in HIV patients because of either virus-specific factors or ARV treatment
Aziz et al. (2012) [61]	Low serum vitamin D values in HIV-infected women are associated with low T $CD4^+$ counts 24 months after starting ART

micronutrients might contribute not only to depletion and dysfunction of $CD4^+$ T cells but also to accelerated disease progression and suboptimal response to ART [55]. Several studies showing the role of micronutrient deficiencies in progression of HIV/AIDS disease are summarized in Table 21.1.

Zayas et al. assessed the nutritional status of 1,000 people with ages between 24 and 59 years that lived in Cuba with HIV/AIDS, and were assisted by the ambulatory care system. They found that 66% of the sample was affected by anemia, regardless of the clinical stage and time of evolution of HIV infection. Average energy and macronutrient intakes were acceptable when compared against current recommendations [62], but poor intakes of dietary riboflavin, iron, and zinc were found in asymptomatic people [63].

Insufficient knowledge of HIV-infected patients regarding their nutritional requirements has been identified as a liability for balanced, sufficient, and complete feeding that is the key for their health and welfare. In addition, geographic scattering of many communities and barriers in the access to health services, among others, impede the consolidation of an adequately decentralized institutional presence; all of these factors limit and weaken the comprehensive, quality-level care these patients should receive [64].

In a study performed in Cuba to assess what people living with HIV/AIDS know about the role of food and nutrition in the prevention of wasting syndrome, it was found that malnutrition affected one-fifth of the respondents in an institution caring for people living with HIV/AIDS in the town of San Luis (1,100 km eastward from Havana City, Cuba). More than one-half of the participants did not know the essentials of food management and preservation, hygiene safety measures for food preparation and cooking, guidelines for a healthy diet, and indications for artificial nutritional support in HIV/AIDS [65]. Also, the completed semi-structured survey revealed that people living with HIV/AIDS had different taboos regarding alimentary habits [65].

The first step for securing the presence of all nutrients required for satisfying nutritional needs of people living with HIV/AIDS is to consume as many varied, healthy foods as possible. Sufficient water intake should be part of nutrient and food recommendations for HIV/AIDS patients. Some of the food recommendations for HIV/AIDS patients are given in Table 21.2.

Several factors need to be taken into account when planning food menus that are recognized as modifiers of HIV/AIDS patients' nutrient requirements, such as previous nutritional status and the presence of malnutrition, obesity, and lipodystrophy; metabolic disorders, intestinal malabsorption, stage of HIV infection, associated opportunistic infections, other concurrent diseases such as hypothyroidism, diabetes, dyslipidemias, and hyperuricemia; type of collateral effects and toxicity of ART; drug–nutrient interactions; available economical resources; physical activity; age; and childbearing and breastfeeding status (among others).

HIV/AIDS patients should be encouraged to be physically active and to engage in physical exercise. Several studies have dealt with the benefits of physical exercise for the general population as well as for chronically ill patients. Physical exercise might increase appetite and, thus, better food intake. Physical exercise might also serve to preserve metabolically active lean tissues, particularly skeletal muscle tissue. In addition, physical exercise might improve quality of life and self-esteem. Finally, physical exercise might protect the patient from ART-related complications such as dyslipidemias, fat deposition at waist level, and insulin resistance, which are events integrated into the core of the so-called metabolic syndrome [67].

Despite a well-prescribed diet providing all the required nutrients for maintaining the patient's health status and that patient's adherence to it, nutrient supplementation might be necessary [55]. Nutritional assessment of HIV/AIDS patients has repeatedly shown not only weight loss and tissue depletion but also low serum values of vitamin B12, zinc, and selenium; all these events are associated with decreased immunity and disease progression [55]. Nutrient supplementation might boost health status and energy, provide immune system support, increase effectiveness

TABLE 21.2 Some Food Recommendations for HIV/AIDS Patients

- Choose carbohydrates wisely: Certain breads, cereals, rice, and pastas are good choices of carbohydrates rich in nutrients and fiber. Combined with carbohydrates taking from fruits and vegetables, they might help to provide a substantial portion of the energy you need every day [64].
- Symptomatic people require between 20% and 30% more of daily food energy, whereas those that are symptoms-free might need 10% more of daily food energy, in order to maintain an adequate body weight. These same increases in the amount of food energy are also recommended for ARV-treated people [64].
- Enjoy a wide variety of vegetables and fruits daily. Vegetables and fruits are an important part of a healthy and balanced diet. They provide vitamins and minerals that preserve the body and boost the immune system. They are particularly important food for people living with HIV/AIDS to fight infection [66].
- Consume enough proteins: Food proteins are essential for a healthy body and a strong immune system. Choose from a wide variety of foods, including low-fat meats, poultry, fish, legumes, eggs, nuts, grains, milk, yogurt, and cheese [64]. The exact amount to consume might require to be adjusted based on individual needs. However, food proteins quantities for a HIV/AIDS patient are not different from those recommended for a noninfected patient. Food proteins should amount to between 15% and 20% of total food energy content. This equals (approximately) 1.5 g/kg of body weight [64].
- Be cautious about fat intakes: Fat should not exceed 30% of total food energy content. It is advised to limit the intake of fats in general, with particular attention to fats from animal origin, saturated fats, and cholesterol. Consumption of vegetable oils as source of monounsaturated fatty acids, and essential fatty acids such as polyunsaturated fatty acids, is better. Some antiretroviral drugs might raise blood lipids values and increase the risk of cardiovascular diseases such as dyslipidemias [64].
- In people living with HIV/AIDS, it is necessary to insist on variety, emphasizing on diet components with antioxidant effects such as vitamins C, E, A, or beta carotene. To get a varied diet, food from the seven basic groups should be selected daily: Group I (cereals and tubers), Group II (vegetables), Group III (fruits), Group IV (meat, poultry, fish, eggs, and beans), Group V (milk, yogurt, and cheese), Group VI (fats), and Group VII (sugar and sweets). Food from Groups I, II, and III can be enjoyed in greater numbers; those from Groups IV and V in moderate amount; and finally those from Groups VI and VII in limited quantities [62].

of ancillary medical treatment, improve general quality of life and appetite, and support the healing process [55].

In a double-blind randomized trial, 201 HIV-infected South African children aged 4–24 months were assigned to receive either multi-micronutrient supplements or placebo daily for 6 months. Weight-for-height improved significantly among supplemented children, without further impact on height-for-age, and number of monthly episodes of diarrhea and respiratory symptoms were reduced [68].

Probiotics could be of value in nutrient supplementation of HIV/AIDS patients. Regarding immune function of HIV patients, Hummelen et al. assessed the impact of supplementation of *Lactobacillus rhamnosus* GR-1 strain and yogurt, either plain or fortified with micronutrients [69]. Additional probiotic supplementation was well-tolerated, without any adverse events. Incidences of diarrhea or clinical symptoms were independent of nutrient supplementation. Improvement of Hb levels was observed in all subjects. Addition of probiotics to a micronutrient-fortified yogurt was well-tolerated but was not associated with a further increase in CD4 count after 1 month of treatment [69].

Despite this, evidence supporting the benefits of nutritional supplementation for patients placed on ART in settings with limited resources is lacking. Investigators showed the effect of a nutritional supplement taken concurrently with ART for 6 months on BMI and body composition as well as on laboratory and biochemical markers. Participants in a study aimed at assessing the effect of nutrient supplementation taken concurrently with ART on body weight and composition (as well as other nutritional markers) were provided with and instructed to consume high-protein, high-energy meals, along with vitamins, minerals, amino acids, and omega-3 fatty acid supplements [55]. After 6 months, supplemented patients showed higher CD4 counts, higher average percentage changes in body weight and BMI values, and increased absolute CD4 counts and Hb values [55]. Supplemented patients also had a higher mean percentage fat-free mass, total body water, intracellular water, and basal metabolic rate values. Supplemented patients also showed an improvement in physical activity 6 months after starting ART [55]. These encouraging results suggest that nutritional supplements taken concurrently with ART can promote weight gain and improve immune response and physical activity in HIV-positive patients who start ART with weight loss [55].

21.4 THE CUBAN EXPERIENCE IN THE PROVISION OF FOOD AND NUTRITION CARE TO PEOPLE WITH HIV/AIDS

Based on data accumulated until September 2013, there were 18,883 HIV-positive cases in Cuba [70]. HIV prevalence rate estimated from the Cuban sexually active population is one of the lowest in the world [70].

Since 1983, when the first case of HIV had not yet been reported in Cuba, Cuban sanitary authorities stopped importing blood derivatives from countries that had reported positive cases, and an epidemiologic surveillance system for Kaposi sarcoma, repetitive pneumonias, and any other entity that could make one to think of AIDS was deployed in hospital institutions of the country [71].

The first kits for HIV diagnosis were purchased and introduced in the National Health System in 1985. Later, the Cuban medical industry was able to produce and distribute proprietary diagnostic kits for use in laboratories and blood banks, and also for distribution to third countries.

The year 1985 marked the report of the first case of AIDS in Cuba, and sexual intercourse was determined as the main cause of HIV infection. By the end of 1985, the National Program for Control and Prevention of HIV/AIDS was drafted. Existing experiences in the control of sexually transmitted diseases (STD) were taken into account to establish massive screening of at-risk groups, epidemiological assessment of every infected subject, a health education component aimed at the Cuban population, and commitment of all diagnosed with HIV to a sanatorium. The existing National Health System, being accessible and free to all Cuban population, regardless of sex, skin color, religion, political standpoint, or economical power, allowed the country to deploy the drafted program for prevention and control of HIV/AIDS [71].

The first sanatorium for HIV/AIDS patients was founded in 1986 in the town of Santiago de las Vegas, approximately 50 km east of Havana. By 1991, sanatoria had been implemented in most of the provinces of the country. In the early years, commitment to a sanatorium was mandatory to educate and train persons to live with HIV/AIDS, and also to provide them with psychological and medical assistance and the care required to cope with the impact of the diagnosis on their future life.

After 1994, and given the experience acquired after the deployment of the program and the operation of sanatoria, an Ambulatory Care System was established. This system enabled the reincorporation of HIV-positive people into the Cuban society after being deemed fit to live with the virus and to take care of their lives, as well as of the other's, by themselves. People diagnosed with HIV were allowed to continue studying and/or working under Cuban present legislation [71]. The former sanatoria were transformed into Comprehensive Care Centers for People with HIV and perform an important number of activities and functions. In addition, there is an Enhanced National Response (ENR) to the HIV epidemic in Cuba, with participation and active mobilization of all the sectors at the community level and preventive actions taken through education and training in all the country's workplaces [72].

Comprehensive care of HIV patients in Cuba involves all levels of the National Health System, from the community to third-level research institutes and national reference centers. Being the main beneficiary of the national health programs, the community is the reason for the existence of the system, the place where health problems are identified and prioritize, and where actions for intervention, control, and assessment are taken, thus responding to the society's interests and needs [73].

At the community level, health areas are considered the main frame for the assistance and provision of care to HIV patients, for starting and managing ART, and for the conduction of actions aimed to foster adequate therapeutic adherence.

Care goals for HIV-infected individuals in Cuba comprise access to comprehensive care, prevention and timely treatment of complications, provision of ART, adequate clinical and laboratory follow-up (keeping with the particularities of each case), and comprehensive rehabilitation of HIV-infected patients.

Regarding of ART history, evolution of HIV/AIDS in Cuba can be divided into three main stages: the first one, from 1986 to 1996, when there was no ART and one could only hope that someday such drugs would appear; the second one, from 1996 to 2001, when there were just a few of these drugs, but Cuba simply could not afford them for all patients; and the third one, from 2001 onward, when the Cuban state decided to start locally manufacturing generic drugs similar to those commercially available in the international market [74], allowing total and free access to medications for all patients in need. Use of Cuban generic drugs has proven to be effective after observing improvements in immune and viral indicators, prolonged survival of patients, and reduction of appearance of opportunistic diseases and number of deaths by HIV/AIDS [75]. We have also been able to show that these generic drugs were not associated with an increased risk of cardiovascular disease, at least regarding blood lipids and lipoproteins values [40].

Currently, the Nutrition and Food Hygiene Institute conducts the Food and Nutrition Care Program for HIV/AIDS People in Cuba aimed to secure adequate nutritional care for these patients, as well as to foster national-reaching policies on these issues. A primordial task of this program has been the creation of nutritional support teams (NSTs) as the vehicle to convey information regarding nutrition issues to these patients to produce significant changes in their food and nutrition habits.

Although creation and operation of NST is not a new idea, its role in the identification and intervention of nutritional disorders and deficiencies in HIV patients in Cuba is a complete novelty. NST integrated by physicians, nurses, dietitians, psychologists, and HIV patients have been constituted throughout the country, and they are responsible for disseminating sound nutritional recommendations among communities, patients, and the general population. Integrating HIV/AIDS patients directly into NST activities allows them to have a more active role in improving their health status and quality of life [63].

NST have been entrusted with the tasks of organizing and conducting workshops and other forms of education and training in food and nutrition issues for people living with HIV/AIDS at the country level. Workshops are aimed at people with HIV and health personnel involved in their care to achieve a multidisciplinary and coherent performance, and also to raise the level of knowledge of these health actors in these disciplines required for better treatment and management of nutritional disorders in these patients.

NST also act as supervising bodies of nutritional policies advanced by sanitary and regulatory agencies, securing constant interdisciplinary cooperation as a way to improve the level of medical care provided to people living with HIV/AIDS in Cuba. In addition, NST are fundamental in assessing the impact of the policies on the outcomes of medical and pharmacological treatment of HIV/AIDS.

21.5 CONCLUSIONS

The nutritional situation of HIV/AIDS patients in Cuba is no longer dominated by malnutrition and macronutrient deficiencies, as implied from the aforementioned results. Cuban researchers have observed a significant trend in those with HIV/AIDS living in Cuba toward overweight and obesity. This can be the most obvious result of the Food and Nutrition Care Program for HIV/AIDS People in Cuba, along with universal access to generic antiretroviral drugs and close follow-up by locally acting medical care teams and NST. Increase in body weight, although desirable as a protection factor from HIV/AIDS-associated cachexia, might place the subject at increased risk for cardiovascular disease and other comorbidities comprising the metabolic syndrome. Excess body weight is nevertheless accompanied by micronutrient disorders such as anemia and B complex vitamin deficiency. New policies are needed to address the emerging problem posed by excess body weight and obesity, along with the sanitary, epidemiological, and nutrition transition in Cuba. Studies are required to reveal the extent of the situation and to assess the impact of interventions on body fat size, distribution, and activity.

References

[1] Freijo S, Mengoni A. Estado nutricional al ingreso de los pacientes internados con VIH. Dieta 2010;28(130):37–44.

[2] López Herce JA. Alteraciones nutricionales en la infección por el virus de la inmunodeficiencia humana (VIH). An Med Interna 2001;18(12):617–8.

[3] Linares M, Bencomo J, Santana S, Barreto J, Ruiz M. Aplicación del método chang en la evaluación nutricional de individuos VIH/sida. J Bras Doenças Sex Transm 2005;17(4):259–64.

[4] Cade Fields G. Compendio de conocimientos sobre la infección por el VIH y temas relacionados con nutrición. Nutrición, Inmunidad, Infección por el VIH. VIH y Nutrición [online]; 2006; p. 1–47. Available from: <http://www.wishh.org/nutrition/papers-publications/wishh_hiv-aids_nutrition_compendium-en_espanol.pdf> [accessed 12.11.12].

[5] Mokori A, Kabehenda MK, Nabiryo C, Wamuyu MG. Reliability of scored patient generated Subjective Global Assessment for nutritional status among HIV infected adults in TASO, Kampala. Afr Health Sci 2011;11(Special Issue):586–92.

[6] Benavente GB. Estado nutricional y hábitos alimentarios de pacientes con VIH. Rev Peru Epidemiol 2011;15(2):113–7.

[7] Kotler DP, Tierney AR, Wang J, Pierson RN. Magnitude of body cell-mass depletion and the timing of death from wasting in AIDS. Am J Clin Nutr 1989;50:444–7.
[8] Castro KG, Ward JW, Slutsker L, Buehler JW, Jaffe HW, Berkelman RL. 1993 Revised classification system for HIV infection and expanded surveillance case definition for AIDS among adolescents and adults. National Center for Infectious Diseases Division of HIV/AIDS [online]; 1992; 41(RR-17). Available from: <http://www.cdc.gov/mmwr/preview/mmwrhtml/00018871.htm> [accessed 19.11.12].
[9] Thiébaut R, Malvy D, Marimoutou C, Davis F. Anthropometric indices as predictors of survival in AIDS adults. Aquitaine cohort, France, 1985–1997. Groupe d'Epidémiologie Clinique du Sida en Aquitaine (GECSA). Eur J Epidemiol 2000;16(7):633–9.
[10] Malvy E, Thiébaut R, Marimoutou C, Dabis F. Groupe d'Epidemiologie Clinique du Sida en Aquitaine. Weight loss and body mass index as predictors of HIV disease progression to AIDS in adults. Aquitaine cohort, France. Am Coll Nutr 2001;20(6):609–15.
[11] Romero Corral A, Somers VK, Sierra Johnson J, Thomas RJ, Collazo-Clavell ML, Korinek J, et al. Accuracy of body mass index in diagnosing obesity in the adult general population. Int J Obes 2008;32(6):959–66.
[12] Langford SE, Ananworanich J, Cooper DA. Predictors of disease progression in HIV infection: a review. AIDS Res Ther 2007;4:11.
[13] Maas JJ, Dukers N, Krol A, Van Ameijden EJC, Van Leeuwen R, Roos MTL, et al. Body mass index course in asymptomatic HIV-infected homosexual men and the predictive value of a decrease of body mass index for progression to AIDS. J Acquir Immune Defic Syndr Hum Retrovirol 1999;7(3):4456–62.
[14] Castetbon K, Anglaret X, Toure S, Chene G, Ouassa T, Attia A, et al. Prognostic value of cross-sectional anthropometric indices on short-term risk of mortality in human immunodeficiency virus-infected adults in Abidjan, Cote d'Ivoire. Am J Epidemiol 2001; 154(1):75–84.
[15] Koethe JR, Heimburger DC. Nutritional aspects of HIV-associated wasting in sub-Saharan Africa. Am J Clin Nutr 2010;91(4):1138S–1142S.
[16] Maia LH, De Mattos AB. Progression to overweight, obesity and associated factors after antiretroviral therapy initiation among Brazilian persons with HIV/AIDS. Nutr Hosp 2010;25(4):635–40.
[17] Tate T, Willig AL, Willig JH, Raper JL, Moneyham L, Kempf MC, et al. HIV infection and obesity: Where did all the wasting go? Antivir Ther 2012;17(7):1281–1289.
[18] Zachariah R, Fitzgerald M, Massaquoi M. Risk factors for high early mortality in patients on antiretroviral treatment in a rural district of Malawi. AIDS 2006;20(18):2355–60.
[19] Boodram B, Plankey MW, Cox C, Tien PC, Cohen MH, Anastos K, et al. Prevalence and correlates of elevated body mass index among HIV-positive and HIV-negative women in the women's interagency HIV study. AIDS Patient Care STDS 2009;23(12):1009–16.
[20] Koethe JR, Lukusa A, Giganti MJ. Association between weigh gain and clinical outcomes among malnourished adults initiating antiretroviral therapy in Lusaka, Zambia. J Acquir Immune Defic Syndr 2010;53(4):507–13.
[21] Madec Y, Szumilin E, Genevier C, Ferradini l, Blkan S, Pujades M, et al. Weight gain at 3 months of antiretroviral therapy is strongly associated with survival: evidence from two developing countries. AIDS 2009;23:853–61.
[22] León MA, Linares EM. La regresión logística binaria como instrumento para la predicción de deterioro inmunológico a partir de indicadores nutricionales en personas con VIH/sida. Investigación Operacional 2014;35(1):35–48.
[23] Cogill B. Anthropometric indicators measurement guide. Food and nutrition technical assistance. Revised Edition [online]; 2003;8–12. Available from: <http://www.fantaproject.org/downloads/pdfs/anthro_1.pdf> [accessed 23.10.12].
[24] Gustafson P, Gomes VF, Vieira CS, Samb B, Nauclér A, Aaby P, et al. Clinical predictors for death in HIV-positive and HIV-negative tuberculosis patients in Guinea-Bissau. Infection 2012;16(5–7):e337–43.

[25] Linares Guerra EM, Acosta Nuñe N, Hernández Rodríguez Y, Sanabria Negrín J, Jerez Hernández E, Plá Cru A. Adiposidad abdominal y riesgo de morbilidad en personas de la provincia de Pinar del Río que viven con VIH/sida. RCAN Rev Cubana Aliment Nutr 2008;18(1):43–52.

[26] Lee GA, Rao MN, Grunfeld C. The effects of HIV protease inhibitors on carbohydrate and lipid metabolism. Curr HIV/AIDS Rep 2005;2(1):39–50.

[27] Paton NI, Sangeetha S, Earnest A, Bellamy R. The impact of malnutrition on survival and the CD4 count response in HIV-infected patients starting antiretroviral therapy. HIV Med 2006;7:323–30.

[28] Ogbe PJ, Idoko OA, Ezimah AC, Digban KA, Oguntayo BO. Evaluation of iron status in anemia of chronic disease among patients with HIV infection. Clin Lab Sci 2012;25(1):7–12.

[29] Anastos K, Quihu S, French AL, Levine A, Greenblatt RM, Williams C, et al. Total lymphocyte count, hemoglobin, and delayed-type hypersensitivity as predictors of death and AIDS illness in HIV-1-infected women receiving highly active antiretroviral therapy. J Acquir Immune Defic Syndr 2004;35(4):83–92.

[30] Obirikorang C, Yeboah FA. Blood haemoglobin measurement as a predictive indicator for the progression of HIV/AIDS in resource-limited setting. J Biomed Sci 2009;16:102.

[31] Míguez MJ, Baum MK, Posner GS. Nutrición e inmunidad en VIH/SIDA. Asociación Colombiana de infectología. Bogotá 1996:14–18.

[32] Linares EM, Bencomo JF, Pérez LE, Torres O, Barrera O. Influencia de la infección por VIH/SIDA sobre algunos indicadores bioquímicos del estado nutricional. Revista RCAN Cubana Aliment Nutr 2002;16(2):119–26.

[33] Campbell LJ, Dew T, Salota R, Cheserem E, Hamzah L, Ibrahim F, et al. Total protein, albumin and low-molecular-weight protein excretion in HIV-positive patients. BMC Nephrol 2012;13:85.

[34] Romo García J, Salido Rengell F. SIDA: manejo del paciente con HIV. Segunda edición. México, DF: Editorial El Manual Moderno; 1997.

[35] Tabarsi P, Chitsaz E, Moradi A, Baghaei P, Farnia P, Marjani M, et al. Treatment outcome, mortality and their predictors among HIV-associated tuberculosis patients. Int J STD AIDS 2012;23(9):e1–4p.

[36] Forrellat M, Gautier du Défaix H, Fernández N. Metabolismo del hierro. Rev Cubana Hematol Inmunol Hemoter 2000;16(3):149–60.

[37] Santana S, Barreto J, Martínez C, Espinosa A, Morales L. Evaluación nutricional. Acta Méd 2003;11(1):59–75.

[38] Leite JF, Antunes CF, Monteiro JC, Pereira BT. Value of nutritional parameters in the prediction of postoperative complications in elective gastrointestinal surgery. Br J Surg 1987;74(5):426–9.

[39] Masaisa F, Gahutu JB, Mukiibi J, Delanghe J, Philippé J. Transferrin polymorphism and opportunistic infections in HIV-infected women in Rwanda. Acta Haematol 2012;128(2):100–6.

[40] Linares Guerra EM, Jeréz Hernández E, Pla Cruz A, Acosta Nuñez N, Hernández Alfonso M. Cambios provocados por la terapia antirretroviral sobre indicadores bioquímicos del estado nutricional en personas con VIH/sida. Rev Cienc Méd 2011;15(4):8–21.

[41] Lau B, Gange SJ, Phair JP, Riddler SA, Detels R, Margolick JB. Use of total lymphocyte count and hemoglobin concentration for monitoring progression of HIV infection. Jaids J Acquir Immune Defic Syndr 2005;39(5):620–5.

[42] Gange SJ, Lau B, Phair J, Riddler SA, Detels R, Margolick JB, et al. Rapid declines in total lymphocyte count and hemoglobin in HIV infection begin at CD4 lymphocyte counts that justify antiretroviral therapy. AIDS 2003;17(1):119–21.

[43] Balakrishnan P, Solomon S, Kumarasamy N, Mayer KH. Low-cost monitoring of HIV infected individuals on highly active antiretroviral therapy (HAART) in developing countries. Indian J Med Res 2005;121(4):345–55.

[44] Santana Porbén S. ¿Cómo saber que el paciente quirúrgico está desnutrido? Nutrición Clínica [México] 2004;7(4):240–50.

[45] Santana Porbén S. Utilidad de algunos indicadores bioquímicos del estado nutricional del paciente con enfermedad colorrectal maligna. Nutrición Clínica [México] 2006; 9(1):5–12.

[46] Overton ET. Metabolic complications of HIV infection and its therapies. Top Antivir Med 2014;22(3):651–4.

[47] Dubé MP, Cadden JJ. Lipid metabolism in treated HIV infection. Best Pract Res Clin Endocrinol Metab 2011;25(3):429–42.

[48] Linares EM. Combination antiretroviral therapy and the risk of lipid disorders in HIV-infected adults [Electronic poster]. Proceedings of the XVIII international AIDS conference on AIDS 2010. Vienna; 2010.

[49] Santana Porbén S, Comentario al artículo Detsky AS, McLaughlin JR, Baker JP, Johnston N, Whittaker S, et al. What is Subjective Global Assessment of nutritional status? JPEN J Parenter Enteral Nutr 1987;11:8–13. Nutrición Hospitalaria [España] 2008;23:395–407.

[50] Chang RWS, Richardson R. Nutritional assessment using a microcomputer. 2. Programme evaluation. Clin Nutr 1984;3:75–82.

[51] Detsky AS, McLaughlin JR, Baker JP, Johnston N, Whittaker S, Mendelson RA, et al. What is Subjective Global Assessment of nutritional status? J Parenter Enteral Nutr 1987;11:8–13.

[52] Polo R, Gómez-Candela C, Miralles C, Locutura J, Álvarez F, et al. Recomendaciones de SPNS/GEAM/SENPE/AEDN/SEDCA/GESIDA sobre nutrición en el paciente con infección por VIH. Madrid: Ministerio de Sanidad y Consumo Secretaría General Técnica Centro de Publicaciones [online]; 2006 [accessed 21.12.12]. Available from: <http://www.gesida-seimc.org/pcientifica/fuentes/DcyRc/DcyRc_RecomendacionesNutricionVIHSep_2006.pdf>.

[53] Linares EM, Santana S, Carrillo O, León MA, Sanabria JG, Acosta N, et al. Estado nutricional de las personas con VIH/sida. Su relación con el conteo de las células T CD4+ . Nutrición Hospitalaria [España] 2013;28(6):2197–207.

[54] Ketch JA, Paterson M, Maunder EW, Rollins NC. Too little, too late: comparison of nutritional status and quality of life of nutrition care and support recipient and non-recipients among HIV-positive adults in KwaZulu-Natal. South Africa. Health Policy 2011;99:267–76.

[55] Evans D, McNamara L, Maskew M, Selibas K, Amsterdam D, Baines N, et al. Impact of nutritional supplementation on immune response, body mass index and bioelectrical impedance in HIV-positive patients starting antiretroviral therapy. Nutr J 2013;12:111.

[56] Giraldo R. Terapia nutricional para el tratamiento y la prevención del sida. Conferencia presentada en la reunión con los Ministros de Salud de 14 países de la Comunidad para el Desarrollo del Sur del África (SADC). Johanesburgo; 2003.

[57] Anish TS, Vijaykumar K, Simi SM. Determinants of rapid progression to immunodeficiency syndrome among people infected with human immunodeficiency virus, Kerala, India. Indian J Sex Transm Dis 2011;32(1):23–9.

[58] Allavena C, Dousset B, May T, Dubois F, Canton P, Belleville F. Relationship of trace element, immunological markers, and HIV1 infection progression. Biol Trace Elem Res 1995;47(1–3):133–8.

[59] Delmas-Beauvieux MC, Peuchant E, Couchouron A, Constans J, Sergeant C, Simonoff M, et al. The enzymatic antioxidant system in blood and glutathione status in human immunodeficiency virus (HIV)-infected patients: effects of supplementation with selenium or beta-carotene. Am J Clin Nutr 1996;64(1):101–7.

[60] Lake JE, Adams JS. Vitamin D in HIV-infected patients. Curr HIV/AIDS Rep 2011;8(3):133–41.

[61] Delmas-Beauvieux MC, Peuchant E, Couchouron A, Constans J, Sergeant C, Simonoff M, et al. The enzymatic antioxidant system in blood and glutathione status in human immunodeficiency virus (HIV)-infected patients: Effects of supplementation with selenium or beta-carotene. Am J Clin Nutr 1996;64(1):101–7.

[62] Zayas GM, Álvarez A, Mujica E, Villalón MB, Blanco J, Pineda S, et al. Nutrición y SIDA. Manual para la atención alimentaria y nutricional en personas viviendo con VIH/SIDA. La Habana; 2004.

[63] Zayas GM, Castanedo R, Domínguez Y, González DI, Herrera V, Herrera X, et al. Estado nutricional de las personas con VIH/SIDA asistidas por el sistema de atención ambulatoria. Rev Cubana Aliment Nutr 2009;19(1):106–14.

[64] ONUSIDA. Manual de alimentación y nutrición para el cuidado y apoyo de personas adultas viviendo con VIH o sida. Bogotá; 2010.

[65] Domínguez R, Ortega RN, Llorente YB, Ramírez MC. Estado de los conocimientos sobre alimentación y nutrición de las personas que viven con VIH/sida. Influencia en la prevención del síndrome de desgaste. RCAN Rev Cubana Aliment Nutr 2011;21(2):263–74.

[66] OMS/FAO. Aprendiendo a vivir con VIH. Manual sobre cuidados y apoyo nutricionales a los enfermos de VIH/SIDA. Roma; 2003.

[67] Jaggers JR, Prasad VK, Dudgeon WD, Blair SN, Sui X, Burgess S, et al. Associations between physical activity and sedentary time on components of metabolic syndrome among adults with HIV. AIDS Care 2014;26(11):1387–92.

[68] Mda S, Raaij JM, Villiers F, Kok FJ. Impact of multi-micronutrient supplementation on growth and morbidity of HIV-infected South African children. Nutrients 2013; 5(10):4079–92.

[69] Hummelen R, Hemsworth J, Changalucha J, Butamanya NL, Hekmat S, et al. Effect of micronutrient and probiotic fortified yogurt on immune-function of anti-retroviral therapy naive HIV patients. Nutrients 2011;3(10):897–909.

[70] UNAIDS 2013. GLOBAL REPORT. UNAIDS report on the global AIDS epidemic [online]. Available from: <https://unaids.org/en/media/unaids/contentassets/documents/epidemiology/2013/gr2013/UNAIDS_Global_Report_2013_en.pdf>.

[71] Aragonés López C, Campos Díaz JR, Sánchez Valdés L, Pérez Ávila J. Grupos de prevención del SIDA (GPSIDA): 15 años de trabajo sostenido en la prevención del VIH/sida. Rev Cubana Med Trop [on line]. 2007 Dic [citado 2014 July 08]; 59(3):0-0. Available from: <http://scielo.sld.cu/scielo.php?script=sci_arttext&pid=S0375-07602007000300014&lng=es>.

[72] República de Cuba. PLAN ESTRATEGICO NACIONAL ITS/VIH/SIDA 2007–2011. Available from: <http://files.sld.cu/sida/files/2011/07/plan_estrategico_nacional-2007-2011.pdf>.

[73] MINSAP. Programa nacional de prevención y control de las ITS/VIH-sida 2009. PAUTAS PARA LA ATENCIÓN INTEGRAL AL PACIENTE CON INFECCIÓN POR VIH/SIDA EN CUBA. Available from: <http://www.who.int/hiv/pub/guidelines/cuba_art.pdf>.

[74] Tarinas A, Tápanes RD, Pérez LJ. Terapia antiviral para VIH/SIDA. Rev Cubana Farm 2000;34(3):207–9.

[75] Pérez J, Pérez D, González I, Díaz Jidy M, Orta M, Aragonés C, et al. Perspectives and practices in antiretroviral treatment: approaches to the management of HIV/AIDS in Cuba. Case study. Geneva: World Health Organization; 2004. (cited on: June 20, 2007). Available from: http://www.who.int/hiv/pub/prev_care/cuba/en/index.html.

Index

Note: Page numbers followed by "*b*", "*f*," and "*t*" refer to boxes, figures, and tables, respectively.

C

D

T

U

V

W